FILING PATENTS ONLINE

PATENTS

ONLINE

A Professional Guide

FILING PATENTS ONLINE

A Professional Guide

Sarfaraz K. Niazi

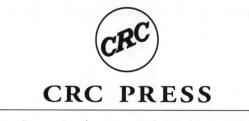

CRC PRESS

Boca Raton   London   New York   Washington, D.C.

Library of Congress Cataloging-in-Publication Data

Niazi, Sarfaraz, 1949-
  Filing patents online : a professional guide / by Sarfaraz K. Niazi.
      p. cm.
  Includes index.
  ISBN 0-8493-1624-3 (alk. paper)
    1. Patents—United States—Data processing. 2. Patent practice—United States— Data
  processing. 3. Patents—Data processing. 4. Patent practice—Data processing. 5. United
  States. Patent and Trademark Office—Data processing. 6. World Intellectual Property
  Organization—Data processing. I. Title.

  KF3125.C5 N53 2003
  346.7304'86'0285—dc21

                                                                            2002041307

Visit the CRC Press Web site at www.crcpress.com

© 2003 by CRC Press LLC

No claim to original U.S. Government works
International Standard Book Number 0-8493-1624-3
Library of Congress Card Number 2002041307
Printed in the United States of America 1 2 3 4 5 6 7 8 9 0
Printed on acid-free paper

Preface

With over a million patents filed every year around the world and the number increasing rapidly, patent offices worldwide have become increasingly burdened with the responsibility of evaluating and awarding patents in a timely manner. The world patent bodies have taken bold steps to develop online filing systems, overcoming the many strategic and logistic problems associated with matters of authentication (validating filer identity), integrity (data were not modified during transmission), nonrepudiation (data have been delivered), and confidentiality (application is read only by authorized entities). The U.S. Patent and Trademark Office was the first to begin accepting patent applications online in 1999, followed by the European Patent Office in 2000; the World Intellectual Property Organization will begin accepting applications in 2003. It is anticipated that other major consortiums and countries will follow suit.

The benefits of online filing of patents include cost savings to patent offices (estimated to be in the billions of dollars) and time saving and thus faster issuance of patents, which will help both the inventor and the consumer. Unfortunately, the necessary complexities involved in preparing and transmitting patent files electronically have produced software programs that are cumbersome, intricate, and difficult to master. This has kept a majority of patent law practitioners and *pro se* inventors from adopting electronic writing and online filing of patents as their method of choice; paper still rules. The reluctance in adopting online filing systems comes not only from perceived uncertainties but also from the attitude of a less Internet-friendly generation that still cannot visualize a paperless system.

The power of the Internet in the development of intellectual property is unquestioned today. Using a desktop computer, one can search the entire world to prove the patentability of an idea; patent examiners now have the same tools and thus anyone who does not fully exploit the value of Internet power faces stiff resistance in securing rights to intellectual property. An issued patent is not above challenge and it is not a seal of approval by the patent office; more such challenges will be forthcoming because of the accessibility of information that can be used to invalidate claims. Therefore, it behooves patent practitioners and inventors to adopt the new cyber tools if they want to stay competitive. Using these tools may not just be good business practice; it may be the only way to file patents in the future.

Filing Patents Online: A Professional Guide is the first comprehensive treatise written to help patent law practitioners and *pro se* inventors write electronically and file patents online to patent offices worldwide. Using a step-by-step approach, it teaches how to harness the unlimited power of the Internet in three important ways: (1) evaluating patentability, (2) writing patent applications electronically (using the software prescribed by worldwide patent offices), and (3) filing patent applications online at a fraction of cost in time and money, compared to what it took just a few years ago. With over a million patents filed every year worldwide and the number increasing rapidly, patent offices are rapidly switching to electronic management of patents, and it is likely that online filing may be the only way to file patents in the future. Additional help with issues relating to patent law, patentability of inventions, status updates on online filing software, and a discussion group are available at http://www.eUSPTO.com. The reader is encouraged to make this Web site the starting point for all patent-related work.

Whereas I have tried to ensure that the information contained in the book is current and verified, mistakes are inevitable, particularly as the state of the art is changing rapidly. I would appreciate any omissions on my part brought to my attention (mail to: niazi@niazi.com) so that corrections can be made in future editions of this book.

I am highly indebted to Rich O'Hanley at Auerbach Publications (a division of CRC Press) for his vision in directing this project, and to Sara Kreisman at CRC Press for her invaluable assistance in the technical writing of the manuscript, and to scores of other friends and associates who critiqued the book and advised on improving the presentation. The patent offices around the world extended extensive help in the writing of this book; I am particularly thankful to USPTO Commissioner for Patents, Nicholas P. Godici; Manuel Desantes of the International Affairs Section at the EPO; and Karl Kalejs, Project Manager, PCT Electronic Filing Unit at WIPO, for directing me to the PCT-SAFE systems to be initiated in 2003. Nevertheless, any mistakes remaining are altogether mine.

Sarfaraz K. Niazi, Ph.D.
Deerfield, Illinois
March 2003

About the Author

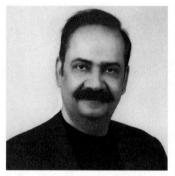

Professor Sarfaraz K. Niazi has been teaching for over 30 years at major universities. He has published over 100 refereed research articles, numerous books including textbooks, and hundreds of syndicated articles. He is recipient of many fellowships of learned societies as well as recognition awards from institutions, and a frequent invited speaker worldwide on a variety of topics such as intellectual property, poetry, and American art. He is also an inventor with scores of patents and a licensed agent to practice patent law at the U.S. Patent and Trademark Office and has several years of experience in filing electronic and online patent applications worldwide.

Acknowledgment

The patent system added the fuel of interest to the fire of genius.

—Abraham Lincoln

The information contained in this book has been obtained from noncopyrighted sources and no intentional inclusion is made of any information that may be proprietary, confidential, or protected by a copyright. Where possible, proprietary products are identified by a registered (®) symbol, errors and omissions excepted. The author extends his gratitude to the United States Patent and Trademark Office, the European Patent Office, and the World International Property Organization for allowing use of the documents prepared by these agencies in describing the electronic and online filing of patents to their offices; additional specific assistance granted by these offices is further acknowledged.

Acknowledgment

The author wishes to thank ...

To My Always-On Line of Help, Anjum

Table of Contents

Chapter 4

Chapter 5

Chapter 6

1 The Patent Filing Systems

INTRODUCTION

For 200 years, millions of inventors have sought to protect their inventions through the American patent system. These patented inventions include Thomas Edison's electric lamp, Alexander Graham Bell's telegraphy, Orville and Wilbur Wright's flying machine, John Deere's steel plow, George Washington Carver's use of legume oils to produce cosmetics and paint, and Edwin Land's Polaroid camera. Today, more than six million patents later, the world is a much better place to live because of inventions that have improved our lives, from the making of Po.tash (Figure 1.1) to gene therapy.

Inventions alone do not accrue benefits to mankind, however; it is the commercialization of useful products at an affordable price that improves quality of life. Sovereign nations around the world, particularly capitalist societies, ensure protection of inventions by allowing the inventor to reap the profits for a limited time by preventing others from exploiting an invention so that in the long run it can be made competitively available to the public. Awarding patents to inventors accomplishes this goal because the inventor is obliged to disclose fully the gist of his invention in a manner that allows others to reproduce it after the expiry of patent. The commercial potential of inventions drives the world's capitalist systems and thus the race to secure inventions through patents is fast and getting faster, causing patent offices worldwide to creak under the pressure of paperwork. One of the most remarkable inventions of the twentieth century, which was not patented, comes to the rescue of the patenting system: the Internet. Going paperless and filing patents online is the future of intellectual property management, one whose time has arrived. *Filing Patents Online: A Professional Guide* takes the reader to the very far edge of available technology to stay ahead of the revolution taking place in inventing and patenting inventions.

A BRIEF HISTORY OF THE INTERNET

1957: The U.S.S.R. launches Sputnik, the first artificial Earth satellite. In response, the U.S. forms the Advanced Research Projects Agency (ARPA) within the Department of Defense (DoD) to establish U.S. lead in science and technology applicable to the military.

1962: Paul Baran of the RAND Corporation (a government agency) is commissioned by the U.S. Air Force to conduct a study of how it can maintain command and control over its missiles and bombers after a nuclear attack. This is to be a decentralized military research network that can survive a nuclear strike, so that if locations (cities) in the U.S. are attacked, the military can still control nuclear arms for a counterattack.

1968: The ARPA awards the ARPANET contract to Bolt, Beranek and Newman (BBN). BBN selects a Honeywell minicomputer as the base on which to build the switch. The physical network is constructed in 1969, linking four nodes: the University of California at Los Angeles, Stanford Research Institute, the University of California at Santa Barbara, and the University of Utah. The network is wired together via 50 kbps circuits.

1972: The first e-mail program is created by Ray Tomlinson of BBN. The ARPA is renamed the Defense Advanced Research Projects Agency (DARPA). ARPANET is currently using the Network Control Protocol (NCP) to transfer data. This allows communications between hosts running on the same network.

1973: Development begins on the protocol later to be called TCP/IP; it is developed by a group headed by Vinton Cerf from Stanford and Bob Kahn from DARPA. This new protocol is used to allow diverse computer networks to interconnect and communicate with each other.

1984: ARPANET is divided into two networks: MILNET and ARPANET. MILNET is to serve the needs of the military and ARPANET is to support the advanced research component; the DoD continues to support both networks. Upgrade to CSNET is contracted to MCI. New circuits will be 1.5 Mbps T1 lines, which are 25 times faster than the old 56 kbps lines. IBM will provide advanced routers and Merit will manage the network. The new network is to be called NSFNET (National Science Foundation Network), and old lines continue to be called CSNET.

1985: The National Science Foundation begins deploying its new T1 lines, which will be finished by 1988.

1986: The Internet Engineering Task Force (IETF) is created to serve as a forum for technical coordination by DARPA contractors working on ARPANET, U.S. Defense Data Network (DDN), and the Internet core gateway system.

1987: BITNET and CSNET merge to form the Corporation for Research and Educational Networking (CREN), another work of the National Science Foundation.

1988: Soon after the completion of the T1 NSFNET backbone, traffic increases so quickly that plans are made immediately to begin upgrading the network.

1990: Merit, IBM, and MCI form a not-for-profit corporation called ANS (Advanced Network and Services), which is to conduct research in high-speed networking. It soon comes up with the concept of the T3, a 45-Mbps line. NSF quickly adopts the new network, and by the end of 1991 all of its sites are connected by this new backbone. While the T3 lines are being constructed, the DoD disbands the ARPANET and replaces it with the NSFNET backbone. The original 50-kbps lines of ARPANET are taken out of service. Tim Berners-Lee and CREN in Geneva implement a hypertext system to provide efficient information access to the members of the international high-energy physics community.

1991: CSNET (which consists of 56-kbps lines) is discontinued after fulfilling its important early role in the provision of academic networking services. A key feature of CREN is that its operational costs are fully met through dues paid by its member organizations. The NSF establishes a new network, named NREN, the National Research and Education Network, the purpose of which is to conduct high-speed networking research. It is not to be used as a commercial network, nor to send much of the data that the Internet now transfers.

1992: The Internet Society is chartered. World Wide Web is released by CREN. NSFNET backbone is upgraded to T3 (44.736 Mbps).

1993: InterNIC is created by NSF to provide specific Internet services: directory and database services (AT&T), registration services (Network Solutions Inc.), and information services (General Atomics/CERFnet). Marc Andreessen, NCSA, and the University of Illinois develop a graphical user interface to the Web, called Mosaic for X.

1994: No major changes are made to the physical network; the most significant thing that happens is the growth. Many new networks are added to the NSF backbone. Hundreds of thousands of new hosts are added to the Internet during this time period. Pizza Hut offers pizza ordering on its Web page. First Virtual, the first cyberbank, opens. ATM (Asynchronous Transmission Mode, 145 Mbps) backbone is installed on NSFNET.

1996: Most Internet traffic is carried by backbones of independent ISPs, including MCI, AT&T, Sprint, UUnet, BBN Planet, ANS, and others. The Internet Society, the group that controls the Internet, is trying to figure out new TCP/IP to enable billions of addresses rather than the current limited system.

January 1999: The World Intellectual Property Organization (WIPO) releases PCT-EASY, a software program to compile (but not file) a patent application electronically.

December 1999: The U.S. Patent and Trademark Office (USPTO) Electronic Filing System (EFS) receives its first electronic filing of a new utility patent application.

July 2002: The European Patent Office (EPO) receives its first electronic filing.

Mid-2003: The WIPO is set to begin accepting online filing of PCT applications, first at the International Bureau and then later in the year at the receiving offices.

U.S. LAWS AND SYSTEMS

In the U.S., the law that governs patents is Title 35 of the United States Code, commonly cited as 35 USC. It incorporates the Patent Cooperation Treaty (PCT, managed by the World Intellectual Property Organization, a UN agency) and changes made for conformity to the intellectual property provisions of the General Agreement on Tariffs and Trade (GATT). Most industrialized nations have their own patent registration rules, and several treaties provide joint patent protection agreements between various countries, most significantly the European Patent Convention, the Paris Treaty, and the Patent Cooperative Treaty.

There are about one million patent publications filed every year around the world. The filings of U.S. patent applications were projected to increase to 350,000 in FY2002, an increase of over 35% since FY1997. However, USPTO staff resources will not increase at the same rate. Even with planned increases in the number of examiners, manually processing the physical volume of paper represented by this number of applications will tax the agency's ability to store and process applications while maintaining a high level of service to applicants. The USPTO recognizes this problem and has formulated a strategy for implementing an electronic workplace. It is anticipated that within the next 5 years, more than 50% of all patent applications will be filed electronically, eventually converting to a paperless patenting system.

> The Twenty-first Century Strategic Plan is the USPTO's road map for creating, over the next five years, an agile and productive organization fully worthy of the unique leadership role the American intellectual property system plays in the global economy. The Plan is predicated on behavioral changes within the USPTO and a willingness to embrace change among all players in the intellectual property system.
>
> **—James E. Rogan**
> *Undersecretary of Commerce for Intellectual Property and Director of the USPTO*
> *before the Subcommittee on Courts, the Internet, and Intellectual Property Committee*
> *of the Judiciary*
> *U.S. House of Representatives, July 18, 2002*

These forward-looking statements amply describe the resolve of the U.S. government in harnessing the power of the Internet to support long-term plans to cope with the paper onslaught at the government level.

The online filing system of the USPTO is called the Electronic Filing System (EFS), and has been operational for more than 2 years; it facilitates users in filing most types of applications with only a few exceptions. Emulating the bold steps taken by the USPTO, the EPO also began accepting applications electronically in mid-2002. The online and fully electronic international application (WIPO's PCT) will be available for filing by mid-2003; currently, the WIPO provides software to write part of the PCT application electronically and then submit it on electronic media, not online. The financial impact of online filing of patents is remarkable; for example, the EPO estimates that a saving of three days of work on each application will net the EPO a savings of over 600 million deutsche marks. The savings at the USPTO will be in billions of dollars, in addition to faster approval of patents, which will be more robust as a result of the improved prosecution process.

The utility of the Internet in making online filing of patent applications worldwide is a reality today that will grow exponentially in the years to come. This book will:

- Help you to understand the requirements for online filing of patents worldwide
- Demonstrate actual examples
- Teach you how you can avoid errors
- Assist you in fully exploiting the power of the Internet in searching for intellectual property evaluation online

The focus of this book is not to advise you on patentability issues, or the art and science of writing patent applications, or the details involved in complying with worldwide legislation on prosecuting patents. You are expected to be familiar with patent laws and well versed in traditional patent-filing modes; however, a summary of patent application essentials is provided in Chapter 2. You will find a much-expanded version of the following discussion at the author's Web site (http://www.eUSPTO.com).

INTERNATIONAL PATENT LAWS, PROCESSES, AND SYSTEMS

THE PARIS CONVENTION

One of the oldest patent-related treaties, adhered to by 140 countries including the U.S., is known as the Paris Convention for the Protection of Industrial Property. It provides that each country guarantees to the citizens of the other countries the same rights in patent and trademark matters that it grants to its own citizens. The treaty provides also for the right of priority in the case of patents, trademarks, and industrial designs (design patents). These rights mean that, on the basis of a regular, first application filed in one of the member countries, the applicant may, within a certain period of time, apply for protection in all the other member countries. These later applications then are regarded as if they had been filed on the same day as the first application. Thus, these later applications will have priority over applications for the same invention that may have been filed during the same period of time by other persons. Moreover, these later applications, being based on the first application, will not be invalidated by any acts accomplished in the interval such as, for example, publication or exploitation of the invention, the sale of copies of the design, or use of the trademark. The period of time within which the subsequent applications may be filed in other countries is 12 months in the case of first applications for patents and 6 months in the case of industrial designs and trademarks.

PATENT COOPERATION TREATY

Another treaty, known as the Patent Cooperation Treaty (PCT), was negotiated at a diplomatic conference in Washington, D.C., in June 1970. The treaty came into force on January 24, 1978, and is presently adhered to by over 115 (and growing) countries, including the U.S. The treaty facilitates the filing of applications for patent on the same invention in member countries by providing, among other things, centralized filing procedures and a standardized application format. The Patent Cooperation Treaty permits an inventor to file what is called a PCT patent application. An international patent application does not, however, lead to an "international patent"; it merely leads to the ability to file patent applications in designated countries over a wider range of permissible times than if no international patent application were filed. Other tangible results of filing an international patent application include a PCT publication, a Search Report from the International Searching Authority, and optionally, a Written Opinion from the International Preliminary Examining Authority (IPEA).

For an applicant who has filed a patent application in a particular country, a PCT application offers a way to postpone having to make decisions about filing patent applications in other countries. If there were no such thing as the Patent Cooperation Treaty, then the only opportunity to postpone making decisions about foreign filing would be the opportunity provided by the Paris Convention. Under the Paris Convention, someone who files an application in one country is forced to make a decision, within one year, as to whether to file patent applications in other countries, which would claim priority from the first application. A PCT application offers a way to extend the time during which a decision must be made about foreign patent filings for a longer period than the decision-postponement period provided by the Paris Convention. By filing a PCT application, the applicant can postpone for 30 months (rather than 12 months under the Paris Convention) the decision about whether to spend the money for foreign patent filings in many countries. In addition, assuming that the first application is filed in a country that has adhered to Chapter II of the Patent Cooperation Treaty, it is possible to perform a step called "demanding preliminary examination," which entitles the applicant to receive an International Preliminary Examination Report (IPER), which may be helpful in assessing the likelihood of patentability. (In a PCT patent application in which the applicant has demanded Preliminary Examination, the application must be examined by a competent IPEA, generally the USPTO or the EPO. The applicant chooses the particular IPEA that will search the PCT application.)

Another possible advantage of a PCT application is that it proceeds on a fixed timetable. The applicant may be sure of receiving a Search Report from the International Searching Authority no later than 15 months after the priority date of the application. If the applicant demands Preliminary Examination, the IPER will be received no later than 26 months after the priority date of the application. An ordinary U.S. patent application, depending on the backlog in the examining group handling the application, can sometimes go for more than 2 years before a first Office Action is received. The PCT applicant can thus get faster feedback from a patent office.

There are instances where a PCT filing may not be advisable. For example, not everyone knows for sure at the time of the first patent filing which, if any, foreign countries should have patent applications filed. After a year or two, the inventor may have more information about whether to do foreign filings, and the invention may prove to have great commercial potential in some foreign countries and not others. In particular, the inventor who benefits from having filed a PCT application is the one who discovers between 12 and 30 months after the filing date that it is no longer desirable to perform foreign filing. In this case, when the decision is made to drop the foreign filings the inventor will have saved all the money that would have been spent on those filings.

The laws of many countries differ in various respects from the patent law of the U.S. In most foreign countries, publication of the invention before the date of the application will bar the right to a patent. Maintenance fees may be required, and there may be a requirement to manufacture the patented invention in a particular country after a certain period, usually 3 years. If there is no manufacture within this period, the patent may be void in some countries, although in most countries the patent may be subject to the grant of compulsory licenses to any person who may apply for a license.

There are several mutual treaties between countries and the costs of filing international applications can be prohibitive. Recent changes in laws allow you to "buy" a 30-month window to decide if you should file an application; unfortunately, you have only 12 months (or before the issuance of patent, whichever is earlier) to buy this protection. Because the rights granted by a U.S. patent extend only through-out the territory of the U.S. and have no effect in a foreign country, an inventor who wants patent protection in other countries must apply for a patent in each of the other countries or in regional patent offices. Almost every country has its own patent law, and a person desiring a patent in a particular country must make an application for patent in accordance with the requirements of that country.

EUROPEAN PATENT CONVENTION

The European Patent Convention (EPC) has given rise to the European Patent Office (EPO), which grants European patents for the contracting states to the EPC signed in Munich, October 5, 1973, and entered into force October 7, 1977. It is the executive arm of the EPO, an intergovernmental body set up under the EPC, whose members are the EPC contracting states. The organization's administrative council, composed of delegates from the contracting states, supervises the activities of the EPO. The EPO offers a way to file a single patent application, which can lead to patent coverage in all the European countries that belong to the EPC. While the EPO has its historical origins in the European Union (EU), it is interesting to note that its formalities can lead to patent coverage in countries that do not belong to the EU. For example, as this book is being written Switzerland is not a member of the EU, and yet it is possible to secure Swiss patent protection through the EPC and the EPO.

The countries that belong to the EPO include Austria, Belgium, Denmark, France, Germany, Greece, Ireland, Italy, Liechtenstein, Luxembourg, Monaco, The Netherlands, Portugal, Spain, Sweden, Switzerland, and the United Kingdom.

For an inventor, the main decision that has to be made is whether to file directly with the country or countries in Europe in which patents are desired, or to do a single filing with the EPO. As a first approximation, if it is only desired to get patent coverage in one or two countries of Europe, it may be more economical to file directly with the patent offices in those countries. On the other hand, if the number of countries of Europe in which patent protection is desired is greater than just one or two, then it probably would be economical to file directly with the EPO.

ONLINE AND ELECTRONIC FILING REQUIREMENTS

There are three types of patent application preparations: (1) paper; (2) electronic, which means preparing the application for transmission on media, such as is currently done for PCT filings and an option for U.S. filings; and (3) electronic/online, which means preparing an electronic application and transmitting it directly to the patent office either though a proprietary network setup or through the Internet.

The patent applications can be filed online to the USPTO and soon to the WIPO for PCT (mid-2003). It is inevitable that online filing of patents will replace paper filing as the increasing load of paper handling becomes unmanageable; the Internet is ideally suited to accomplish this.

The main concerns of online patent filing relate to authentication of the filer, assurance of perfect transmission, and confidentiality of data submitted; these issues have been resolved through digital signature and the use of cryptographic software. The USPTO has taken the lead and has developed one of the most comprehensive and debugged systems. Recently, the USPTO has awarded contracts to private organizations to develop and offer online filing software compatible with its requirements; the intent is to simplify and streamline online filing and to privatize the domain of technology involved in online filing of patents. The EPO has developed its own specifications, having chosen a format different than the U.S. system, and the WIPO has yet to offer online filing although it does offer electronic preparation of applications.

Throughout this book, a detailed description of the use of proprietary software is described and whereas the hardware requirements are spelled out in the instructions that accompany the software, it is assumed that the user has at least a Pentium II PC with 128 Mb RAM and a hard drive of sufficient capacity. Whereas any Internet connection will suffice, it is noted that slow connections such as 56k modems often prove problematic if the transmission is interrupted, creating havoc in the transferred record. The use of DSL or ASDL connection is therefore advised; higher-speed connections are preferred. It is advisable also to back up the data, particularly the electronic keys that are created to authenticate the signatures. Whereas European system authentication is hardware based, the U.S. system now and the WIPO system in the future will rely on software with extremely sensitive codes requiring great precaution in password entry. It is further recommended that filers develop a backup for all systems involved in online filing of patents. Further caution is directed to legal requirements in the use of software; for example, it is illegal to download the USPTO software prior to the registration process, although there is no filter to check it.

In addition to providing details on filing patents online, this book details also the techniques of online search for patentability, a function highly critical to patent law practitioners which requires fast Internet connection to enhance efficiency of search time. A large number of URLs are listed in the book and were tested before the book went to press; however, there is a possibility that some addresses may have changed. If an error message results from entering a URL, first make sure that you have entered the address correctly (the most common error); one way to ensure a correct URL address is through the links at http://www.eUSPTO.com. At this Web site also you will find many features and resources such as a searchable MPEP

(*Manual of Patent Examining Procedure, 8th Edition*), an updated listing of online search resources, forms required for registering to file online, computer software that is allowed to be distributed (freeware), and a discussion group to resolve problems you might face in online filing of patents.

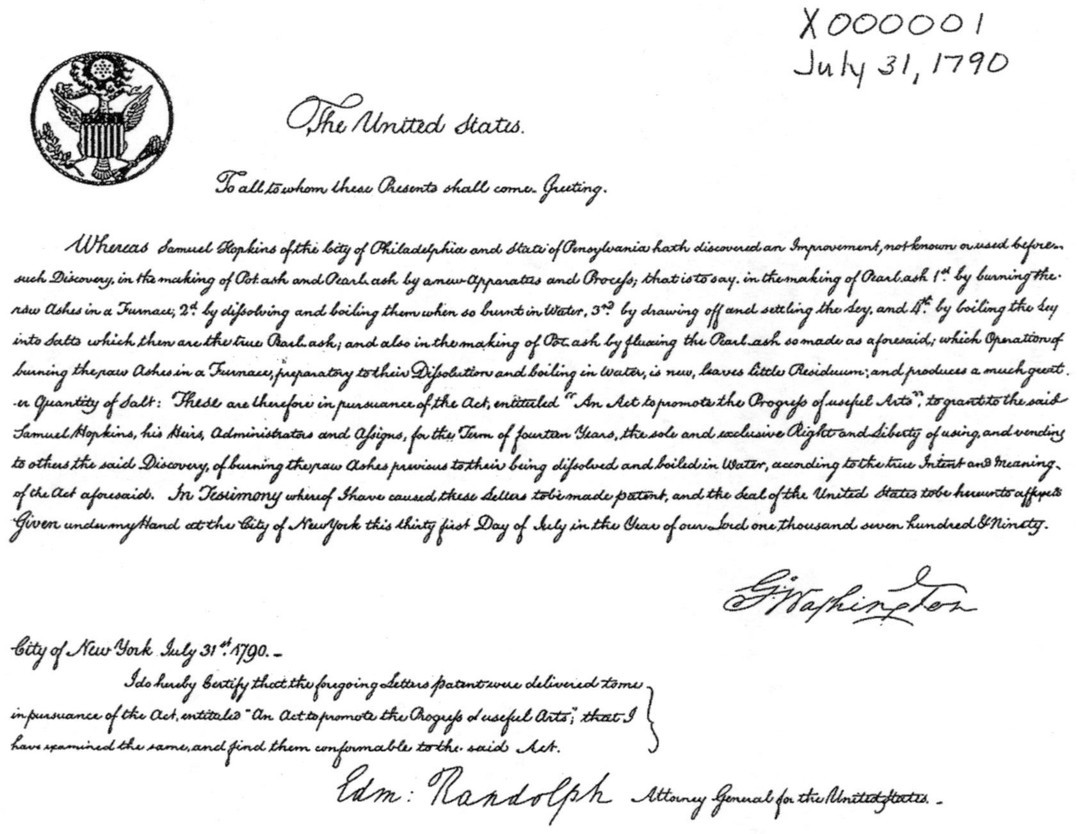

X000001
July 31, 1790

The United States.

To all to whom these Presents shall come. Greeting.

Whereas Samuel Hopkins of the City of Philadelphia and State of Pensylvania hath discovered an Improvement, not known or used before such Discovery, in the making of Pot ash and Pearl ash by a new Apparatus and Process; that is to say, in the making of Pearl ash 1st by burning the raw Ashes in a Furnace, 2d by dissolving and boiling them when so burnt in Water, 3d by drawing off and settling the Ley, and 4th by boiling the Ley into Salts which then are the true Pearl ash; and also in the making of Pot ash by fluxing the Pearl ash so made as aforesaid; which Operation of burning the raw Ashes in a Furnace, preparatory to their Dissolution and boiling in Water, is new, leaves little Residuum, and produces a much greater Quantity of Salt: These are therefore in pursuance of the Act, entituled "An Act to promote the Progress of useful Arts", to grant to the said Samuel Hopkins, his Heirs, Administrators and Assigns, for the Term of fourteen Years, the sole and exclusive Right and Liberty of using, and vending to others the said Discovery, of burning the raw Ashes previous to their being dissolved and boiled in Water, according to the true Intent and Meaning of the Act aforesaid. In Testimony whereof I have caused these Letters to be made patent, and the Seal of the United States to be hereunto affixed. Given under my Hand at the City of New York this thirty first Day of July in the Year of our Lord one thousand seven hundred & Ninety.

G. Washington

City of New York July 31st 1790. –

I do hereby Certify that the foregoing Letters patent were delivered to me in pursuance of the Act, entituled "An Act to promote the Progress of useful Arts"; that I have examined the same, and find them conformable to the said Act.

Edm: Randolph Attorney General for the United States. –

FIGURE 1.1 The first U.S. Patent signed by President George Washington.

2 Patent Application Essentials

INTRODUCTION

Whereas the focus of this book is electronic preparation and filing of patent applications, the choice of various application filing modules depends greatly on the type and scope of the patent application. This chapter summarizes patentability requirements as a primer to the field of patenting and in determining the essential features of an application, particularly in the U.S. Abbreviated definitions are provided with the assumption that the reader is well versed in the field of patent law. Further details and explanations of these laws and rules are available through the U.S. Patent and Trademark Office at http://www.uspto.gov.

A patent for an invention is the grant of a property right to the inventor issued by the USPTO or by other patent offices around the world. The term of a new U.S. patent is 20 years from the date on which the application for the patent was filed or, in special cases, from the date an earlier related application was filed, subject to the payment of maintenance fees. U.S. patent grants are effective only within the U.S., its territories, and its possessions.

The right conferred by the patent grant is, in the language of the statute and of the grant itself, "the right to exclude others from making, using, offering for sale, or selling" the invention in the U.S., or "importing" the invention to the U.S. What is granted is not the right to make, use, offer for sale, sell, or import, but the right to exclude others from doing so. Similar to a real property, patent deeds can be assigned or sold.

In the U.S., the inventor must file the patent either on his own or through a patent agent or patent attorney licensed by the USPTO. Patent applications can be filed on behalf of the dead or the mentally insane as well. Just about anything under the sun can be patented as long as it is useful and does not claim to defy the laws of nature or is itself not a law of nature or an abstract thought.

Patent law specifies the general field of subject matter that can be patented and the conditions under which a patent may be obtained. In the language of the statute, any person who "invents or discovers any new and useful process, machine, manufacture, or composition of matter, or any new and useful improvement thereof, may obtain a patent," subject to the conditions and requirements of the law.

- The term *process* is defined by law as a process, act, or method, and primarily includes industrial or technical processes.
- The term *machine,* as used in the statute, needs no explanation.

- The term *manufacture* refers to articles that are made, and includes all manufactured articles.
- The term *composition of matter* relates to chemical compositions, and may include mixtures of ingredients as well as new chemical compounds.

These classes of subject matter taken together include practically everything that is made by man and the processes for making the products. The Atomic Energy Act of 1954 excludes the patenting of inventions useful solely in the utilization of special nuclear material or energy for atomic weapons.

Patent law specifies that the subject matter must be "useful." The term *useful* in this connection refers to the condition that the subject matter has a useful purpose, and also includes operativeness, i.e., a machine that does not operate to perform the intended purpose would not be considered useful, and therefore would not be granted a patent.

Interpretations of the statute by the courts have defined the limits of the field of subject matter that can be patented, thus it has been held that the laws of nature, physical phenomena, and abstract ideas are not patentable subject matter. A patent cannot be obtained on a mere idea or suggestion; the patent is granted on the new machine, manufacture, etc., as has been said, and not on the idea or suggestion of the new machine. A complete description is required of the actual machine or other subject matter for which a patent is sought.

Ordinarily, there is nothing that prohibits a patentee from making, using, offering for sale, selling, or importing his own invention, unless he thereby infringes the prior, in-force rights of others. For example, a patent for an improvement of an original device already patented would be subject to the patent on the device.

A patentee may not violate the federal antitrust laws, such as by resale price agreements or entering into combination in restraints of trade.

According to the law in the U.S., only the inventor may apply for a patent, with certain exceptions. If a person who is not the inventor applies, the patent (if obtained) is invalid. The person applying in such a case who falsely states that he is the inventor would be subject to criminal penalties. If the inventor is dead, legal representatives, i.e., the administrator or executor of the estate, may make the application. If the inventor is insane, a guardian may make the application for patent. If an inventor refuses to apply for a patent or cannot be found, a joint inventor or a person having a proprietary interest in the invention (if there is no joint inventor available) may apply on behalf of the nonsigning inventor. If two or more persons make an invention jointly, they apply for a patent as joint inventors. A person who makes only a financial contribution is not a joint inventor and cannot be joined in the application as an inventor. It is possible to correct an innocent mistake in erroneously omitting an inventor or in erroneously naming a person as an inventor. Officers and employees of the USPTO are prohibited by law from applying for a patent or acquiring, directly or indirectly, except by inheritance or bequest, any patent or any right or interest in any patent. Unlike U.S. patent laws, foreign countries allow patent filing by assignees or corporations.

Under U.S. law it is necessary, in the case of inventions made in the U.S., to obtain a license from the Director of the USPTO before applying for a patent in a foreign country. The license is required if the foreign application is to be filed before an application is filed or within 6 months after filing an application in the U.S. unless a filing receipt with a license grant was issued earlier. The filing of an application for patent constitutes the request for a license and the granting or denial of such request is indicated in the filing receipt mailed to each applicant. After 6 months from the U.S. filing, a license is not required unless the invention has been ordered to be kept secret; if such is the case, the consent to the filing abroad must be obtained from the Director of the USPTO during the period the order of secrecy is in effect.

KEY DEFINITIONS

The terminology of patenting language is presented in the Glossary. Following are some common terms used frequently throughout this book:

Design: The emphasis of this type of patent is on the design of the invention, not on its functionality. The important aspect of this type of patent is the invention's unique ornamental and aesthetic properties.

Invention: An invention is the conception of a new and useful article, machine, composition, or process.

Patent: Right of ownership granted by the government that gives the owner the right to exclude others from making, selling, or using the claimed invention.

Patent application: A document submitted to a patent office with the aim of obtaining a patent on an invention. The patent application describes an invention in detail.

Plant: This type of patent includes new varieties of asexually reproduced plants.

Prior art: Knowledge that is in existence or publicly available before the date of an invention or more than one year prior to the first patent application date.

Reduction to practice: An in-depth description of how the invention works, described in concrete terms.

Utility: This is the most common type of patent. It includes inventions that operate in a new and useful manner.

MISCONCEPTIONS

The patenting of inventions is a complex process that historically has been confusing, particularly for inventors who may not be practitioners of patent law. For example:

- Patents are valuable only if they can be used to protect a profit stream by excluding others from making, using, or selling whatever is covered by the patent's claims.
- A patent does not mean that the invention works as verified by the government; it is left for the licensors to evaluate; it is suspected that as

many as 10% of all issued patents are invalid for being nonfunctional as claimed.

- You cannot get a provisional patent. You can file a Provisional Patent Application for a small fee that allows you 12 months to file a regular application while protecting your priority. A Provisional Application is not simply "describing the idea"; it is a complete application without the required claim(s). You may not change anything in the body of the application when you file the regular application if you want to take priority advantage.

- You cannot get a patent for an idea or a mere suggestion. Patents are granted to people who (claim to) "invent or discover any new and useful process, machine, manufacture, or composition of matter, or any new and useful improvement thereof," to quote the essence of the U.S. statute governing patents. Complete and enabling disclosure also is required.

- A patent can be enforceable from the time it is issued until it expires, not necessarily a 20-year term. New rules provide some guarantee that the enforceable term of a utility patent will be at least 17 years and that some royalties may be collectable when a patent is published before it issues. Design patents are good only for 14 years and cover only the ornamental appearance of the item, not its structure or functionality.

- A patent right is exclusory only. A patent does not give the owner the exclusive right to make, use, or sell an invention; it gives its owner the right to exclude others from making, using, or selling exactly what is covered by the patent claims. A holder of a prior patent with broader claims may prevent the inventor whose patent has narrower claims from using the inventor's own patent.

- A U.S. patent is enforceable only in the U.S. It can be used to stop others from importing into the U.S. what the patent covers, but people in other countries are free to make, use, and sell the invention anywhere else in the world that the inventor does not have a patent. This is the reason one must consider filing a PCT application and following it up with either individual state filings or a consortium filing such as the European Patent Office (EPO).

- A patent does not protect an invention because only a patent in conjunction with a legal opinion of infringement will give the owner(s) of the patent the right to sue in a civil case against the alleged infringer. The U.S. government does not enforce patents (however, the Customs Service can help block infringing imports), and infringement of a patent is not a crime. The responsibility and expense of enforcing the rights granted by a patent (and securing Customs Service help) lie with the patent owner(s).

- Filing for a patent is not the only way to protect an invention. When properly used, the USPTO Disclosure Document Program ($10), Nondisclosure Agreements (free), and Provisional Applications for Patent ($80), along with maintaining good records and diligent pursuit, can keep your patenting rights intact until you file for a patent.

- A patent attorney or agent is not needed to file your patent; an inventor may choose to file *pro se* (on his own). However, given the complexity of the law, advice from professionals often proves invaluable.

INTRODUCTION TO PATENT PRACTICE

PURPOSE OF PATENT

The purpose of the patent is to award the patentee with the right in the U.S. to exclude others from making, using, selling, offering to sell, or importing the patented invention. A patent is not a right to practice an invention. Society benefits after patent expiry, allowing for improvement of the invention and designing around the claims.

LAWS GOVERNING PATENTS

The U.S. Constitution gives Congress the power to enact laws relating to patents in Article I, section 8, which reads: "Congress shall have power ... to promote the progress of science and useful arts, by securing for limited times to authors and inventors the exclusive right to their respective writings and discoveries." Under this power Congress has from time to time enacted various laws relating to patents. The first patent law was enacted in 1790. The patent laws underwent a general revision which was enacted July 19, 1952, and which came into effect January 1, 1953. It is codified in Title 35, United States Code. Additionally, on November 29, 1999, Congress enacted the American Inventors Protection Act of 1999 (AIPA), which further revised the patent laws. The Constitution establishes the laws 35 USC contains; 37 CFR (Code of Federal Regulations) contains the rules; MPEP (*Manual of Patent Examining Procedure*) governs the applications of law; modifications and treaties modify the regulations and applications of law continuously; case law defines the limits of legal definition.

IMPORTANT DATES

1. *December 8, 1993/January 1, 1996:* Dates that may be relied on to establish a date of invention (by an applicant or patentee) in NAFTA (North American Free Trade Agreement) and WTO (World Trade Organization) countries, respectively; dates claimed prior to these dates are shifted down to these dates.
2. *June 8, 1995:* Provisional application allowed; 20-year term from filing date forward of this date.
3. *November 29, 1999:* 12 months to convert provisional to nonprovisional even if provisional is abandoned. If provisional application's anniversary falls on holiday or weekend, the due date for filing claimed nonprovisional application is moved to the following business day; all of it is effective retroactive to June 8, 1995. 35 USC 103 was amended to add a safe haven for 102(e)/103(f) and (g) events when common assignee is the beneficiary. 102(g) amended (added section 1): dates of invention permitted to

constitute as prior art only when established in an interference in PTO or in U.S. District Court.

4. *May 29, 2000:* RCE (Request for Continued Examination) may be filed on an application for which prosecution is closed (that is not a continuing application) if filed on and after June 8, 1995; CPA (Continued Prosecution Application) may not be validly filed on and after May 29, 2000 except for designs and patent applications filed before May 29, 2000 (if filed, it will be treated as RCE); patent term guarantee (response times, issuance period, total time pending) 14–4–4–4–36 month obligations of PTO with offsets for dilatory applicant prosecution.

5. *November 29, 2000:* Preissuance publication of application 18 months postfiling, which publications become prior art as of the application filing date (not the publication date).

6. *April 2, 2002:* Time to enter national stage after Chapter I filing extended to 30 months; no change in Chapter II filing deadlines; applicable to Chapter I filings due for 20-month Chapter II filing after April 2, 2002.

PARTS OF A PATENT

DRAWINGS (35 USC 113)

- Drawings are required when necessary, most likely in mechanical or electrical and some chemical applications
- Drawings must show all of the claimed elements
- Filing date is not assigned if drawings are not provided at the OIPE (Office of Initial Patent Examination) level of evaluation
- Examiner may require drawings but filing date is not affected
- Drawings may be added later by amendment if already described in the specification or claim as originally filed
- No need for manufacturing drawings (such as tolerances or in-process controls)

SPECIFICATION (35 USC 112)

The written description, the manner and process of making and using should be in such full, clear, concise, and exact terms as to enable any person skilled (with ordinary skills) in the art to which it pertains, or with which it is most nearly connected, to make and use the invention and setting forth the best mode contemplated by the inventor for carrying out the invention. There are three requirements: description, enablement, and best mode.

1. Description
   - Must describe what is claimed clearly
   - Focus is on the claimed invention only

- Scope commensurate with scope of claim(s); disclosure of a single species may or may not support a generic claim
- Critical or essential element must be recited in claim(s)
- The vantage point is one of ordinary skill in the art
- The inventor may be his own lexicographer; spell out but not befuddle, not use in a manner contrary to what is commonly acceptable
- Theory need not be set forth; if theory is wrong, the error is not fatal (unless theory is claimed invention)
- Manner of invention (how the invention was made) is not important

2. Enablement
   - A person of ordinary skills can make and use
   - Without undue experimentation
   - Not necessarily for commercial production
   - This requirement is different than §101 requirement of being useful
   - Claim not reciting the essential matter may be rejected for lack of enablement; failing to claim the subject matter that the applicant regards as the invention
   - Publications after filing date may be used to defeat enablement (such as by examiner)
   - Scope of enablement must be commensurate with scope of claim(s)
   - Amount of disclosure required depends on the state of the art and predictability; the more that is known and the greater the predictability, the less disclosure is required

3. Best mode
   - What inventor considers best mode may not be what anyone else considers best and not what is best objectively
   - At the time application is filed; need not and cannot be updated by amendment (as it will be considered new matter) even in a division or continuation, but can be updated in CIP (Continuation-in-Part) if it pertains to a new claim made
   - Must be disclosed although not necessarily identified as such; embodiment disclosed is automatically considered as the best mode; several embodiments may be disclosed without identifying which one is the best

112 ¶1 REQUIREMENT: DESCRIPTION, ENABLEMENT, AND BEST MODE

Description, enablement, and best mode for each claim as filed or else claim is rendered invalid if contested. Mythical person is one of ordinary skills in the art, not a layperson. Need to disclose what is considered as required knowledge of one of ordinary skill. Any one or more of these specific portions of an application can satisfy each of these three requirements: specification, drawing(s), and claims as originally filed. Unclaimed inventions need not satisfy this requirement.

112 ¶2 Requirement: Parts of a Claim

- Preamble sets the tone for the invention's technical environment and class (composition, process, or apparatus, etc.: *a method of, apparatus for, a composition*). It is not limiting if it merely states the purpose of the invention; however, if it breathes life and meaning into the claim (such as if it is essential to tell what is claimed if the body of claim refers to it as antecedent support), it can become limiting.
- Transitional phrase connects the body of the claim to the preamble: *comprising, consisting of, consisting essentially of*, etc. Three types: (1) open-ended (*comprising, including, containing, characterized by*, etc.), (2) closed (*consisting of, also composed of, having, being*, etc., some of these can be interpreted differently), and (3) partially closed (*consisting essentially of*), wherein it allows only those additional elements that do not affect the basic and novel characteristics of the invention without introducing synergism. The applicant has burden of proof to show that additional elements in prior art would materially change the characteristics of the invention. If ABCD is known and ABC is claimed, absence of D must be demonstrated to materially affect the invention.
- Body is a list of elements such as ingredients of a composition, or components of an apparatus; all elements must be interconnected (there must a reason to recite a component, not merely to list it).

READING A CLAIM

Claim reading is an exercise to find out if what a claim states is present in an invention or a written statement.

- Prior art to prove validity of claim
- A device or process to indicate infringement
- Owner specification satisfies §112 ¶1 requirements

Claim does not read on prior art with elements ABCD if the claim is ABC and closed (*consisting of*); however, it reads if the transitional phrase is open (*comprising*) and may or may not read if it is partially closed (*consisting essentially of*).

Punctuation of Claim

A claim consists of one sentence with a comma after the preamble and a colon after a transitional phrase. Each element gets its own paragraph; a semicolon at the end of each paragraph; *and* between the last two elements. More than one period means more than one sentence and thus an indefinite claim (§112 ¶2).

DEFINITENESS OF CLAIM

- Without proper antecedent basis, a claim is rendered indefinite. *A* or *an* introduces an element for the first time except in a means-plus-function format. *Said* or *the* refer back to previously introduced elements or limitations, or refer to inherent properties (not required to be recited for antecedent purpose; e.g., *the surface of said element* when *surface* is not defined earlier).
- Inferential claiming where interconnectivity of elements is not certain; does not tell if the element is part of combination.

NARROWING OF CLAIM

A claim is narrowed by adding an element or limitation to a previously recited element; a narrow claim can be dependent or independent. Adding a step narrows a claim; adding an element to a closed claim (see Markush Group discussion) broadens a claim.

Dependent Claims (§112 ¶3–4)

- Claim can be dependent or independent; a dependent claim incorporates by reference all the limitations of the claims to which it refers and is always narrower; must depend from a preceding claim, not a following claim (numbering of claims is readjusted during prosecution).
- *Further comprising* or *further including* used to narrow a claim by adding another element or step.
- Claim narrowed by further defining an element or the relationship between elements. Transitional element *wherein* used to add limitation. Narrowing can be both adding an element and further defining the relationship.
- Defining a step further narrows method claim.

Multiple Dependent Claims (§112 ¶5)

- A claim referring to more than one previously set forth claim but only in the alternative (*or*) and narrows the claim from which it depends.
- Cannot serve as a basis for another multiple dependent claim; may refer to other dependent claim and a dependent claim may depend on a multiple dependent claim.
- Incorporates by reference all the limitations of the particular claim in relation to which it is being considered (individually and not collectively).
- It takes place of writing several dependent claims in its spirit.
- A flat special fee is charged at the time of filing application if multiple dependent claim or claims are included.

Dominant–Subservient Claims

Dominant (subcombination, genus) combinations (subservient, species) need two members (species) to create a genus, which is illustrated by the selection of species; genus is an inherent commonality among embodiments (species).

Means-Plus-Function Clauses (§112 ¶6)

- Claim defining an element by its function. Means for performing a function. Interpreted by the literal function recited and corresponding structure or materials described in specification and equivalents thereof. Does not cover all structures for performing the recited function.
- A claim reciting only a single means-plus-function clause without any other element is impressible.
- Must have the phrase *means for*, which then must be modified by functional language but not modified by the recitation of structure sufficient to accomplish the specific function.
- If specification does not adequately disclose the structure corresponding to the "means" claimed, the claim fails to comply with ¶2 requirement for "particularly pointing out and distinctly claiming" the invention.
- If disclosure is implicit (for those skilled in the art), an amendment may be required or stated on record of what structure performs the function.
- Equivalents: examiner must explain rationale; prior art must perform, not excluded by explicit definition in the specification for an equivalent, prior art supported by:
  - Identical function, substantially same way, substantially same results
  - Art-recognized interchangeability
  - Insubstantial differences
  - Structural equivalency

Process Claims

A method for making a product or using a specified or known material (*comprising the steps of*); recitation of at least one step required and a single-step method claim is proper.

Step-Plus-Function Clauses

- Functional method claims reciting a particular result but not the specified act, i.e., techniques used to achieve results such as adjusting pH, raising temperature, reducing friction, etc.
- No recital of acts in support required.
- Typically introduced by *whereby, so that,* or *for.*
- Addition of a functional description alone is not sufficient to differentiate claim; rejected under §102.

- Functional language without recitation of structure, which performs the function, may render the claim broader (rather than narrower) and rejected under §112 ¶1.

Ranges

Commonly used for temperature, pressure, time, and dimensional limitations. *Up to* means from zero to the top limit; *at least* means not less than (does not set upper limit, which must be fully disclosed in specification); specification must support eventual ranges. A dependent claim cannot broaden the range. Range within range is indefinite in a claim but acceptable in specification.

Negative Limitations

Permissible if boundaries set forth definitely, such as free of an impurity or a particular element or incapable of performing a certain function. Absence of structures cannot be claimed as structural elements (holes, channels, etc.).

Relative and Exemplary Terminology

Imprecise language may satisfy definiteness requirement (for one of ordinary skill). *So dimensioned* or *so spaced* can be definite if it is as accurate as the subject will permit; *about* is clear and flexible but rendered indefinite if specification or prior art does not provide indication about the dimensions anticipated. *Essentially, substantially,* and *effective amount* are definite if one of ordinary skills would understand.

Exemplary terminology is always indefinite; *such as, or like material,* and *similar* are all rejected.

Markush Group

- Closed form. Two forms: (1) wherein P is a material selected from a group consisting of A, B, C, and D; or (2) wherein P is A, B, C, or D. Members must belong to a recognized class, possess properties in common as disclosed in specification and these properties mainly responsible for their function or the grouping is clear from their nature or the prior art that all members possess the property.
- Adding members broadens claim.
- Prior art with one of the members anticipates the claim.

Markush Alternates

- *Or* terminology if choices are related: *one or several pieces; made entirely or part of; red, blue or white.* If unrelated choices, the use of *or* will lead to indefinite interpretation.
- *Optionally* if definite; if there are no ambiguities in the scope of claim as a result of choices offered.

Jepson-Type Claims, Improvement Claims

Preamble defines what is conventional; transitional phrase: *wherein the improvement comprises.* Body builds on preamble; can add element or modify element in preamble. Preamble is limiting.

Mixed-Class Claims

Mixed elements are improper; methods claims should have no structural elements, apparatus claims should have no step elements. Limitations can be mixed, such as method step may include a structural limitation and an apparatus may include a process limitation.

Product-by-Process Claims

A product claim that defines the claimed product in terms of the process by which it is made: *a product made by the process comprising of steps.* Patentability based on product itself and not on method of production. If the product is the same (as prior art), using another process does not make it patentable. If examiner shows that product appears to be the same or similar, the burden shifts to applicant; USPTO bears lesser burden of proof in making out a case of *prima facie* obviousness.

One-step method claims acceptable but claims where body consists of single "means" elements are not acceptable.

NOVELTY AND LOSS OF RIGHT TO PATENT: §102

DATE OF INVENTION

Conception is the formation in the mind of the inventor of a definite and permanent idea of the complete and operative invention as it is thereafter to be applied in practice. An invention date is the date when diligence began and leads to reduction to practice. §104 prohibited evidence outside of the U.S. prior to December 8, 1993 except for filing of a PCT or foreign application or acts domiciled in the U.S. but serving outside of the U.S. on government business after December 8, 1993 but prior to January 1, 1996, NAFTA countries included, and on or after January 1, 1996, all countries of WTO included. If there were events prior to these dates, they are taken to the dates the privileges became available. This is important for overcoming 102(a) rejections.

STATUS OF INVENTION

Actual means constructing the machine or article, synthesizing the composition or performing the method, and testing sufficiently to demonstrate that the invention works for its intended purpose. Testing is not required if one of ordinary skill in the art would recognize that it will work. *Constructive* means filing U.S. patent application in compliance with first paragraph of §112. *Diligence* is working on reducing the invention to either practice, or else it is considered abandoned.

TYPES OF §102 EVENTS

An event means a physical happening related to disclosure.

*   Novelty-defeating events occurring prior to invention: 102(a), (e), and (g): age
*   Time-barring events occurring more than fixed time (e.g., 1 year) prior to U.S. filing date: 102(b) and (d): absolute time bar
*   Miscellaneous: 102(c) and (f): others

§102(a)

*   Events by others; public knowledge and use only in the U.S. or patented or printed publication anywhere in the world — all prior to date of invention. By definition, the inventor himself cannot trigger a 102(a) event. Applicant's own publication is not but if someone else describes applicant's invention without learning anything from the applicant then it is a 102(a) event if it happened prior to date of invention.
*   *Knowledge* means the claimed invention must have been publicly known to a sufficiently large segment of the public, the size depending on the number of persons skilled in the art that have such knowledge — the more likely it is then for the invention to be in public knowledge.
*   *Use by others* means in use before date of invention and by more than one person and the use must have been accessible to the public without deliberate attempt to keep the use secret, although it need not be visible to the public — such as a hidden device.
*   *Printed publication* is a reference only for what it discloses and enables (it cannot be a passing remark); the effective date of publication is when the document is indexed or cataloged in a library or disseminated by mail — the test being if one of ordinary skill would have had access to the document with reasonable diligence to locate it. The number of copies distributed, whether recipients constitute a significant portion of those interested in the subject matter and whether the disclosure was an oral paper only at a conference, determines publication status. It need not be in a classic printed form — the key is public accessibility, even if stored in a remote location in a remote library, even if no one read the document in the library. Electronic publication such as online databases or Internet resources are printed publications if accessible.
*   *Patent* is a reference to the date it becomes enforceable, but if it is kept secret (as in some countries), then it is the date it becomes sufficiently accessible to the public; if patent is published before its rights are exercisable, the date is when it becomes exercisable, not the date of publication. The published patent is treated as "printed publication" and not a patent until such time. The patented subject matter includes, in addition to claimed subject matter, subject matter disclosed in the specification that is covered by the claims; unclaimed species are covered by a genus claim. Specification that relates to the subject matter also is "patented"

matter. The disclosure need not be enabling, quite unlike the requirements for a "printed publication."

- Priority can be claimed to avoid 102(a) rejection based on earlier filed applications which include foreign, continuation, provisional, or nonprovisional applications. Claiming priority is necessary to establish the 'effective' filing date. However, this can only be done if the earlier application provides §112 ¶1 support, and provided this application is filed within 1 year (or 6 months for design) of the earlier application on which a priority is claimed.

§102(b)

- Events by anyone (including inventor); public use and on-sale only in the U.S. or patented or printed publication anywhere in the world, more than 1 year before filing date — the earliest U.S. filing date of application; also called "the critical date." If anniversary date of the critical date falls on a weekend or a federal holiday, the application may be filed on the next business day to avoid statutory bar. §102(b) is a statutory time bar; it cannot be removed or antedated, regardless of date of invention or who was responsible.
- A §102(b) event anticipates a claim if and only if all elements and limitations recited in the claim (under application) are present in the subject matter of the event, i.e., if the claim reads on the subject matter of the event.
- A single public use of the claimed invention by a single person is sufficient for this bar. Hidden from sight but public uses are sufficient. Intentionally concealing (making it available on a restricted basis and confidentiality obligation) is not public use. Misappropriated use is still a public use. Experimental use is not public use (where necessary to demonstrate the workability and where the profit was incidental to the experimental use). Experimentation must be the primary purpose (control by the inventor, confidentiality agreements, record of performance and progress report kept, necessity of public testing, length of test period, whether payments were made, changes made as a result of use). Product acceptance by the market is not experimental use.
- On-sale bar applies when offered for sale in the U.S. and the invention was "ready for patenting," reduced to actual practice or the inventor had prepared drawings or other descriptions of the invention sufficient to enable a person skilled in the art to practice the invention. The product sold need not be on hand or in physical existence. The sale offer can be made by anyone (inventor, assignee, or third party). Published abstracts may qualify for on-sale rejection if they identify product's vendor, contain information useful for potential buyers (contact, price, warranties, etc.), along with date of product release or installation before the critical date. *Note:* It can be a §102/103 bar as well (obviousness based on sale activity). A sale can be conditional, secret (phone or discrete), without profits, an offer from the U.S. to an offeree abroad or vice versa, offer originating

but not received prior to critical date, an offer that never reaches, rejected offer, not consummated, single sale, sale between two related entities not controlled by each other, or even sale made without inventor's consent or in violation of any confidentiality agreement. Not a sale event: incidental sale to experimental use is not a sale even if yields profit provided the primary purpose was experimental study (see above for conditions); assignment of rights is not an on-sale event, the *res* (substance) of invention must be sold.

- Patents on the date of their availability become §102(b) bar. A foreign filing within 12 months of §102 event and then filing U.S. patent within 1 year of the foreign filing does not remove §102(b) bar. It must be filed in the U.S. within 12 months either as provisional or nonprovisional. Foreign priority does not remove this bar, the U.S. priority does. A continuation application is governed by its ancestral filing date and thus it can avoid §102(b) bar.

§102(c)

- Events by inventor — abandonment of invention, expressed, implied, by action or by inaction.
- Unreasonable delays in filing the U.S. patent, developing invention, coupled with other evidence such as spurring into activity if someone else has commercialized or is about to commercialize the product of invention. Delay alone is not sufficient to demonstrate abandonment.
- Disclosing but not claiming a distinct embodiment; can be overcome by filing another application claiming the disclosed embodiment within 1 year of the issue date of the patent or filing a broadening reissue application within 2 years of the patent.
- Abandoned invention may be recaptured by proceeding diligently to obtain a U.S. patent prior to another's invention of the same subject.

§102(d)

- Events by inventor or affiliate (as allowed in foreign filings) — filing abroad more than 1 year (6 months for design) before U.S. filing date and patent must issue before U.S. filing date (unlike §102(a) and (b), the date of patent is the date rights attach even if the patent is kept secret).
- The same invention must be involved but not necessarily claimed in the U.S. application; a different aspect of the invention might be claimed.

§102(e)

- The default date of invention of a pending application is its filing date (constructive reduction to practice) unless otherwise proven.
- Events by others; published application in the U.S. or in English if PCT and designating U.S. or an issued U.S. patent filed before the date of

invention of application in question. *Note:* The only date the USPTO has for a pending application is the filing date of application (constructive reduction to practice), which must then be challenged through affidavits if contested, if rejection is based on §102(e). "Another" means an inventive entity different from the application's inventive entity. An inventive entity is different if not all inventors are the same; a Rule 1.132 declaration can be used to establish this.

- §102(e)(2)[A]. A U.S. patent to "another" stemming from a domestic application (not a PCT filing designating U.S.) has the effective date as a reference as of its U.S. filing date (with claim extending to its provisional or continuation application if applicable) as a prior art reference but NOT its foreign priority date, where applicable, against a pending U.S. application. On the contrary, the pending U.S. application against which the reference is used can use its foreign priority date as a shield, provided the reference's U.S. filing date is later than the foreign filing date of the application. This is applicable even if the reference has a foreign filing date prior to the foreign filing date of the application because the foreign filing date of the reference is immaterial. However, if the reference has a domestic priority date prior to the applicant's foreign priority date, then the foreign priority date of applicant cannot be used to overcome §102(e)(2)[A] rejection.

- §102(e)(2)[B]. A U.S. patent to "another" stemming from a national stage PCT application has the priority date depending on the filing dates of the pending applications against which it is used. If the application under examination was filed:

  - For a pending USPTO application filed prior to November 29, 2000 and not voluntarily published, the priority date of the U.S. patent as a reference is the date when the PCT application for this reference patent entered the national stage in the U.S.
  - For a pending USPTO application filed before November 29, 2000 and published voluntarily, the U.S. patent stemming from a national stage PCT filing has no effect on this application (meaning that the U.S. patent reference has no effective filing date; it does not exist).
  - For a pending USPTO application filed on or after November 29, 2000, the U.S. patent stemming from a national stage PCT filing has no effect on this application (meaning that the U.S. patent reference has no effective filing date; it does not exist).

- §102(e)(1)[A]. Published domestic U.S. patent application is an anticipatory reference as of its filing date, even if it were subsequently abandoned. The §102(e) reference must contain an enabling disclosure relative to the application claim against which it is applied; an issued U.S. patent has a statutory presumption of validity, a published application does not. If the reference is not enabling, it cannot be a §102 event but can still be a §103 event.

- §102(e)(1)[B]. Published PCT patent application (by WIPO or by USPTO — entering national stage) is a reference as of the PCT filing date if it did designate U.S. and was published by WIPO in English. The USPTO-published national stage is a reference as of its PCT filing date but only if the PCT application was published by WIPO in English. If a PCT application does meet these requirements, it can be a §102(a) or (b) event but not §102(e).

§102(f)

The inventor is the one who conceives the invention, and does not derive it from someone else (disclosed by or getting the idea from someone else).

§102(g)

- §102(g)(2). A patent bar arises if the invention was made in this country by another inventor who did not abandon, suppress, or conceal it. An interference proceeding or an *ex parte* examination decides and thus §102(g) becomes applicable only after these evaluations. Five conditions apply: (1) the invention must have been made, i.e., reduced to practice, (2) in this country (§104, invention in foreign countries, does not apply), (3) by another, (4) before the applicant's date of invention, and (5) the other did not abandon, suppress, or conceal it. Reasonable diligence is a major key to these decisions.
- §102(g)(1). Applies only in an interference proceeding to establish that the invention was made within the limits of §104 — NAFTA country after December 7, 1993 or WTO country after December 31, 1996. Other conditions of abandoning, suppressing, and concealing apply as above. Countries outside NAFTA or WTO are not considered regardless of date of activity in those countries. Even in NAFTA and WTO countries the latest date of activity is the date given above when they entered the jurisdiction; all prior dates are shifted to these dates.

§102 Special Forms

- Abandoned applications: If an issued patent refers to an abandoned application, the contents of that application become evidence of public knowledge [§102(a)]. If an issued application expressly incorporates the disclosure of an abandoned application by reference, then the contents become part of the disclosure effective as of the patent's filing date under §102(e)(2).
- Material cancelled from an application is not part of the patent for the purposes of §102(e)(2); however, the prosecution history becomes available to the public as of the issue date of the patent and becomes a §102(a) event.

- Incipient §102(e) references: Unpublished applications cannot be cited as prior art under §102(e); however, claims in a later-filed application may be provisionally rejected over an earlier application under §102(e) if the two applications have a common inventor or assignee.
- Oral testimony alone, without at least some documentary corroboration, is generally insufficient to prove invalidity.
- Statutory invention registrations (SIRs) examined in compliance with §112 ¶1 are treated the same as a patent for §102(e)(2) purpose — defensive purpose.
- Doctrine of forfeiture: A commercial, purposely hidden use of a process or a machine by an applicant (but not by a third party) more than 1 year before the filing date of the application, coupled with a sale of the *res* precludes the application from obtaining a patent.

OBVIOUSNESS/NONOBVIOUSNESS (§103)

§103(A)

If the difference between the claimed invention and the prior art are such that the invention as a whole would have been obvious at the time of invention to a person having ordinary skill in the art to which said subject matter pertains, a patent will not be granted.

MANNER OF INVENTION

The manner in which the invention is made does not negate patentability (e.g., an invention made by someone not familiar with the field of invention or making an accidental invention).

GRAHAM V. JOHN DEERE: FUNDAMENTAL INQUIRY

Graham v. John Deere, 383 U.S. 1, 148 USPQ 459 (1966) is one of the most famous cases that establishes what is considered prior art that makes the invention obvious. The Patent Office follows the factual inquiry based on this case to:

(A)   Determine the scope and contents of the prior art
(B)   Ascertain the differences between the prior art and the claims at issue
(C)   Resolve the level of ordinary skill in the pertinent art
(D)   Evaluate evidence of secondary considerations

- The scope and content of the prior art
- The difference between the prior art and the claims at issue
- The level of ordinary skill in the pertinent art
- Secondary considerations, i.e., objective indicia of unobviousness:
  - Commercial success
  - Long-felt but unresolved needs
  - Failure of others, etc.

- Recognition of problem
- Failure to resolve problem
- Competitors' prompt copying
- Licensing of patent to industry
- Teaching away (when a disclosure asserts that what the invention represents cannot or should not be done)
- Unexpected results
- Disbelief and incredulity

PRIMA FACIE OBVIOUSNESS

It is the level of showing that the PTO must make in order to shift to the applicant the burden of going forward with production of evidence or arguments tending to prove nonobviousness. The examiner, on the basis of prior art, proposes a combination that would be possible for one of ordinary skills to make. To protect the applicant:

- Hindsight is impermissible.
- Examiner must step back before invention.
- Knowledge of applicant's disclosure is put aside.
- Only the facts gleaned from the prior art may be used.

Examiner bears the initial burden of supporting *prima facie* conclusion; otherwise, the applicant has no obligation to submit evidence of nonobviousness. Once so produced, the burden shifts to the applicant to submit additional evidence, e.g., commercial success, unexpected results, etc.

PRIMA FACIE REQUIREMENTS

- There must be some suggestion or motivation, either in the references themselves or in the knowledge generally available to one of ordinary skill in the art, to modify the references or to combine reference teachings. *Prima facie* does not hold if it is shown that:
  - Teachings can be modified or combined.
  - Prior art does not suggest the desirability of combination.
  - One of ordinary skill is merely capable of combining the teachings.
  - Modifications or combinations destroy the intended function.
  - There is a change in the principle of operation of the prior art.
  - Modification or combination of prior art teaches away from such modification or combination.
  - Applicant's invention is the discovery of problem or the source of problem.
- There must be a reasonable, not absolute, expectation or predictability of success of the proposed modification or combination of the prior art at the time invention was made, not when the examiner evaluates it.

- The prior art reference(s) must teach or suggest *all* the claim limitations. This includes indefinite limitations (not meeting §112 ¶2) and limitations unsupported by the specification in the application. (Thus there may be rejection on the basis of §112 but not §103 in these situations.) Unclaimed features are not germane to the obviousness determination.
- The prior art must be "analogous" to invention — either in the field of invention or reasonably pertinent to it.
- Only the teachings of prior art, which must be combinable; it is not necessary that the specific structure be physically combinable; *prima facie* obviousness is not negated for business reasons not to combine; the issue is technologic combination.
- Prior art need not suggest same advantage or results as the invention; motivation to modify or combine the prior art may be stimulated by a purpose different from that of the claimed invention, or the solution of a problem different from that solved by the claimed invention.
- Routine manipulative steps cannot be *prima facie* obvious when the claimed material it uses or produces is patentable, i.e., where either the starting or the ending material is patentable.

§102(E), (F), AND (G) EVENTS AS §103 PRIOR ART

- §103: Prior art under §102(e), (f), and (g) may be modified or combined to establish obviousness, except when the subject matter of prior art and the invention claimed in the application under examination were, at the time the claimed invention was made (not when it was filed), owned by the same person or subject to an obligation of assignment to the same person.
- With respect to §102(e), §103(c) is effective as of November 29, 1999 (American Inventors Protection Act, AIPA). Rejections on the basis of §102(e)/§103 can be obviated using an affidavit if ownership is the same by an affidavit for an application filed after November 29, 1999. For applications filed prior to this date, a continuation application may be filed to take advantage of this ruling change.
- Whereas references in §103 are as of the date of invention, an exception arises when using a §102(e) event are applied, wherein the prior art is applied as of the date of the filing of the application vis-à-vis the filing date of the reference.

ADMISSION AS PRIOR ART UNDER §103

If an applicant admits a reference as prior art it cannot be reversed in a traversal; admissions include labeling drawings as prior art and any written admission during prosecution in addition to whatever has been submitted in the specification. A Jepsen claim, however, can be rebutted.

RIGHTS AND PROCEDURES UNDER THE PATENT COOPERATIVE TREATY (PCT)

DEFINITIONS

Contracting state: PCT member countries
U.S./RO: U.S. Receiving Office
IB: International Bureau (Geneva)
National application: 35 USC 111(a) nonprovisional application
International PCT application: 35 USC 351 application
National stage application: 35 USC 371(c) application

STRATEGIES

- **Multiple concurrent national filings:** This can be done in any state (country or a group of countries such as European, Eurasian, African Regional Industrial Property Organization (ARIPO), African Intellectual Property Organization (OAPI), where one application suffices for all member countries) of choice simultaneously at a great initial cost particularly because at this stage the patentability of an invention is not certain.
- **Paris Convention national filings:** First file in U.S. (priority application) followed by individual country filings within 12 months — cost optimized because some idea about patentability is ascertained.
- **File international application (PCT):** New laws effective April 2002 now allow up to 30 months with a single filing to defer filing in other countries.
  - One application is filed designating all states (countries) where patent is desired — the International Application. This is similar to filing national application in several countries although PCT does not result in issuance of patent.
  - Filed in one of the official languages accepted by the Receiving Office — which can be home patent office or the International Bureau (new rules mandate home filing).

PCT PROCESS

An international application is a license to defer national filing and consists of two stages:

1. Stage one is called Chapter I, which is the Search stage. An initial application of PCT goes through many distinct steps including: correction of defect(s), foreign filing assessment (granted or not), determination of unity of invention (single general inventive concept or not; cf. restriction in U.S. filing), payment of extra fee if for more than one inventive concept or payment of fee and filing the protest; these steps are followed by an international search that results in a report and prior art reporting;

at this time the applicant may withdraw or withdraw conditionally; offer amendment to claims only and comments; following this stage is the publication of application which includes application plus international search and amendment, generally within 18 months.

2. Stage two reaches the 19th month when the applicant may decide to file Chapter II or Demand, which until April 2002 allowed deferment of national filing to 30 months; now this is not necessary. However, one may continue with this practice optionally; there are some clear advantages to proceeding through Demand. Chapter II (examination) includes prelimi-nary amendment (voluntary at applicant's option), unity of invention determination where, if there is more than a single inventive entity, extra fee payment is required (that can be done with or without protest); Written Opinion is now issued regarding defects, novelty, and inventive steps which allow for amendment (drawing, description, and claims), and com-ments by applicant; this then leads to International Preliminary Examina-tion with respect to defects, novelty, and inventive steps, and a report is issued in the 28th month. There is just enough time left then for the 30th month national filing. Going through Chapter II voluntarily now gives a better idea about patentability at a much lower cost. Election of state is required for Chapter II.

At the 30th month, the applicant must file a national application — this date is not extendible.

PCT Application

- First-filed national application serves as priority application, if filed; no U.S.-type design or national security applications allowed.
- A U.S. provisional application is accepted for priority; however, there are no claims in the provisional application that can create problems.
- U.S. system works on relative novelty (who discovered first rather than who filed first), while the rest of the world works on absolute novelty (who filed first); appropriate consideration regarding priority should be taken here.
- Within 12 months of priority application filing date, the PCT must be filed — there is no provision for extension of time for any reason (absolute bar). This is a Paris Convention clause.
- PCT application designates states; one applicant must reside in U.S. or be a U.S. national.
- Can designate application as continuation or CIP.
- Use A4 paper and verify no missing components.
- At 30th month, file a copy of the international application, unless it has been previously communicated by the International Bureau or unless it was originally filed in the USPTO with the basic national fee (this must be paid and it is not extendible); translation, if required, and declaration need not be filed at this time; the USPTO will notify applicant of omitted

papers and set time for the filing of the omitted papers; time period is extendible.

- If an international application goes abandoned as to U.S. filing because of missing the dates for filing the "missing parts," one can petition (PTO/SB61/PCT for unavoidable abandonment or PTO/SB64/PCT for unintentional abandonment). *Note:* It does not apply to 30th month filing and payment of fee. In ordinary national filing, payment of fee is not required to get a filing date.
- The question of unity of invention may arise again in the U.S. national filing and be subject to restriction requirements of 35 USC 121 (divisional).
- Applicant designation in an international application can be a "legal entity" to which the invention has been assigned; in the U.S., this must be the applicant; thus if U.S. is a designated state, then all applicants must be identified in the international application (this cannot be changed at the time of U.S. national stage filing).

Significant §102(e) Issues

Pre-AIPA (Filed November 29, 2000 or Earlier)

An international filing date is considered an actual filing date in each designated state according to PCT articles; however, for the purpose of §102(e), it is the date when the national stage application was filed in the U.S. (complete requirements, which include copy of international application, fee, and oath or declaration).

Post-AIPA (Filed November 29, 2000 or Later)

Complicated situations arise when considering whether an application gets a priority date (as a shield against other applications and patents), and whether an application or patent is an §102(e) event (a sword against other applications).

§102(e)(1)
- **Published U.S. application:** Takes shield priority to the date of earliest U.S. filing and acts as a sword against others on the date of its publication.
- **Published PCT application:** If designated U.S. and published in English, then priority date is the publication date of application.

§102(e)(2)
- **U.S. patent:** Earliest effective U.S. filing date. It is possible that patent issues before 18-month publication of application and applicant certifies no foreign filing; in such instance, it is the earliest filing date that governs.
- **U.S. patent from PCT application:** Does not have an effective filing date (and thus reference date) and so it is issue date that counts. The assumption involved here is that the application might have published under PCT (see above).

3 Online Patentability Search

INTRODUCTION

A patent application begins with a thorough search of the inventive idea:

- Knowing whether a patent is patentable based on its statutory class
- Getting a general idea of how an application and patent is structured to help in the preparation of your own application
- Learning more about a new field for market information
- Tracking competitors
- Tracking technology

The goal in conducting a patentability search is to ensure that the invention falls into one of five statutory classes if applying for a utility patent:

1. Process: Includes conventional processes (e.g., the method for making plastics) and software processes
2. Machines: Includes conventional machines, those with moving parts (e.g., a telephone) and software machines
3. Manufactured products: Inventions with nonmoving parts (e.g., books)
4. Compositions of matter: Examples include chemicals, alloys, and pharmaceuticals
5. New uses of any of the above

Other goals of a patentability search are to determine if the invention

- Is useful, even if that use is only for amusement purposes
- Satisfies also the novelty requirement; in other words, it must be original or something that has never been seen before
- Meets the nonobviousness requirement, meaning it would have been unobvious to the people skilled in the area of the invention

Although "anything under the sun" can be patented, there are inventions that are not patentable:

1. Superior material for inferior
2. Change in size, form, or shape

3. Mere adjustability
4. Diminution of parts
5. Omission of parts
6. Use of old art for another purpose
7. Mere aggregation
8. Laws of nature
9. Physical phenomena
10. Abstract ideas
11. Literary, dramatic, musical, and artistic works (these should be copyright protected, not patented)
12. Inventions that are against the laws of nature (e.g., perpetual motion machines)
13. Inventions whose only use is for illegal purposes (e.g., torture devices, terrorist tools, forgeries, etc.)

ANATOMY OF A PATENT

In determining the patentability of an invention, it is not just the claims made in other patents that are important to consider, but the body of issued patent as well. For example, it is possible that your invention may not be reading on claims of other patents but other disclosures in the patent may provide suggestions for your invention. The following brief description is important to understanding the various parts of a patent or a published application (see Figure 3.1):

(10) Patent No.: The number assigned to the issued patent is the best place to branch out your search, particularly the patent numbers quoted in the front page of the patent that served as a related reference.

(12) Publication Type and Inventor's Family Name or Surname.

(45) Date of Patent: The patent becomes effective on the date it is issued (always on a Tuesday); however, the date when the application was published under the new rules determines if the inventors of an issued patent are eligible to claim royalties to a marketed invention if it reads on the patent claims. This date also tells you the period of exclusivity remaining in the patent.

(54) Title: Patent title describes the broadest area of invention description; it is often misleading but very useful in determining the broadest classification of the invention. Most often the title is chosen for the express purpose of making a random search difficult to reveal the content of a patent.

(76) Inventor: Inventor's name and address can be a very useful lead if you know your competitor; often, the same inventor files a series of patents on an invention; this information also helps track down reissues and reexamined patents. Given under the inventor information is a notice with an asterisk indicating patent term extension or reduction granted during prosecution delays by either the U.S. Patent and Trademark Office (USPTO) or the applicant; almost invariably this entry would include any additional patent term extensions granted, based on regulatory delays in the approval

US006447820B1

(12) **United States Patent**
Niazi

(10) **Patent No.:** **US 6,447,820 B1**
(45) **Date of Patent:** **Sep. 10, 2002**

(54) **PHARMACEUTICAL COMPOSITION FOR THE PREVENTION AND TREATMENT OF SCAR TISSUE**

(76) Inventor: **Sarfaraz K Niazi,** 20 Riverside Dr., Deerfield, IL (US) 60015

(*) Notice: Subject to any disclaimer, the term of this patent is extended or adjusted under 35 U.S.C. 154(b) by 0 days.

(21) Appl. No.: **09/681,137**

(22) Filed: **Jan. 22, 2001**

(51) Int. Cl.[7] A61K 35/78; A61K 9/00; A61K 9/50; A01N 25/00

(52) U.S. Cl. 424/767; 424/400; 424/502; 424/725; 514/946; 514/947

(58) Field of Search 424/400, 502, 424/725, 767; 514/946, 947

(56) **References Cited**

U.S. PATENT DOCUMENTS

5,405,608 A * 4/1995 Xu 424/195.1

6,126,950 A * 10/2000 Bindra et al. 424/401

OTHER PUBLICATIONS

Johnson, T. CRC Ethnobotany Desk Reference, 1999, CRC Press LLC, p. 568.*

* cited by examiner

Primary Examiner—Leon B. Lankford, Jr.
Assistant Examiner—Kailash C. Srivastava
(74) Attorney, Agent, or Firm—Welsh & Katz, Ltd.

(57) **ABSTRACT**

The disclosed is a treatment of existing and prevention of new skin scars in humans and animals using a topical application containing alcoholic extracts of Cortex Phellodendri and Opuntia ficus indica in a specific combination.

5 Claims, No Drawings

FIGURE 3.1

of a health care product, which can be found in the Official Gazette or through other searches, as shown below.

(21) Appl. No.: The Application Number assigned to a patent application can be useful in tracking down its publication prior to issuance of patent to compare any changes made in the application during prosecution (something you may get through file wrapper as well).

(22) Filed: The date the application was filed with the USPTO is a critical date for §102(e) prior art reference (see Chapter 2); this date also tells you approximately how long your competitor has been working on this project; because the patent wrapper (all correspondence between the USPTO and the inventor or whomever is prosecuting the patent) is public information, you may want to request the wrapper, particularly if there was a long delay between the filing and issuance of patent (meaning there was some admission by the filer, which may be of use to you in establishing the patentability of your invention).

(51) Int. Cl.: This is an important field that allows you to do comparable international classification searches (more details later); notice that there is a conversion of classification available between the U.S. and the International systems (see below).

(52) U.S. Cl.: The USPTO uses class and subclass information categories to classify or sort various types of inventions. These numbers are important for any patentability search.

(58) Field of Search: This indicates the class or subclasses that were searched for the purpose of determining patentability.

(56) References Cited: During the prosecution, the examiner may bring several references (patents and publications) that formed the basis of defining the scope of invention; given here are the patent number and class/subclass of patents that were brought up during prosecution. Most likely, you would also want to see the full text of these patents. Other publications also are cited here. It is further indicated if these references were brought up by the examiner (marked with an asterisk). Combined with the information in the file wrapper, these references provide the most-significant data on evaluating the proposed invention. The names of examiner and primary examiner are also given here; chances are that if your invention is similar, you will see correspondence from the same examiner or primary examiner.

(74) Attorney, Agent, or Firm: Identification of who did the prosecuting can be important if you want to track down other patents prosecuted by the same attorney, agent, or firm. If no name is listed here or the category is not listed, this patent was filed as a *pro se* patent.

(57) Abstract: Usually concise, this is one paragraph summarizing the invention in plain English (it is preferable not to use legalese or technical jargon here). Because this appears on the front page of the issued patent, it is the most frequently referenced section of a patent. This is one of the most craftily written pieces of language in the patent; as you prepare patent searches, you will learn how to read between the lines in an abstract.

Drawings: Drawings of the invention from different perspectives; also disclosed here is the number of drawings and claims in the patent. If there are no drawings reported, you may not want to switch to the patent image (unless there are chemical structures or other graphical information). The text format of a patent is more suitable for cutting and pasting in your search document; the patent image is in a noneditable TIFF format.

Background of the Invention: This section discusses any previous inventions related to the patented invention — prior art, in legal terms. Because you are allowed to incorporate other patents by reference, you may include this material in your own application if it suits the purpose as well. A recent patent with an extensive background section provides a wealth of information and saves great effort on the part of the filer. Read it carefully as it may disclose information that later can be used by the patent examiner as §103(e) information.

Summary of the Invention: This is a discussion of the invention that captures its essential functions and features; this must be read before reading the background section.

Brief Description of Drawings: A one-sentence description of each drawing figure is useful in deciding if you want to switch to an image of the patent. It is noteworthy that the USPTO Web site allows searching of patents from 1790 through 1975 only by Patent Number and Current U.S. Classification;

later patents are searchable by text entries. Online patent images were recently made available.

Detailed Description: This section is generally an in-depth discussion of the various aspects of the claimed invention. Detailed references to drawings are made in this section; here you see exactly what is invented.

Claims: Analogous to the boundaries of real estate described in a deed, the claims lay out the legal scope of the patent, going down from the broadest claim to the narrowest claim. This section determines if your invention infringes on a patent (reads onto claims). This section also provides you with the vocabulary you may want to use for your own invention. Often, searches are made of the claims section only to determine patentability.

PATENTABILITY SEARCH ONLINE

The use of the Internet to search and sort through the maze of information can be awe inspiring. Done properly, it can yield remarkable results; otherwise, much time can be wasted. Experienced users develop a knack for surfing the Net to make a good catch; novices end up with useless information. To help busy practitioners and inventors, the author provides online support through http://www.eUSPTO.com. It is highly recommended that you use this facility to make the best use of your time.

- The Web site is continuously updated with current regulations, newer information resources, and news relevant to patent practitioners.
- The Web site includes links to all the resources listed later in this chapter without having to retype the URLs, thereby avoiding entry errors; also, if any URLs have changed, the Web site will have the current information.
- Available at this Web site is a comprehensive book on Patent Practice Essentials, which will allow you to keep your knowledge about patent systems updated (see Figure 3.2).

PATENT OFFICE RESOURCES

The patent offices worldwide have opened their databases to the public. There is no better place to start your search for patentability than with these free databases. The same databases are packaged by other vendors that provide additional services and literature searches.

THE U.S. PATENT AND TRADEMARK OFFICE

The USPTO has created one of the world's largest electronic databases which includes every patent issued; recently published applications are also available in the database. Since 1971, the USPTO began storing the patents in both an image format (TIFF) and in a text format with optical character recognition; however, there were some gaps in the capturing of patents between 1971 and 1975. Thus, the search engine of the USPTO warns you that the patents issued before 1975 can be searched

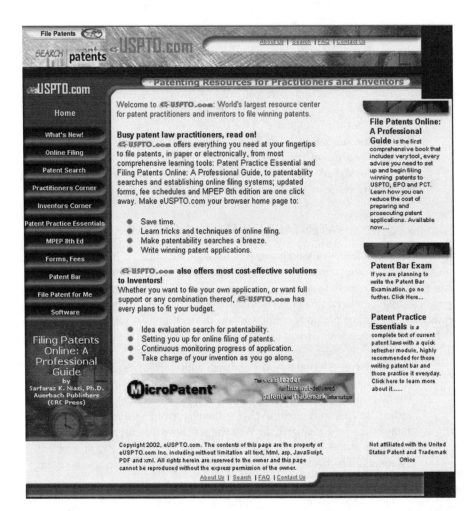

FIGURE 3.2

using patent classification only, and not by text. Whereas older patents do not create the issue of infringement, prior art considerations remain valid and it is not unusual for a patent examiner to pull out a 50-year-old patent as prior art. All paper applications filed with the USPTO undergo an optical character-recognition conversion, which is why filing an electronic application speeds up the process of getting your application docketed more quickly. Whereas the OCR process has substantially improved, errors do occur in converting a paper document to an electronic form, another reason you should consider online filing as the method of choice.

When a database is created, keyword tables are set up to allow your search word to be picked out quickly, and those references where the keyword appears are flagged. The technology involved in designing search engines is mind boggling; you can tunnel through billions of pages in seconds. When you do a manual search, you are trying to compete with the technology in performing this colossal task (a good reason

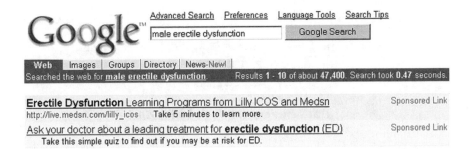

FIGURE 3.3

to no longer turn to the old-fashioned ways). For example, one of the premier search engines at http://www.google.com parses through 2.5 billion Web pages in a fraction of a second. A three-keyword search yielded 47,400 results in 0.47 seconds (Figure 3.3).

Keyword Selection and Searching

The speed of the microprocessor must be complemented by the art of selecting appropriate keywords; otherwise, the information returned can be very unproductive. Selection of keywords begins with defining the invention lucidly. The key determinants are whether the invention is a product or process, and what is claimed about the invention. What does the invention do? What is the end result? How does it work? What is it made of? What is it used for? What problem(s) does it solve? The answers to these questions produce the correct keywords.

> **Wildcards:** A powerful tool used in keyword searching is the wildcard character, such as the dollar sign ($), which is inserted at the end of a word root in place of any number of additional letters, e.g., treat$ would yield treat, treating, treatise, treatment, treats, etc. The keyword therefore requires a careful root selection that will not take the search to unrelated areas as in the example here. There are other wildcards used in different search engines and the reader is referred to the specific database description.
>
> **Boolean Logic:** The USPTO database utilizes Boolean logic as a search technique. Boolean logic uses operators such as AND, OR, and ANDNOT. For example, the Quick Search format (http://patft.uspto.gov/netahtml/search-bool.html) allows you to use two terms and the three operators (Figure 3.4). You may also specify where the search should be made from the Field list box. The AND operator reports only those instances that overlap in the specific fields, narrowing the search considerably, as shown in Figure 3.5.
> - AND will yield only the overlapping domains of the open and shaded circles.
> - OR will yield the domains of both circles.
> - ANDNOT will yield the domains of the shaded circle minus the overlapping range (the two crescents joined).

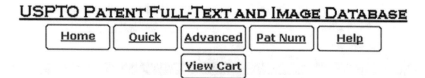

FIGURE 3.4

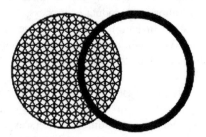

FIGURE 3.5

The Advanced Search page (http://patft.uspto.gov/netahtml/search-adv.htm) offers additional functionality with the use of these operators in a nested form and other search modalities (Figure 3.6).

Nested Search Operators: You can use the Advanced Search page to create and execute quick searches with more than two search terms that use the Boolean operators (OR, AND, ANDNOT). Along with these operators, you can use parentheses to further clarify your search statement. In the absence of parentheses, all operators associate from left to right.

- **Example 1: tennis AND (racquet OR racket).** If you enter this query, you will retrieve a list of all patents that contain the term *tennis* and either *racquet* or *racket* somewhere in the document.
- **Example 2: television OR (cathode AND tube).** This query will return patents containing either the word *television* or both the words *cathode* and *tube*.

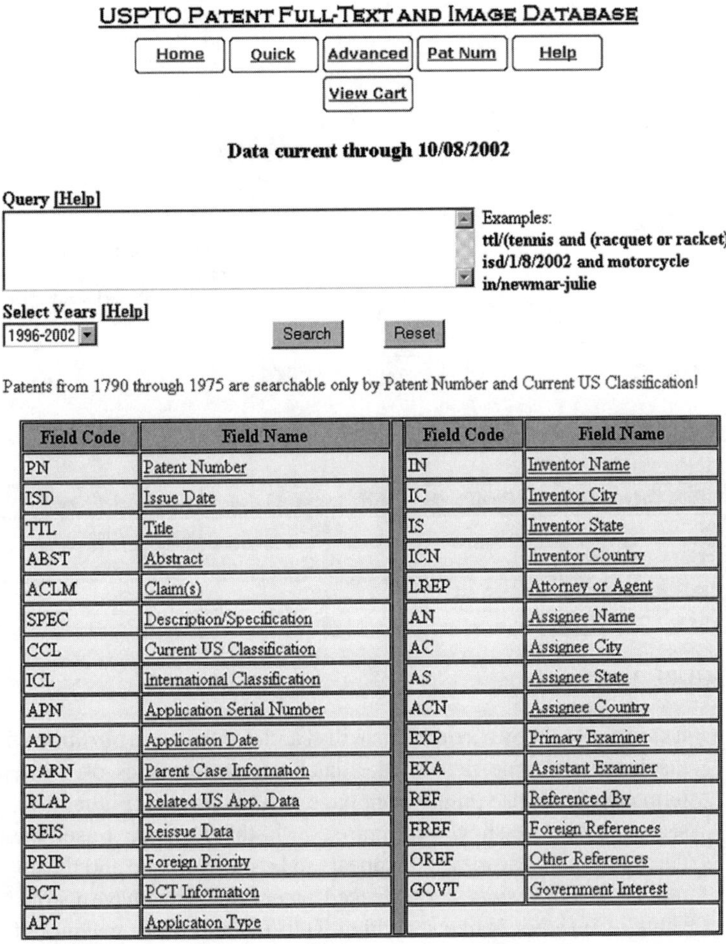

USPTO PATENT FULL-TEXT AND IMAGE DATABASE

| Home | Quick | Advanced | Pat Num | Help |

| View Cart |

Data current through 10/08/2002

Query [Help]

Examples:
ttl/(tennis and (racquet or racket))
isd/1/8/2002 and motorcycle
in/newmar-julie

Select Years [Help]

1996-2002 ▼   Search   Reset

Patents from 1790 through 1975 are searchable only by Patent Number and Current US Classification!

Field Code	Field Name	Field Code	Field Name
PN	Patent Number	IN	Inventor Name
ISD	Issue Date	IC	Inventor City
TTL	Title	IS	Inventor State
ABST	Abstract	ICN	Inventor Country
ACLM	Claim(s)	LREP	Attorney or Agent
SPEC	Description/Specification	AN	Assignee Name
CCL	Current US Classification	AC	Assignee City
ICL	International Classification	AS	Assignee State
APN	Application Serial Number	ACN	Assignee Country
APD	Application Date	EXP	Primary Examiner
PARN	Parent Case Information	EXA	Assistant Examiner
RLAP	Related US App. Data	REF	Referenced By
REIS	Reissue Data	FREF	Foreign References
PRIR	Foreign Priority	OREF	Other References
PCT	PCT Information	GOVT	Government Interest
APT	Application Type		

FIGURE 3.6

- **Example 3: needle ANDNOT ((record AND player) OR sewing).**
  This complex query generates a list of results that contain the word
  needle, but no references to sewing. In addition, none of the results
  will contain the combination of record AND player.

Field Searching: The Advanced Search page allows you to search individual
fields found within patents. You can find a list of all indexed fields in the
table on the bottom of the page. The full names for each field are given to
the right of the column and the corresponding field code is listed on the
left. To narrow your search to hits occurring within a single field, precede
your search term with the field code, followed by a forward slash (/). If
you do not select a specific field, the text of the entire patent will be
searched. If you need help with field searching, you may click on the
specific field listing to see how it is addressed.

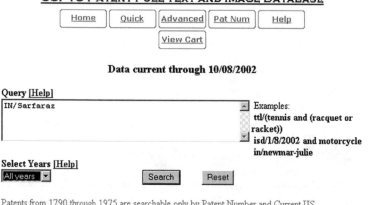

FIGURE 3.7

- **Example 1: IN/Sarfaraz.** This will search for the word *Sarfaraz* within the Inventor Name field of the database. Occurrences of the search term anywhere else on the front page will be ignored (Figure 3.7). The search results are shown in Figure 3.8. In this instance, I used the first name of the inventor, which appears to be more unique and thus brings more relevant results. Experienced patent attorneys have learned the value of Inventor Name searching well. Because most inventors focus on a particular field of invention, inventor search produces much relevant information.
- **Example 2: CLAS/270/31.** This query searches for the class/subclass 270/31, and returns a list of all patents assigned to that class (discussed in more detail later in the chapter).
- **Example 3: AN/MCNC AND TTL/solder.** As this example demonstrates, you can mix field searching with quick searching. This query will retrieve a list of hits that contain MCNC in the Assignee Name field, and the word solder in the Patent Title. Note that field names are associative. Using the search statement ttl/(nasal or nose) is the same as ttl/nasal or ttl/nose.

Phrase Searching: A group of words enclosed in quotation marks (" ") will be treated as a single search term. This allows you to search for a multiword phrase rather than specifying each word as a separate term. The full-text database is incapable of finding multitoken (i.e., multiword) search terms in patents when those terms span a line break in the patent source text;

USPTO PATENT FULL-TEXT AND IMAGE DATABASE

Home	Quick	Advanced	Pat Num	Help

Bottom	View Cart

Searching All Years...

Results of Search in All Years db for:
IN/Sarfaraz: 12 patents.
Hits 1 through 12 out of 12

Jump To	

Refine Search	IN/Sarfaraz

PAT. NO.   Title
1 6,462,083 **T** Suppository base
2 6,447,820 **T** Pharmaceutical composition for the prevention and treatment of scar tissue
3 6,419,963 **T** Composition and method for the treatment of diaper rash using natural products
4 6,365,198 **T** Pharmaceutical preparation for the treatment of gastrointestinal ulcers and hemorrhoids
5 6,338,862 **T** Composition and method of use in treating sexual dysfunction using cGMP-specific phosphodiesterase type 5
                   inhibitors
6 6,312,735 **T** Method for instantaneous removal of warts and moles
7 6,251,421 **T** Pharmaceutical composition containing psyllium fiber and a lipase inhibitor
8 6,235,796 **T** Use of fluorocarbons for the prevention of surgical adhesions
9 6,235,314 **T** Analgesic, anti-inflammatory and skeletal muscle relaxant compositions
10 5,522,963 **T** Method for machining and depositing metallurgy on ceramic layers
11 4,639,368 **T** Chewing gum containing a medicament and taste maskers
12 4,530,936 **T** Composition and method for inhibiting the absorption of nutritional elements from the upper intestinal tract

FIGURE 3.8

thus, searching for multiword text within quotation marks (e.g., "baseball bat") may not return all occurrences of those terms. Note that you cannot truncate within a phrase that is enclosed in quotation marks.

- **Example 1: "bowling balls."** Searching this phrase will return a list of all the patents that have the phrase *bowling balls* anywhere within the indexed text.
- **Example 2: AN/"General Motors."** This query will find all occurrences of the phrase *General Motors* within the Assignee Name field.

Date Range Searching: You can specify a range of dates rather than having to specify a certain day or month to narrow your search. This feature is available only in date fields, such as Issue Date and Application Date. This is done by using the "->" operator between two dates. For example, a query such as ISD/11/1/1997->5/12/1998 will return all patents that were issued on or after November 1, 1997, and on or before May 12, 1998. If the range covers all of the patents issued in a particular year, you will get faster results by selecting just the year instead of all of the dates in the year as a range. *Note:* The selected years must match the range of years you are searching. Both dates in the query must be properly formatted for your search to work. See the help entries on Issue Date and Application Date for details.

Right Truncation: The Advanced Search page supports right truncation in queries. This allows you to use a wildcard on the right side of a search term, to retrieve words that begin with a certain string. If you are searching in a specific field, the string must be at least three characters in length. If you are not searching in a specific field, the string must be at least four characters in length. You cannot truncate within a phrase that is enclosed in quotation marks, e.g., searching AN/"general mot$" will result in an error.

For example, a query such as elec$ will result in a large number of hits, because it will retrieve patents containing the words *electric, electricity, electronic,* etc. To reduce the number of hits, you may want to truncate on a longer string. For example, if you are interested only in patents dealing with electronics, you might truncate electron$ to eliminate electric, electricity, etc. Be aware that the default will search every word in every patent in the year(s) you specify. This can result in very large numbers of hits. It may be preferable to begin by limiting your search to the Title or Abstract fields.

Stopwords: Stopwords are terms that appear so frequently in patent text that they lose their usefulness as search terms. Although they are not indexed as search terms, they will be displayed in the search results: *a, accordance, according, all, also, an, and, another, are, as, at, be, because, been, being, by, claim, comprises, corresponding, could, described, desired, do, does, each, embodiment, fig., figs., for, from, further, generally, had, has, have, having, herein, however, if, in, into, invention, is, it, its, means, not, now, of, on, onto, or, other, particularly, preferably, preferred, present, provide, provided, provides, relatively, respectively, said, should, since, some, such, suitable, than, that, the, their, then, there, thereby, therefore, thereof, thereto, these, they, this, those, thus, to, use, various, was, were, what, when, where, whereby, wherein, which, while, who, will, with, would.*

PATENT IMAGES

In addition to full text searches as described previously, you can view images of each page to see the drawing or other complex formulae and structures included in a patent. The images are in the same format as the ribbon copy of the patent, thus making it easier to print a replica of the ribbon copy. The USPTO's full-page images, nearly 4 TB overall, are stored and delivered at a full 300-dpi (dots per inch) resolution in TIFF format, using CCITT Group 4 compression. This is the format that is required by the international standards to which all patent offices must conform. TIFF is the most "lossless" image format in the world. Unfortunately, due to the volume of image data, available funding, and other technical considerations, the USPTO cannot convert these images to a more-popular format on the Web either permanently or by converting on-the-fly as they are delivered. As a result, in order to view these files on your workstation you must install and use a browser plug-in similar to those required to access Adobe® PDF, RealPlayer®, or Macromedia® Flash files. An alternative method is to use third-party software or services to view these images either directly or after conversion to another format, such as Adobe Acrobat®.

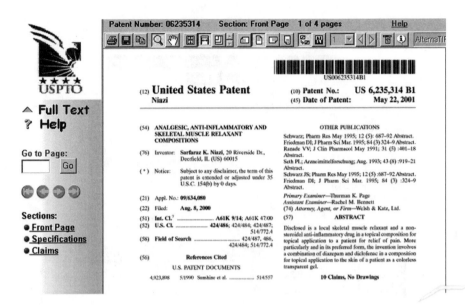

FIGURE 3.9

You cannot use just any TIFF image plug-in. It must be able to specifically display TIFF files using ITU T.6 or CCITT Group 4 compression. The only free, unlimited-time TIFF plug-ins offering full-size, patent viewing and printing unimpeded by advertising on Windows® x86 PCs of which I am aware are AlternaTIFF (http://www.alternatiff.com; tested on Internet Explorer, Netscape, and Opera) and interneTIFF (http://www.innomage.com/interneTIFF.htm; tested on IE and Netscape). For the Macintosh®, Apple's freely distributed QuickTime® version 4.1 or later works with images, but does not provide printing capability. Quicktime is available from the Apple Web site at http://www.apple.com/software. For Linux®, a plug-in called Plugger works nicely with Netscape Communicator®; it is available at http://fredrik.hubbe.net/plugger.html.

The instructions for installing the image viewer are delivered with the plug-in download and are thus not discussed here. Once a plug-in is installed, you will be able to view the images for all patents in the USPTO database (Figure 3.9).

The image viewer offers many navigational functions: you can flip through pages, go directly to claims, save the file, copy the displayed page, and change the image. One of the most-convenient ways to store the image file is to copy each page and paste consecutively in a Microsoft® Word document. This document is easy to forward and use by others who may not have a TIFF-viewing plug-in.

PUBLISHED APPLICATION SEARCH

The screen shown in Figure 3.10 is slightly different than what you see when doing a patent search; this is likely to be modified to look more like the patent search page in the future.

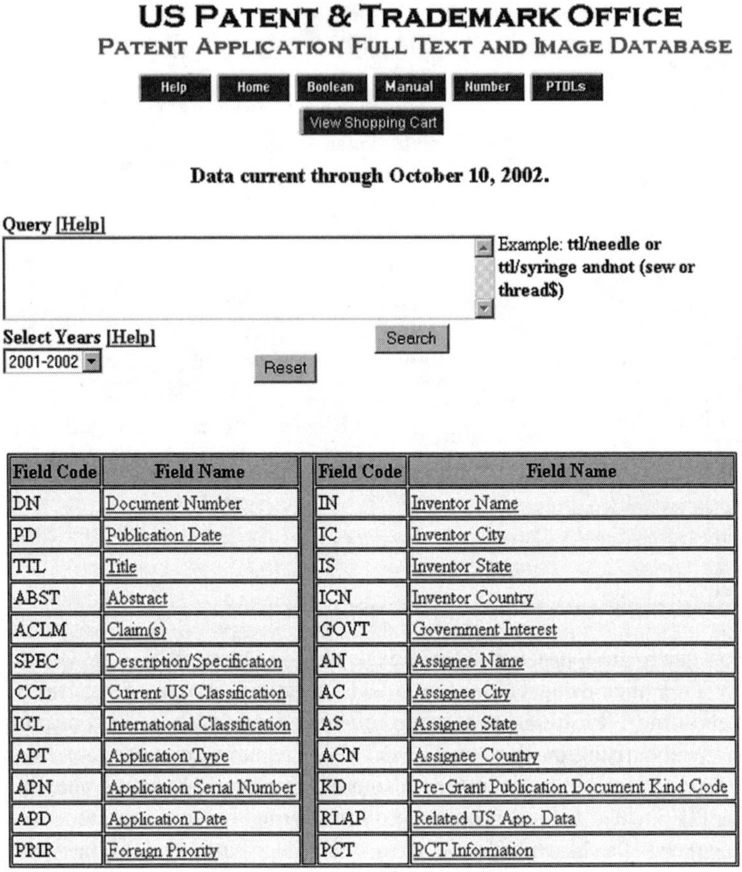

US PATENT & TRADEMARK OFFICE
PATENT APPLICATION FULL TEXT AND IMAGE DATABASE

Help   Home   Boolean   Manual   Number   PTDLs

View Shopping Cart

Data current through October 10, 2002.

Query [Help]

Example: **ttl/needle or ttl/syringe andnot (sew or thread$)**

Select Years [Help]
2001-2002

Search   Reset

Field Code	Field Name	Field Code	Field Name
DN	Document Number	IN	Inventor Name
PD	Publication Date	IC	Inventor City
TTL	Title	IS	Inventor State
ABST	Abstract	ICN	Inventor Country
ACLM	Claim(s)	GOVT	Government Interest
SPEC	Description/Specification	AN	Assignee Name
CCL	Current US Classification	AC	Assignee City
ICL	International Classification	AS	Assignee State
APT	Application Type	ACN	Assignee Country
APN	Application Serial Number	KD	Pre-Grant Publication Document Kind Code
APD	Application Date	RLAP	Related US App. Data
PRIR	Foreign Priority	PCT	PCT Information

FIGURE 3.10

Since March 15, 2001, the USPTO database has included published applications that can be searched the same as the Quick Search of the patent database. Figure 3.11 is an image view of a patent application; notice the similarity of format to patents.

The Kind Code (in this case, A1 in field (10)) listed in the text format does not appear in the image format.

PATENT CLASSIFICATION SEARCH

A patent classification is a code that categorizes the invention. Classifications are typically expressed as "482/1"; the first number, 482, represents the class of invention, the number following the slash is the subclass within the invention class. There are about 450 classes and 150,000 subclasses of invention in the U.S. Patent Classification System (USPC). Classes and subclasses have titles, which provide a short description of the class or subclass. Classes and subclasses also have definitions which provide more detailed explanations. Many classes and subclasses have explicitly defined

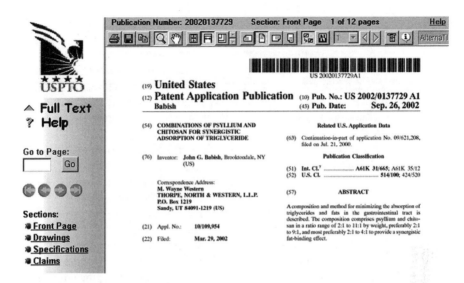

FIGURE 3.11

relationships to one another. Subclasses contain patents. In a sense, classes contain patents also, but for classification purposes patents always are classified at the subclass level. Therefore, one or more classifications (i.e., class/subclass designations) are assigned to each granted patent and each published application. A patent classification also represents a searchable collection of patents grouped together according to similarly claimed subject matter. A classification is used as both a tool for finding patents (patentability searches) and for assisting in the assignment of patent applications for examination purposes. Classifications have definitions and hierarchical relationships to one another.

The USPC index is intended as an initial entry point for users unfamiliar with the USPC and is used by experienced searchers trying to locate an unfamiliar topic. It is a subject matter index such as one finds at the back of a book. The index is an alphabetic listing of technical and common terms. References to actual classes and subclasses of the USPC appear next to each term. The index should not be considered exhaustive. Patent classifiers can update the index when they submit a classification order. Subject headings in the index are not an alphabetical inversion of the Manual of Classification. They are a subjective determination of relevant terms, phrases, synonyms, acronyms, and occasionally even trademarks that have been selected over the years (during reclass activity) as the best identifying description of products, processes, and apparatus of patent disclosures. The index contains product-related entries, whereas the Manual of Classification is descriptive or nonspecific. For example, the index entry for phonograph record molding apparatus is reflected in the Manual of Classification as a "press forming apparatus having opposed press members." Some effort has been made to index current vocabulary usage when the classification system may contain technically general language; e.g., "water bed" or "air mattress" for the concept "fluid-containing mattress."

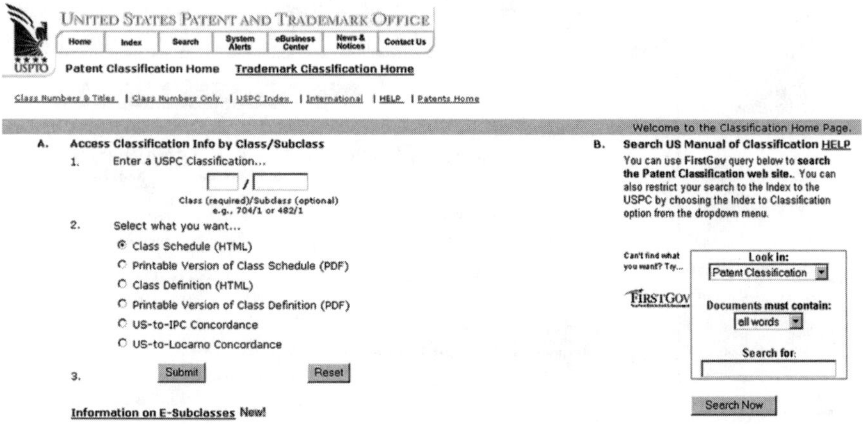

FIGURE 3.12

Begin with this alphabetical subject index to the Manual of Classification. Look for common terms describing the invention and its function, effect, end product, structure, and use. Note class and subclass numbers.

The USPTO provides many useful tools to help you search through this Manual. All the tools needed to begin classification search are available at http://www.uspto.gov/go/classification/ (Figure 3.12).

You have several choices to do the search. You can search a specific classification (Section A), go directly to the Manual (Section B), or look at the classification in different presentations by clicking on one of the links at the top: Class Numbers & Titles, Class Numbers Only, USPC Index, and International.

> **Class Numbers & Titles:** This is the first link on the left. Clicking on this link gives you the opportunity to have all the principal classes listed so that you can search for a schedule listing (in HTML or PDF); a class definition (in HTML or PDF); a conversion from US-to-IPC Concordance; and a conversion from US-to-Locarno Concordance, which refers to International Classification for Industrial Designs under the Locarno Agreement as described at http://www.wipo.int/classifications/fulltext/locarno/enmn01.htm (Figure 3.13).
>
> You have two options at this point: (1) scroll down to see if the invention class is listed or (2) use the page search function from the browser's Edit menu and search for a word on the page. For example, clicking on 424 DRUG, BIO-AFFECTING AND BODY TREATING COMPOSITIONS takes you to Class Schedule or Class Definition, depending on the option you chose in Section 1 of the screen. Choosing Class Schedule as shown in Figure 3.13 will display the screen shown in Figure 3.14.
>
> Again, you can use the page search function (do not invoke a Web site search) to see if your keyword is available. Chances are it will be; however, not necessarily the way you have entered it. For example, a light bulb is listed as an illuminating device rather than as a light.

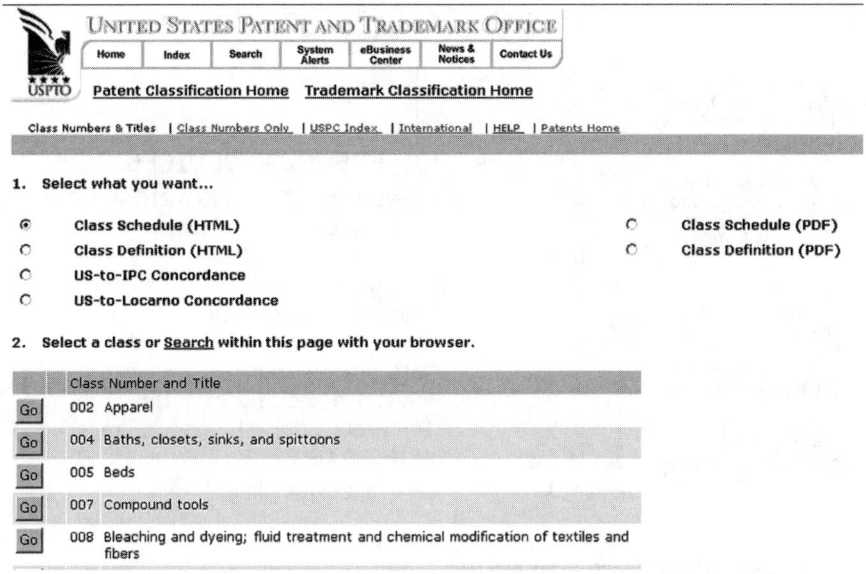

UNITED STATES PATENT AND TRADEMARK OFFICE

| Home | Index | Search | System Alerts | eBusiness Center | News & Notices | Contact Us |

USPTO **Patent Classification Home** **Trademark Classification Home**

Class Numbers & Titles | Class Numbers Only | USPC Index | International | HELP | Patents Home

1. **Select what you want...**

- ⦿ **Class Schedule (HTML)**
- ○ **Class Definition (HTML)**
- ○ **US-to-IPC Concordance**
- ○ **US-to-Locarno Concordance**

- ○ **Class Schedule (PDF)**
- ○ **Class Definition (PDF)**

2. **Select a class or Search within this page with your browser.**

	Class Number and Title
Go	002 Apparel
Go	004 Baths, closets, sinks, and spittoons
Go	005 Beds
Go	007 Compound tools
Go	008 Bleaching and dyeing; fluid treatment and chemical modification of textiles and fibers

FIGURE 3.13

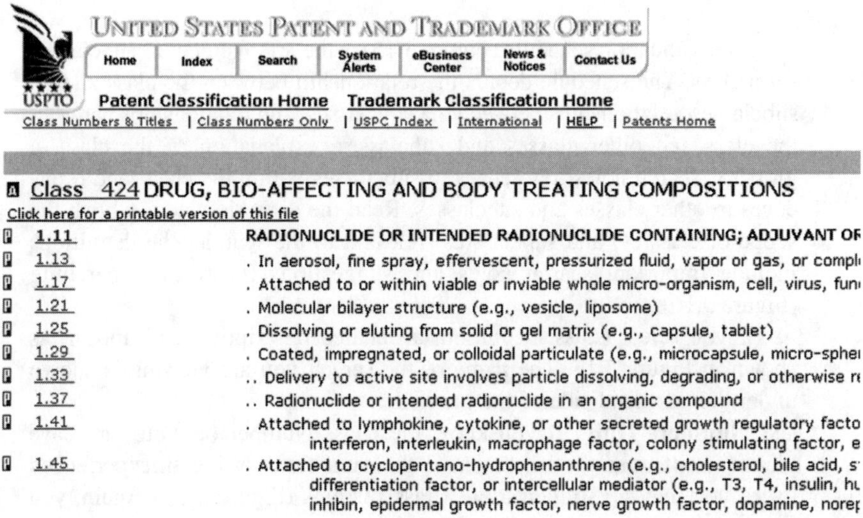

UNITED STATES PATENT AND TRADEMARK OFFICE

| Home | Index | Search | System Alerts | eBusiness Center | News & Notices | Contact Us |

USPTO **Patent Classification Home** **Trademark Classification Home**
Class Numbers & Titles | Class Numbers Only | USPC Index | International | HELP | Patents Home

▣ **Class 424 DRUG, BIO-AFFECTING AND BODY TREATING COMPOSITIONS**
Click here for a printable version of this file

1.11	RADIONUCLIDE OR INTENDED RADIONUCLIDE CONTAINING; ADJUVANT OF
1.13	. In aerosol, fine spray, effervescent, pressurized fluid, vapor or gas, or comple
1.17	. Attached to or within viable or inviable whole micro-organism, cell, virus, fun
1.21	. Molecular bilayer structure (e.g., vesicle, liposome)
1.25	. Dissolving or eluting from solid or gel matrix (e.g., capsule, tablet)
1.29	. Coated, impregnated, or colloidal particulate (e.g., microcapsule, micro-sphe
1.33	.. Delivery to active site involves particle dissolving, degrading, or otherwise re
1.37	.. Radionuclide or intended radionuclide in an organic compound
1.41	. Attached to lymphokine, cytokine, or other secreted growth regulatory facto interferon, interleukin, macrophage factor, colony stimulating factor, e
1.45	. Attached to cyclopentano-hydrophenanthrene (e.g., cholesterol, bile acid, s differentiation factor, or intercellular mediator (e.g., T3, T4, insulin, hu inhibin, epidermal growth factor, nerve growth factor, dopamine, norep

FIGURE 3.14

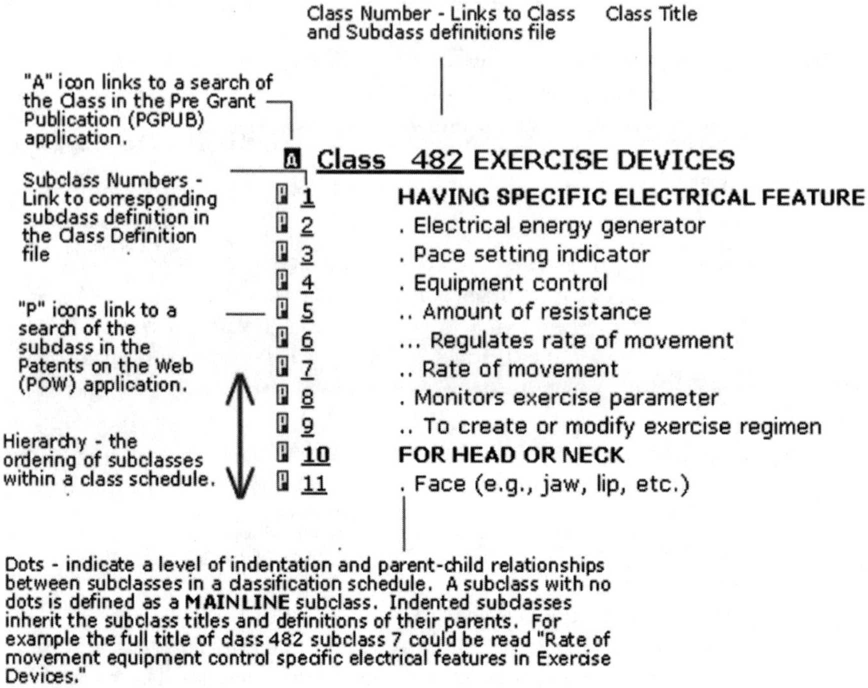

Class Number - Links to Class　Class Title
and Subclass definitions file

"A" icon links to a search of
the Class in the Pre Grant
Publication (PGPUB)
application.

🅰 **Class 482** EXERCISE DEVICES

Subclass Numbers -
Link to corresponding
subclass definition in
the Class Definition
file

"P" icons link to a
search of the
subclass in the
Patents on the Web
(POW) application.

Hierarchy - the
ordering of subclasses
within a class schedule.

🅿 <u>1</u>　**HAVING SPECIFIC ELECTRICAL FEATURE**
🅿 <u>2</u>　. Electrical energy generator
🅿 <u>3</u>　. Pace setting indicator
🅿 <u>4</u>　. Equipment control
🅿 <u>5</u>　.. Amount of resistance
🅿 <u>6</u>　... Regulates rate of movement
🅿 <u>7</u>　.. Rate of movement
🅿 <u>8</u>　. Monitors exercise parameter
🅿 <u>9</u>　.. To create or modify exercise regimen
🅿 <u>10</u>　**FOR HEAD OR NECK**
🅿 <u>11</u>　. Face (e.g., jaw, lip, etc.)

Dots - indicate a level of indentation and parent-child relationships
between subclasses in a classification schedule. A subclass with no
dots is defined as a **MAINLINE** subclass. Indented subclasses
inherit the subclass titles and definitions of their parents. For
example the full title of class 482 subclass 7 could be read "Rate of
movement equipment control specific electrical features in Exercise
Devices."

FIGURE 3.15

A classification schedule (Figure 3.15) is the arrangement of subclasses for a class. The schedule details the relationship between the class and its subclasses, relationships between the subclasses, and relationships between the class and other classes and subclasses, explanation of the class, a glossary, search notes, references to subclasses within the class, and references to other classes and subclasses. Read the definitions to establish the scope of class(es) and subclass(es) relevant to the search. The definitions include important search notes and suggestions for further searching (Figure 3.16).

If you select Class Definition, a detailed description will appear, as shown in Figure 3.17. The name of the screen you are viewing is shown under the left-hand side of the gray bar.

Class Numbers Only: If you know the Class Number (as you may have picked it out from another patent in the same field, or are an experienced user), you may go straight to all Class Listings (Figure 3.18). Again, you have the same output choices as before.

USPC Index: If you are a beginner, most likely you will want to start here. There are two search options: (1) click on the letter that begins your keyword, or (2) enter the keyword in the search box. If you are using the

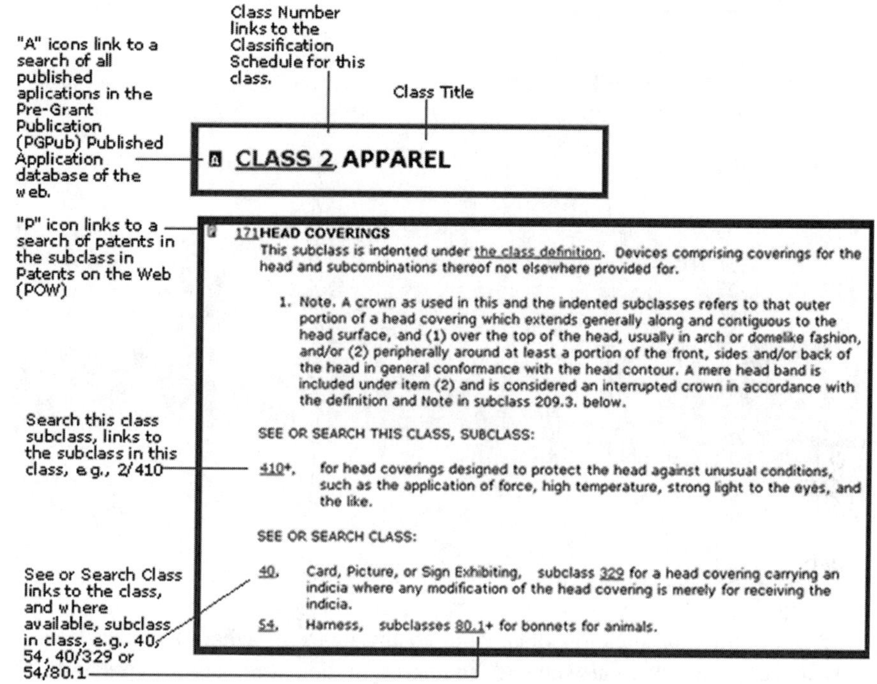

"A" icons link to a search of all published aplications in the Pre-Grant Publication (PGPub) Published Application database of the web.

Class Number links to the Classification Schedule for this class.

Class Title

ⓐ CLASS 2, APPAREL

"P" icon links to a search of patents in the subclass in Patents on the Web (POW)

171 HEAD COVERINGS
This subclass is indented under the class definition. Devices comprising coverings for the head and subcombinations thereof not elsewhere provided for.

1. Note. A crown as used in this and the indented subclasses refers to that outer portion of a head covering which extends generally along and contiguous to the head surface, and (1) over the top of the head, usually in arch or domelike fashion, and/or (2) peripherally around at least a portion of the front, sides and/or back of the head in general conformance with the head contour. A mere head band is included under item (2) and is considered an interrupted crown in accordance with the definition and Note in subclass 209.3. below.

Search this class subclass, links to the subclass in this class, e.g., 2/410

SEE OR SEARCH THIS CLASS, SUBCLASS:

410+, for head coverings designed to protect the head against unusual conditions, such as the application of force, high temperature, strong light to the eyes, and the like.

SEE OR SEARCH CLASS:

See or Search Class links to the class, and where available, subclass in class, e.g., 40, 54, 40/329 or 54/80.1

40, Card, Picture, or Sign Exhibiting, subclass 329 for a head covering carrying an indicia where any modification of the head covering is merely for receiving the indicia.

54, Harness, subclasses 80.1+ for bonnets for animals.

FIGURE 3.16

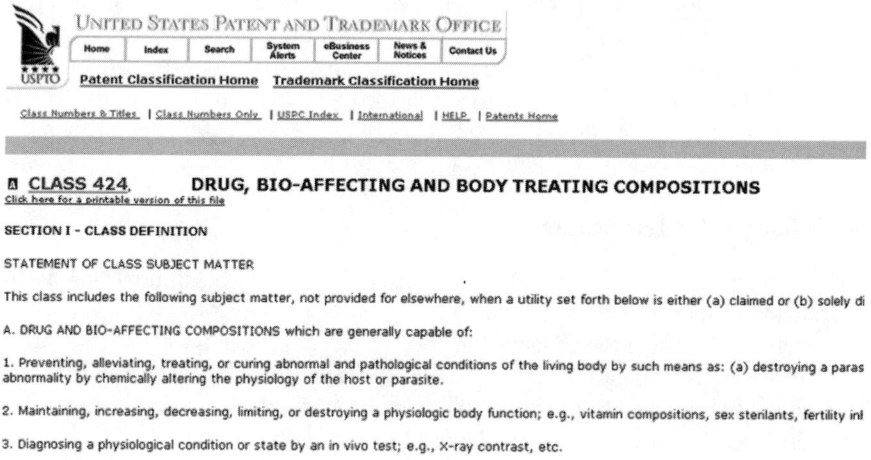

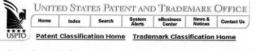

Patent Classification Home   Trademark Classification Home

Class Numbers & Titles | Class Numbers Only | USPC Index | International | HELP | Patents Home

ⓐ CLASS 424, DRUG, BIO-AFFECTING AND BODY TREATING COMPOSITIONS
Click here for a printable version of this file

SECTION I - CLASS DEFINITION

STATEMENT OF CLASS SUBJECT MATTER

This class includes the following subject matter, not provided for elsewhere, when a utility set forth below is either (a) claimed or (b) solely di

A. DRUG AND BIO-AFFECTING COMPOSITIONS which are generally capable of:

1. Preventing, alleviating, treating, or curing abnormal and pathological conditions of the living body by such means as: (a) destroying a paras abnormality by chemically altering the physiology of the host or parasite.

2. Maintaining, increasing, decreasing, limiting, or destroying a physiologic body function; e.g., vitamin compositions, sex sterilants, fertility inl

3. Diagnosing a physiological condition or state by an in vivo test; e.g., X-ray contrast, etc.

FIGURE 3.17

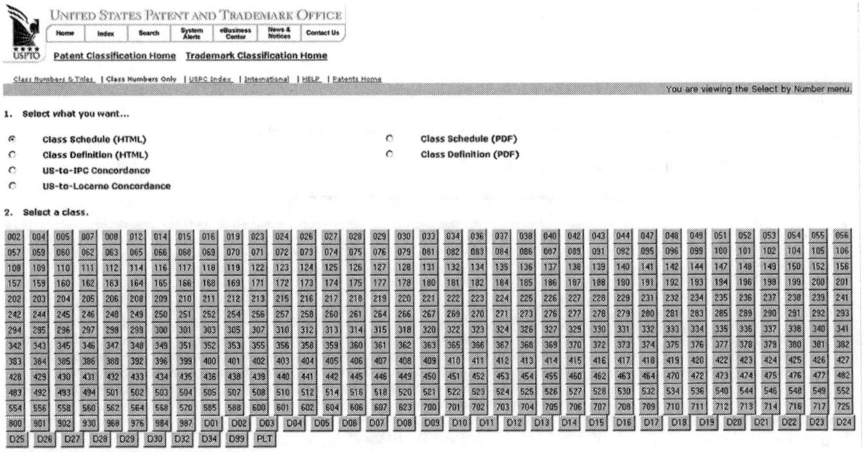

FIGURE 3.18

letter search, you may use the browser's page search function to search for the keyword. If you are using the search box, you can search either the Index to Classification (analogous to the index in a book) or the entire Patent Classification Web site (analogous to the entire book); for example, choosing the keyword *drug* returns 5 entries in the Index to Classification and 91 in the Patent Classification. In the list box, you may also tell the search engine how to treat your entry by choosing "all words," "any words," or "the phrase" (Figure 3.19).

International: Classification home page (http://www.uspto.gov/go/classifi-cation) allows you to convert used codes to international codes. Clicking on the International link will take you to many other resources for international searching of classification. For example, a link is provided to the WIPO listing of classification (http://classifications.wipo.int/full-text/new_ipc/index.htm) that you may want to review before commencing a search for European patents (Figure 3.20).

Searching with Classification

When you have narrowed down the classification, you may begin browsing patent titles and abstracts based on the classification code developed to go a level deeper to subclasses by using the advanced method of patent searching.

Once you have identified the relevant classes and subclasses, obtain a list of all patent numbers granted from 1790 to the present and all published applications from mid-2001 to the present for every class and subclass you want to search.

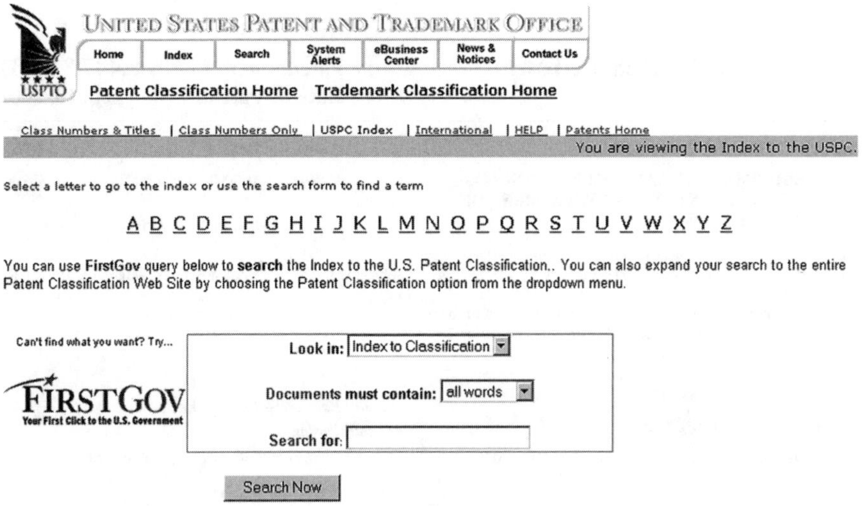

FIGURE 3.19

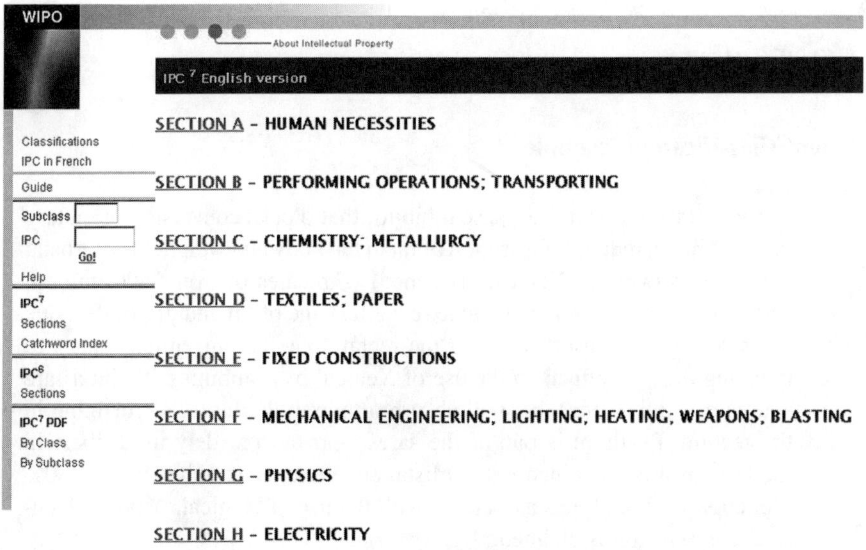

FIGURE 3.20

US006447820B1

(12) **United States Patent**   (10) **Patent No.:**   **US 6,447,820 B1**
Niazi   (45) **Date of Patent:**   **Sep. 10, 2002**

(54) **PHARMACEUTICAL COMPOSITION FOR
THE PREVENTION AND TREATMENT OF
SCAR TISSUE**

(76) Inventor: **Sarfaraz K Niazi**, 20 Riverside Dr.,
Deerfield, IL (US) 60015

(*) Notice: Subject to any disclaimer, the term of this
patent is extended or adjusted under 35
U.S.C. 154(b) by 0 days.

(21) Appl. No.: **09/681,137**

(22) Filed: **Jan. 22, 2001**

(51) **Int. Cl.**[7] **A61K 35/78**; A61K 9/00;
A61K 9/50; A01N 25/00

(52) **U.S. Cl.** **424/767**; 424/400; 424/502;
424/725; 514/946; 514/947

(58) **Field of Search** 424/400, 502,
424/725, 767; 514/946, 947

(56)   **References Cited**

U.S. PATENT DOCUMENTS

5,405,608 A * 4/1995 Xu 424/195.1

6,126,950 A * 10/2000 Bindra et al. 424/401

OTHER PUBLICATIONS

Johnson, T. CRC Ethnobotany Desk Reference, 1999, CRC
Press LLC, p. 568.*

* cited by examiner

Primary Examiner—Leon B. Lankford, Jr.
Assistant Examiner—Kailash C. Srivastava
(74) *Attorney, Agent, or Firm*—Welsh & Katz, Ltd.

(57)   **ABSTRACT**

The disclosed is a treatment of existing and prevention of
new skin scars in humans and animals using a topical
application containing alcoholic extracts of *Cortex Phellodendri* and *Opuntia ficus indica* in a specific combination.

5 Claims, No Drawings

FIGURE 3.21

Patent Classification Example

The Invention: Orlistat is a lipase inhibitor that blocks conversion of dietary fat resulting in reduced absorption of fat in the body and weight loss. Orlistat is sold worldwide as Xenical® (Roche®) with sales of over $500 million. The side effects of Xenical include rectal leakage of oil and discomfort due to presence of unabsorbed fat in the rectal area. The invention relates to reducing the side effects in the use of Xenical by combining it with a safe source of soluble fiber that will absorb or entrap the fat (oil) remaining in the rectum. Psyllium is one of the safest and most widely used fibers in the U.S.; it was combined with Orlistat and patients exhibited a 70 to 80% reduction in side effects associated with the use of Xenical. A pharmaceutical composition is claimed.

Classification: Because the resulting composition is intended to treat a disease, it is considered a drug. A search in the Manual of Classification for *drug* takes you directly to classification numbers 424 and 514: DRUG, BIO-AFFECTING AND BODY TREATING COMPOSITIONS. Because psyllium is of plant origin, it belongs to a subclass under 424 as 725 and under that there is another subclass 738 that refers specifically to psyllium (Plantago). Because the preferred embodiments reported included wafers,

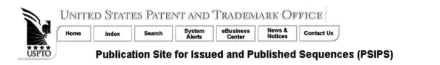

Publication Site for Issued and Published Sequences (PSIPS)

Welcome to the home page for PSIPS. At present, this system stores and allows for retrieval for sequence listings that are at least 300 pages long (roughly 600K) and which have been included in either a granted U.S. patent or a published U.S. patent application. Shorter sequences are accessible via the Patents and Applications on the Web Homepages. You can view individual sequences or download the entire sequence listing for a document. Other large items, such as tables may be downloaded. **More Information**

US Document Format Examples

Utility	Reissue*	Design**	Publication***
6183957	RE000126	D0000126	20010000241

Enter Document ID/Patent ID:

[Submit]   [Reset]

* *(for Reissue insert leading zeros so Document number has 6 digits)*
** *(for Design insert leading zeros so Document number has 7 digits)*
*** *(for Publications 4 digit year and 7 digits sequence number)*

FIGURE 3.22

effervescent formulations, powders, etc., the examiner also included the appropriate subclassification. The two patents that were pulled out as possible prior art were for a very similar application: a combination of an insoluble fiber with Orlistat and a combination of chitosan and Orlistat. The proposed invention did not read onto the claims of these two patents cited by the examiner and claims were allowed (Figure 3.21).

The USPTO now allows you also to search for sequences. You can reach this menu by logging on to http://seqdata.uspto.gov/psipsDIDEntry.html (Figure 3.22).

SEARCHING THE GAZETTE

Go to the Gazette to look for exemplary claim(s) and a representative drawing for all patents on the list(s) to eliminate patents unrelated to the invention. For published applications, see below. The Official Gazette of the USPTO is available online at http://www.uspto.gov/web/patents/patog. The Electronic Official Gazette allows you to browse through the issued patents for the week. The *e*OG:P, as the electronic version of the Gazette is now called, can be browsed by classification or type of patent, e.g., utility, design, and plant. Specific patents can be accessed by class/subclass or patentee name (Figure 3.23).

THE EUROPEAN PATENT OFFICE

The second largest database is accessed through the EPO (http://ep.espacenet.com), where one should conduct a classification search similar to that suggested for the

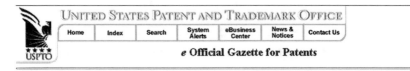

Welcome to the Electronic Official Gazette (eOG:P).

- The Electronic Official Gazette allows you to browse through the issued patents for the week. The *eOG:P* can be browsed by classification or type of patent, for example, utility, design, and plant. Specific patents can be accessed by class/subclass or patentee name.
- Links are provided on the left to the various sections of the *eOG:P*. Click on the section title to use these pages:
  - ○ *Browse by Class/Subclass* page to access patents by a specific classification
  - ○ *Classification of Patents* page with links to patents by a range of classifications
  - ○ *Browse Granted Patents* page to access a patent by patent number or link to patents by type
  - ○ *Index of Patentees* page to browse by names of inventors and assignees in either a cumulative alphabetical index or individual indexes by type of patent. Each patentee listing contains a link to the patent .
  - ○ *Geographical Index of Inventors* to link to patents by the state or country of residence of the first listed inventor
  - ○ *Notices* page containing the text of important notices for the week
  - ○ *Help*
- A link is provided to the full text of the patent in the USPTO Full Text Database from each bibliographic record. Clicking the "Full Text" button in the upper left corner of the patent record will take you to the full text.
- Click **here** for Frequently Asked Questions (FAQ).

Published Issues

Date	Week	Number
October 8, 2002	41	1263-2
October 1, 2002	40	1263-1
September 24, 2002 - Last Issue of Concurrent Paper OG	39	1262-4
September 17, 2002	38	1262-3
September 10, 2002	37	1262-2

FIGURE 3.23

USPTO (Figure 3.24). The EPO offers an Online Patent Register Inspection system (http://register.epoline.org/espacenet/ep/en/srch-reg.htm; Figures 3.25 and 3.26A–H).

THE WORLD INTELLECTUAL PROPERTY ORGANIZATION

WIPO (http://ipdl.wipo.int) offers many useful features, including complete details of the PCT and its gazette. Upon reaching this Web site, you will need to create an account and then click on Search IPDL (Intellectual Property Digital Library) for the following page (Figure 3.27). This is an extremely valuable source of free information because most worthwhile inventions end up as PCT applications (see Chapter 12).

CANADIAN PATENT OFFICE

The Canadian Patent Office Web site is located at http://patents1.ic.gc.ca/srch_bool-e.html (Figure 3.28).

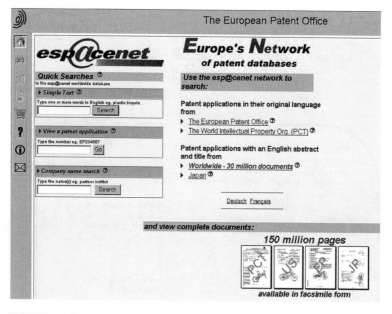

FIGURE 3.24

epoline Online European Patent Register

Publication Number / Date		eg. EP811545 or WO9504154 eg. 19980826
Application Number / Date		eg. EP1988850217 or WO1994JP01239 eg. 19980826
Priority Number / Date		eg. FR19910001995 eg. 19980830
Applicant		eg. Smith George or Phillips
Inventor		eg. Smith George or Phillips
Representative		eg. Smith George or Smith Hellmann and Partner
Opponent		eg. Smith George or Phillips
Classification (IPC)		eg. B62J1/02

Submit Clear Help

Deutsch Legal notices epoline® homepage Français

FIGURE 3.25

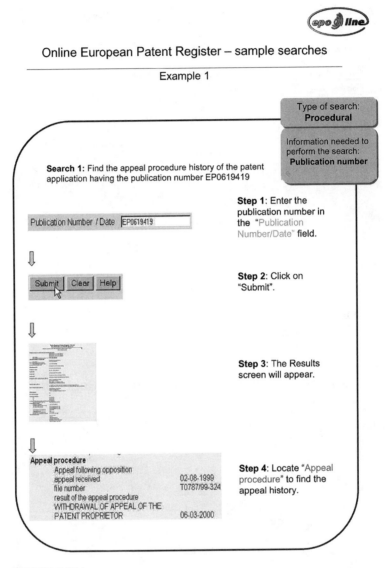

FIGURE 3.26A

Online European Patent Register – sample searches

Example 2

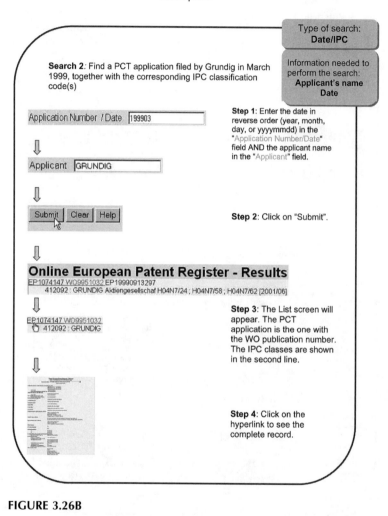

Search 2: Find a PCT application filed by Grundig in March 1999, together with the corresponding IPC classification code(s)

Type of search:
Date/IPC

Information needed to perform the search:
**Applicant's name
Date**

Application Number / Date 199903

Step 1: Enter the date in reverse order (year, month, day, or yyyymmdd) in the "Application Number/Date" field AND the applicant name in the "Applicant" field.

Applicant GRUNDIG

Submit   Clear   Help

Step 2: Click on "Submit".

Online European Patent Register - Results
EP1074147 WO9951032 EP 19990913297
       412092 : GRUNDIG Aktiengesellschaf H04N7/24 ; H04N7/58 ; H04N7/62 [2001/06]

Step 3: The List screen will appear. The PCT application is the one with the WO publication number. The IPC classes are shown in the second line.

EP1074147 WO9951032
      412092 : GRUNDIG

Step 4: Click on the hyperlink to see the complete record.

FIGURE 3.26B

Online European Patent Register – sample searches

Example 3

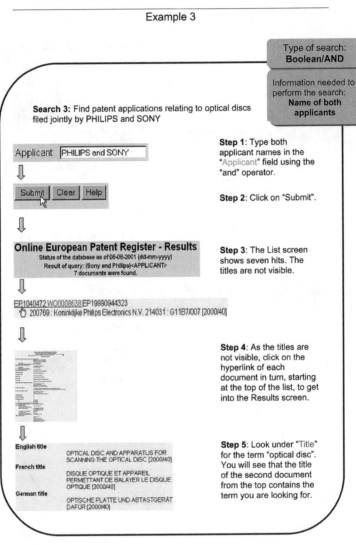

FIGURE 3.26C

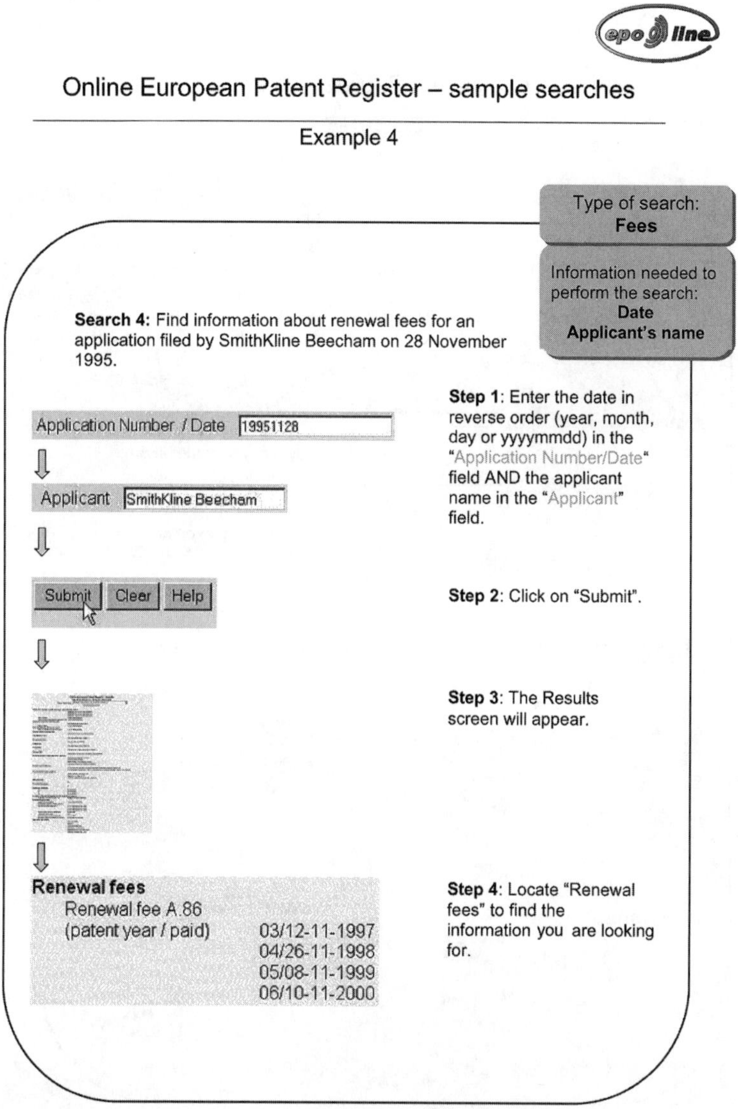

Online European Patent Register – sample searches

Example 4

> Type of search:
> **Fees**

> Information needed to perform the search:
> **Date**
> **Applicant's name**

Search 4: Find information about renewal fees for an application filed by SmithKline Beecham on 28 November 1995.

Application Number / Date [19951128]

⇩

Applicant [SmithKline Beecham]

⇩

[Submit] [Clear] [Help]

⇩

⇩

Renewal fees
    Renewal fee A.86
    (patent year / paid)   03/12-11-1997
                      04/26-11-1998
                      05/08-11-1999
                      06/10-11-2000

Step 1: Enter the date in reverse order (year, month, day or yyyymmdd) in the "Application Number/Date" field AND the applicant name in the "Applicant" field.

Step 2: Click on "Submit".

Step 3: The Results screen will appear.

Step 4: Locate "Renewal fees" to find the information you are looking for.

FIGURE 3.26D

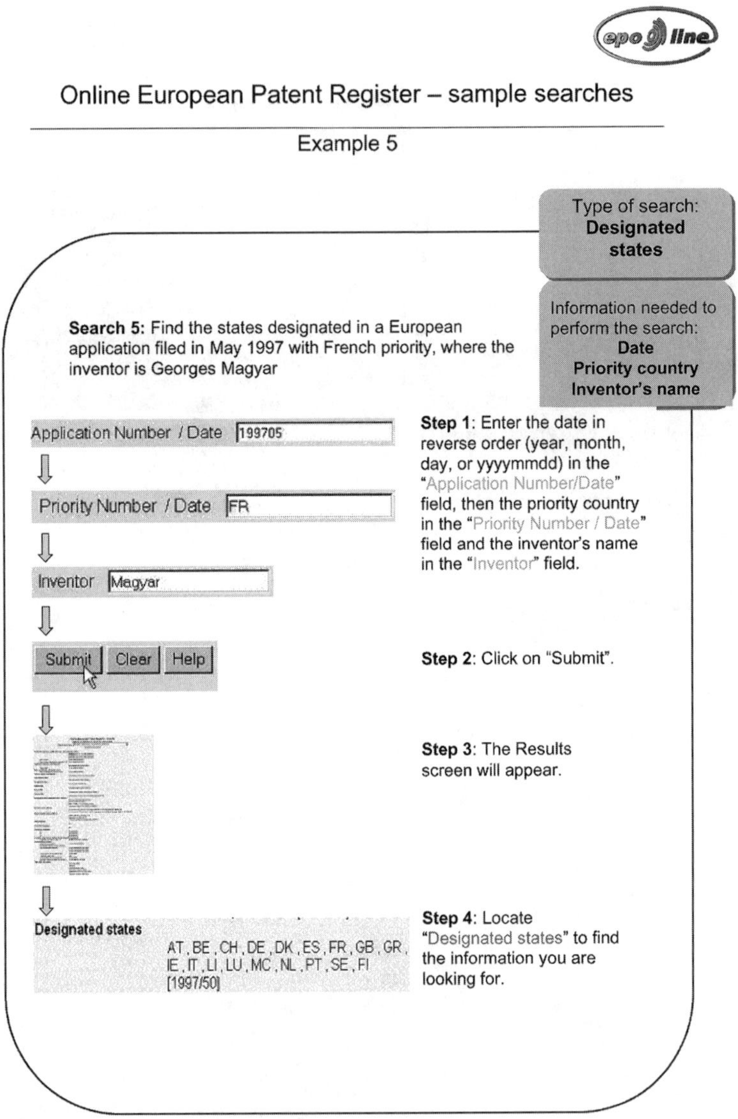

Online European Patent Register – sample searches

Example 5

Type of search:
**Designated
states**

Information needed to
perform the search:
**Date
Priority country
Inventor's name**

Search 5: Find the states designated in a European
application filed in May 1997 with French priority, where the
inventor is Georges Magyar

Application Number / Date 199705

Priority Number / Date FR

Inventor Magyar

Submit | Clear | Help

Designated states
AT , BE , CH , DE , DK , ES , FR , GB , GR ,
IE , IT , LI , LU , MC , NL , PT , SE , FI
[1997/50]

Step 1: Enter the date in
reverse order (year, month,
day, or yyyymmdd) in the
"Application Number/Date"
field, then the priority country
in the "Priority Number / Date"
field and the inventor's name
in the "Inventor" field.

Step 2: Click on "Submit".

Step 3: The Results
screen will appear.

Step 4: Locate
"Designated states" to find
the information you are
looking for.

FIGURE 3.26E

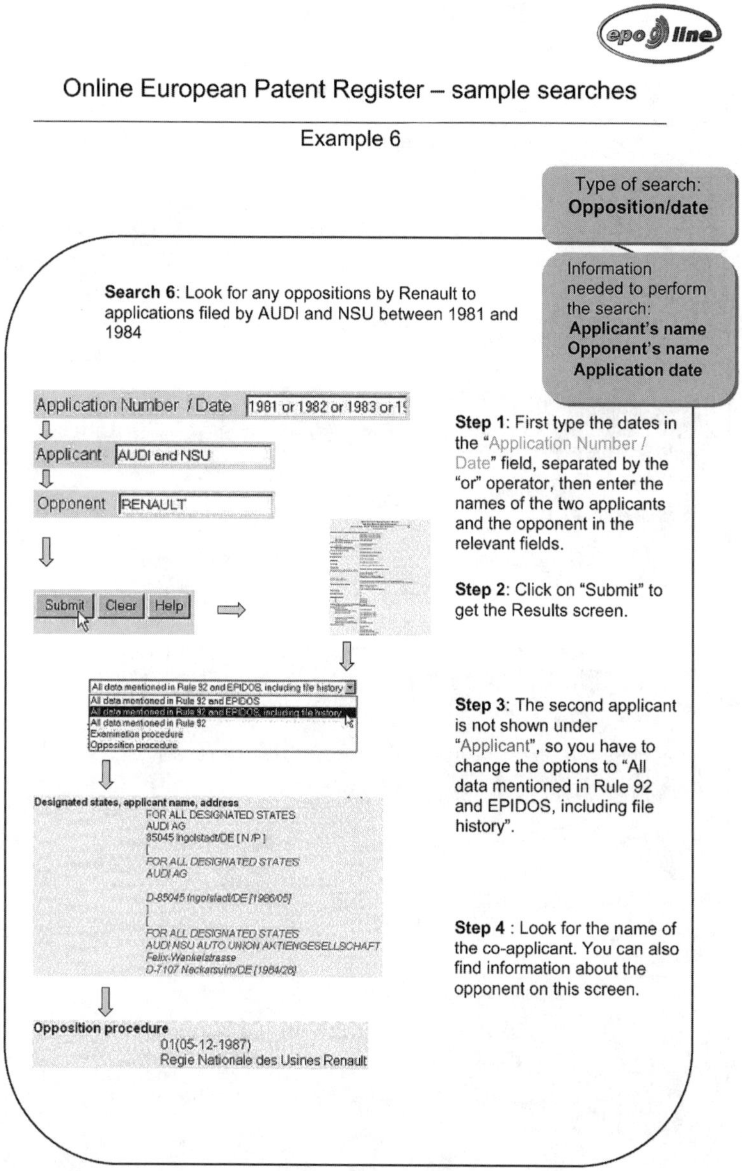

Online European Patent Register – sample searches

Example 6

Type of search:
Opposition/date

Information needed to perform the search:
**Applicant's name
Opponent's name
Application date**

Search 6: Look for any oppositions by Renault to applications filed by AUDI and NSU between 1981 and 1984

Application Number / Date | 1981 or 1982 or 1983 or 19

Applicant | AUDI and NSU

Opponent | RENAULT

Submit | Clear | Help

All data mentioned in Rule 92 and EPIDOS, including file history
All data mentioned in Rule 92 and EPIDOS
All data mentioned in Rule 92 and EPIDOS, including file history
All data mentioned in Rule 92
Examination procedure
Opposition procedure

Designated states, applicant name, address
FOR ALL DESIGNATED STATES
AUDI AG
85045 Ingolstadt/DE [N /P]
[
FOR ALL DESIGNATED STATES
AUDI AG

D-85045 Ingolstadt/DE [1986/05]
[
FOR ALL DESIGNATED STATES
AUDI NSU AUTO UNION AKTIENGESELLSCHAFT
Felix-Wankelstrasse
D-7107 Neckarsulm/DE [1984/26]

Opposition procedure
01(05-12-1987)
Regie Nationale des Usines Renault

Step 1: First type the dates in the "Application Number / Date" field, separated by the "or" operator, then enter the names of the two applicants and the opponent in the relevant fields.

Step 2: Click on "Submit" to get the Results screen.

Step 3: The second applicant is not shown under "Applicant", so you have to change the options to "All data mentioned in Rule 92 and EPIDOS, including file history".

Step 4 : Look for the name of the co-applicant. You can also find information about the opponent on this screen.

FIGURE 3.26F

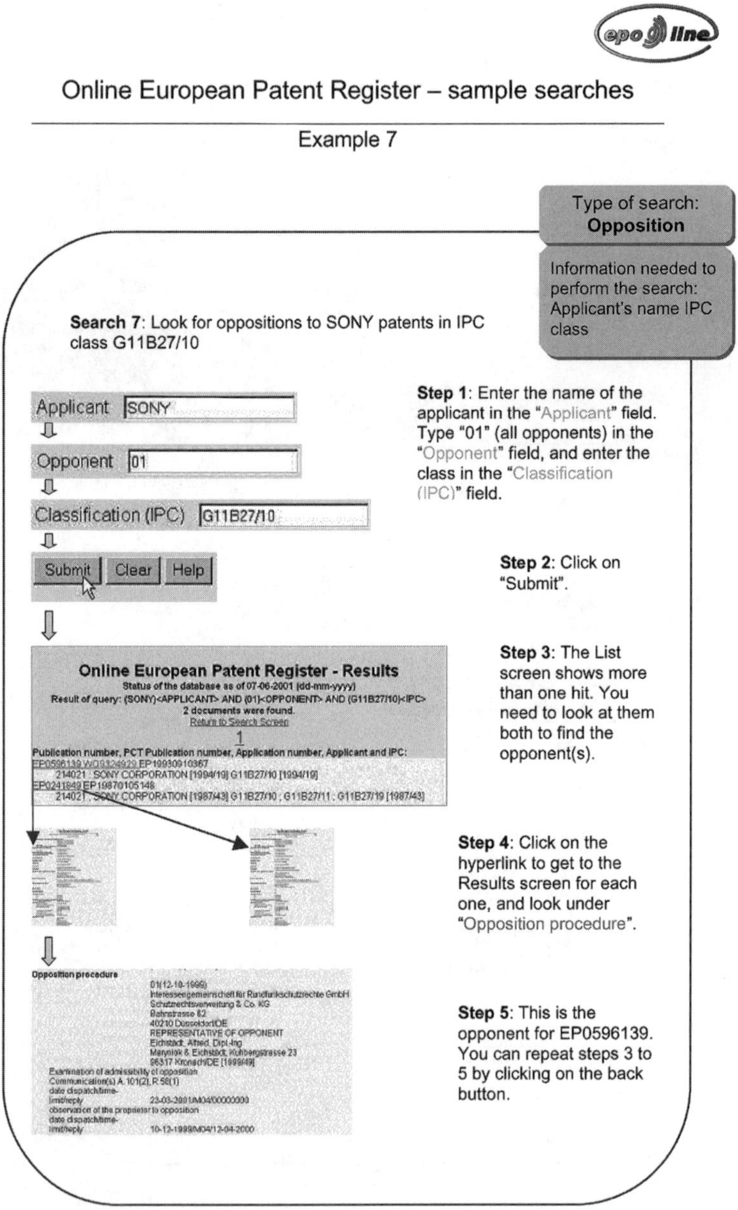

Online European Patent Register – sample searches

Example 7

Type of search:
Opposition

Information needed to perform the search: Applicant's name IPC class

Search 7: Look for oppositions to SONY patents in IPC class G11B27/10

Applicant [SONY]

⇩

Opponent [01]

⇩

Classification (IPC) [G11B27/10]

⇩

[Submit] [Clear] [Help]

⇩

Step 1: Enter the name of the applicant in the "Applicant" field. Type "01" (all opponents) in the "Opponent" field, and enter the class in the "Classification (IPC)" field.

Step 2: Click on "Submit".

Online European Patent Register - Results
Status of the database as of 07-06-2001 (dd-mm-yyyy)
Result of query: (SONY)<APPLICANT> AND (01)<OPPONENT> AND (G11B27/10)<IPC>
2 documents were found.
Return to Search Screen
1
Publication number, PCT Publication number, Application number, Applicant and IPC:
EP0596139 WO9324929 EP19930910367
214021 : SONY CORPORATION [1994/19] G11B27/10 [1994/19]
EP0241849 EP19870105148
214021 : SONY CORPORATION [1987/43] G11B27/10 ; G11B27/11 ; G11B27/19 [1987/43]

Step 3: The List screen shows more than one hit. You need to look at them both to find the opponent(s).

Step 4: Click on the hyperlink to get to the Results screen for each one, and look under "Opposition procedure".

Opposition procedure
01(12-10-1995)
Interessengemeinschaft für Rundfunkschutzrechte GmbH
Schutzrechtsverwaltung & Co. KG
Bahnstrasse 62
40210 Düsseldorf/DE
REPRESENTATIVE OF OPPONENT
Eichstädt, Alfred, Dipl.-Ing
Marynnix & Eichstädt, Kuhbergstrasse 23
96317 Kronach/DE [1999/49]
Examination of admissibility of opposition
Communication(s) A. 101(2), R. 58(1)
date dispatch/time-
limit/reply   23-03-2001/M04/00000000
observation of the proprietor to opposition
date dispatch/time-
limit/reply   10-12-1999/M04/12-04-2000

Step 5: This is the opponent for EP0596139. You can repeat steps 3 to 5 by clicking on the back button.

FIGURE 3.26G

Online European Patent Register – sample searches

Example 8

Type of search:
Applicant/IPC

Information needed to perform the search:
Applicant's name

Search 8: Look for patent applications from NOKIA having the classifications H04M1/03 and H04R1/22

Step 1: Type the applicant's name in the "Applicant" field, then enter the classes in the "Classification (IPC)" field.

Applicant: NOKIA

Classification (IPC) H04M1/03 and H04R1/22   eg. B62J1/02

Submit Clear Help

Step 2: Click on "Submit".

Online European Patent Register - Results

Status of the database as of 23-10-2001 (dd-mm-yyyy)

Result of query: (NOKIA)<APPLICANT> AND (H04M1/03 and H04R1/22)<IPC>

2 documents were found.

Return to Search Screen

1

Publication number, PCT Publication number, Application number, Applicant and IPC:

EP1044592 WO0039880 EP19980969923

997966 : NOKIA MOBILE PHONES LTD. H04R1/22 ; H04R1/10 ; H04M1/03 [2000/42]

EP0929077 EP19980960097

997966 : NOKIA MOBILE PHONES LTD. [1999/16] H04M1/03 ; H04R1/22 [1999/16]

Step 3: The Results screen shows two documents matching the search. Click on the corresponding hyperlink to view each one.

FIGURE 3.26H

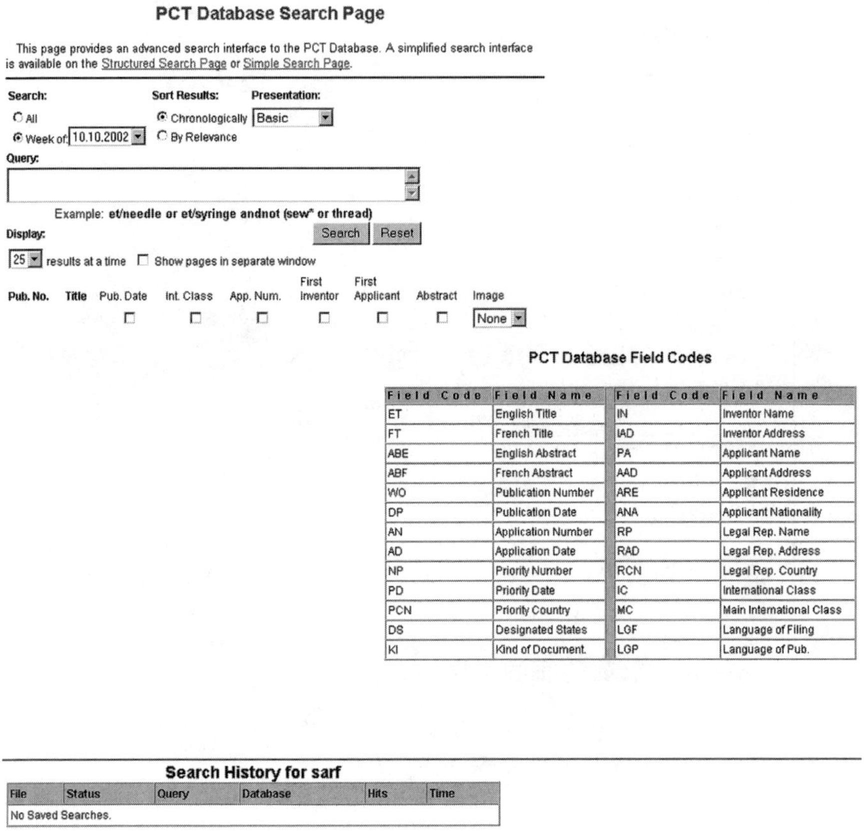

PCT Database Search Page

This page provides an advanced search interface to the PCT Database. A simplified search interface
is available on the Structured Search Page or Simple Search Page.

Search:	Sort Results:	Presentation:
○ All	⦿ Chronologically	Basic ▾
⦿ Week of: 10.10.2002 ▾	○ By Relevance	

Query:

```
                                                                          ▲
                                                                          ▼
```

Example: **et/needle or et/syringe andnot (sew* or thread)**

Display: Search   Reset

25 ▾ results at a time   ☐ Show pages in separate window

Pub. No.	Title	Pub. Date	Int. Class	App. Num.	First Inventor	First Applicant	Abstract	Image
		☐	☐	☐	☐	☐	☐	None ▾

PCT Database Field Codes

Field Code	Field Name	Field Code	Field Name
ET	English Title	IN	Inventor Name
FT	French Title	IAD	Inventor Address
ABE	English Abstract	PA	Applicant Name
ABF	French Abstract	AAD	Applicant Address
WO	Publication Number	ARE	Applicant Residence
DP	Publication Date	ANA	Applicant Nationality
AN	Application Number	RP	Legal Rep. Name
AD	Application Date	RAD	Legal Rep. Address
NP	Priority Number	RCN	Legal Rep. Country
PD	Priority Date	IC	International Class
PCN	Priority Country	MC	Main International Class
DS	Designated States	LGF	Language of Filing
KI	Kind of Document.	LGP	Language of Pub.

Search History for sarf

File	Status	Query	Database	Hits	Time
No Saved Searches.					

FIGURE 3.27

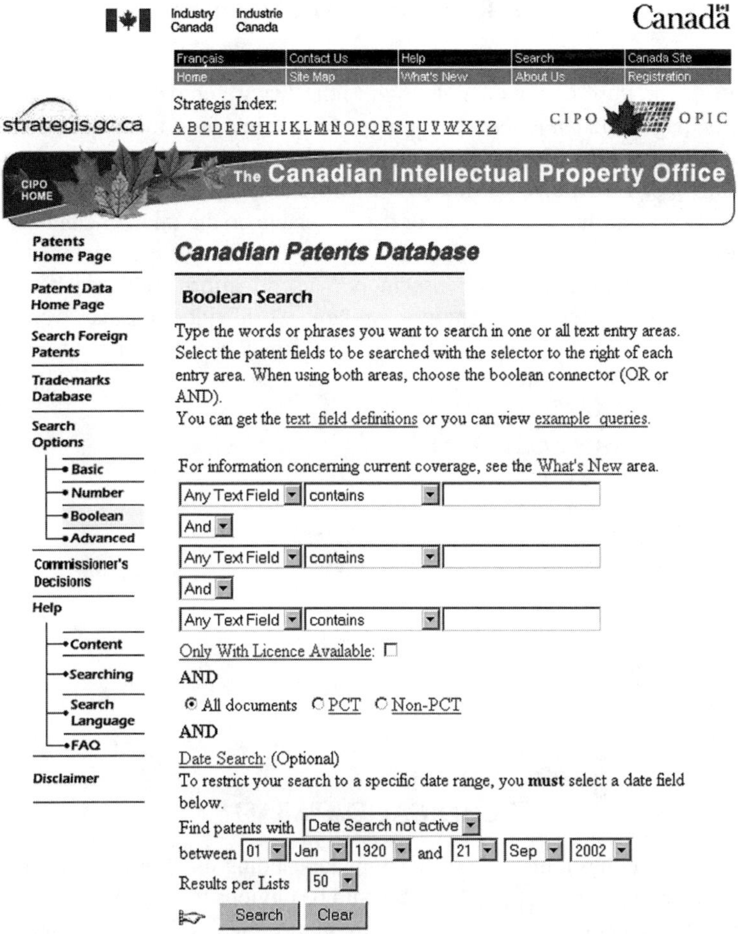

Industry **Industrie**
Canada Canada

Canadä

| Français | Contact Us | Help | Search | Canada Site |
| Home | Site Map | What's New | About Us | Registration |

strategis.gc.ca

Strategis Index:
A B C D E F G H I J K L M N O P Q R S T U V W X Y Z

CIPO OPIC

CIPO
HOME
The **Canadian Intellectual Property Office**

Patents
Home Page

Patents Data
Home Page

Search Foreign
Patents

Trade-marks
Database

Search
Options

→ **Basic**
→ **Number**
→ **Boolean**
→ **Advanced**

Commissioner's
Decisions

Help

→ **Content**
→ **Searching**
→ **Search**
  Language
→ **FAQ**

Disclaimer

Canadian Patents Database

Boolean Search

Type the words or phrases you want to search in one or all text entry areas. Select the patent fields to be searched with the selector to the right of each entry area. When using both areas, choose the boolean connector (OR or AND).

You can get the text field definitions or you can view example queries.

For information concerning current coverage, see the What's New area.

| Any Text Field ▾ | contains ▾ | |

| And ▾ |

| Any Text Field ▾ | contains ▾ | |

| And ▾ |

| Any Text Field ▾ | contains ▾ | |

Only With Licence Available: ☐

AND

⦿ All documents ○ PCT ○ Non-PCT

AND

Date Search: (Optional)
To restrict your search to a specific date range, you **must** select a date field below.

Find patents with | Date Search not active ▾ |

between | 01 ▾ | Jan ▾ | 1920 ▾ | and | 21 ▾ | Sep ▾ | 2002 ▾ |

Results per Lists | 50 ▾ |

☞ [Search] [Clear]

FIGURE 3.28

INTERNET SEARCH ENGINES

An example was given earlier to demonstrate the power of search engines on the Internet; in one third of a second, Google (http://www.google.com) parses through 2.5 billion pages and compiles a list of about 50,000 hits for a three-keyword search. Search technology has come of age and presents a remarkable tool to search for patentability of inventions, particularly as it pertains to issues of obviousness and prior art. However, the large volume of data available on the Internet can make these searches confusing, voluminous, and redundant. If you develop a habit of using a specific search engine and learn its "mood," useful information can be obtained quickly. To learn about search engines available worldwide, you may want to visit http://www.searchenginecolossus.com or http://www.searchengineguide.com. Following is a list of key search engines:

- www.alltheweb.com
- www.altavista.com
- www.excite.com
- www.google.com
- www.infoseek.com
- www.infospace.com
- www.lycos.com
- www.msn.com
- www.webcrawler.com
- www.yahoo.com

TECHNICAL DATABASES

Patentability searches require an in-depth understanding of what is considered prior art. This requires an evaluation of what would be obvious to one with ordinary skills in formulating a similar invention. These are highly specific legal terms that require thorough literature search. The power of the online search shows well here. There are several excellent sources of free information, and a large number of databases and services available to complete this task quickly and comprehensively.

American Chemical Society (http://stneasy.cas.org/html/english/login1.html) offers one of the premier scientific databases from where you can get original papers faxed to you if you urgently need them (Figure 3.29).

Delphion (formerly IBM Intellectual Property database; http://www.delphion.com) offers a low-cost solution for more in-depth search of patents as well as access to many consolidated databases (Figure 3.30).

Derwent (http://www.derwent.com) is one of the most widely used databases, from which the USPTO examiners benefit as well (Figure 3.31).

Dialog (http://www.dialog.com) is a large database that allows you to search without having to register an account; you pay as you go, using your credit card. You cannot do this if you are searching for trademarks (Figure 3.32).

National Institutes of Health (http://www4.ncbi.nlm.nih.gov/PubMed) offers more than 12 million research papers mainly in the biomedical sciences, available through the National Library of Medicine (Figure 3.33). This free database allows download of abstracts in an ASCII format for direct placement into programs such as Microsoft Word to develop a comprehensive bibliography.

Nerac (http://www.nerac.com) offers numerous online databases (Figure 3.34).

PATENT SEARCHES AND IP SERVICES

Investor's Digest (http://www.inventorsdigest.com), a very active site, offers resources for inventors (Figure 3.35).

MIT (http://web.mit.edu/invent/) has provided an elaborate and detailed Web site for invention development; it is worth a detailed look (Figure 3.36).

Patent Café (http://www.patentcafe.com) is a hangout for patent product vendors (Figure 3.37).

PATENT COPIES AND SEARCH FACILITIES

Faxpat: http://www.faxpat.com

Lexis-Nexis: http://www.lexis-nexis.com

Mayall: http://mayallj.freeserve.co.uk

Micropatent (http://www.1790.com/0/patentweb9809.html) is perhaps the most comprehensive service available at a very reasonable cost. The Web site is easy to navigate. Highly recommended (Figure 3.38).

Questel: http://www.questel.orbit.com

Patentec: http://www.patentec.com

STN_Easy_

Home Page

+ Help
+ Account Info
  Price List
  Browser Support
+ Customer Support
  Secure Session
+ More STN Info
  Comments

About STN Easy for
Intranets

Searching for scientific information has never been easier!

What's New

- Search History Available as a RTF Document
- Additional Search and Display Fields Added
- STN Easy Now Has Over 85 Databases
- Six Databases Added to Additional Categories
- STN Easy Search History Available for Four Days
- Patent Lookup Tab Added
- Additional Patent Search Fields Added to Advanced Search
- STN Keep & Share® (Data Re-use and Redistribution Tools) Now Available

Select Language
- ⦿ English
- ○ Deutsch
- ○ Japanese
- ○ French
- ○ Spanish

Login:

Password:

Start Your Session

Open New Account

Free Demo

STN is the Scientific & Technical Information Network. It is operated in cooperation with CAS in North America, FIZ Karlsruhe in Europe, and JST in Japan.

FIGURE 3.29

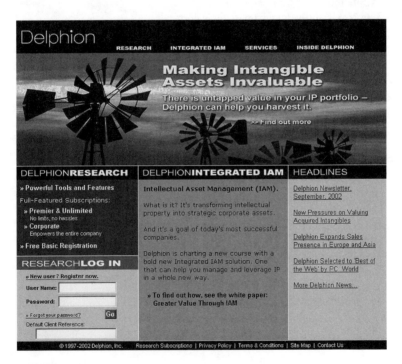

FIGURE 3.30

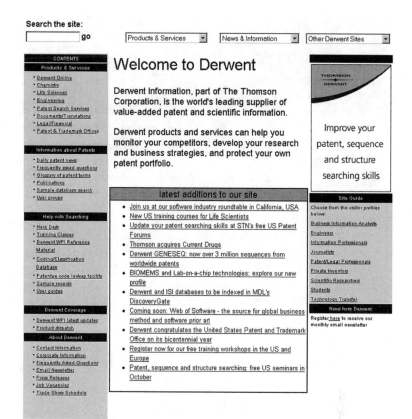

FIGURE 3.31

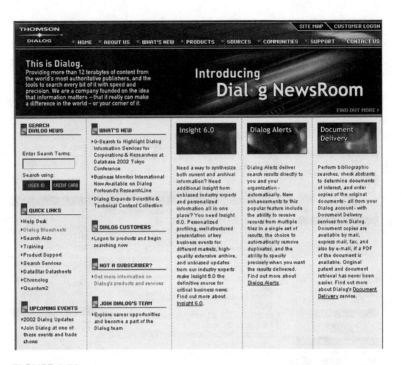

FIGURE 3.32

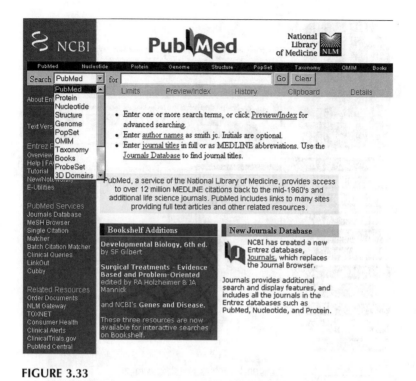

FIGURE 3.33

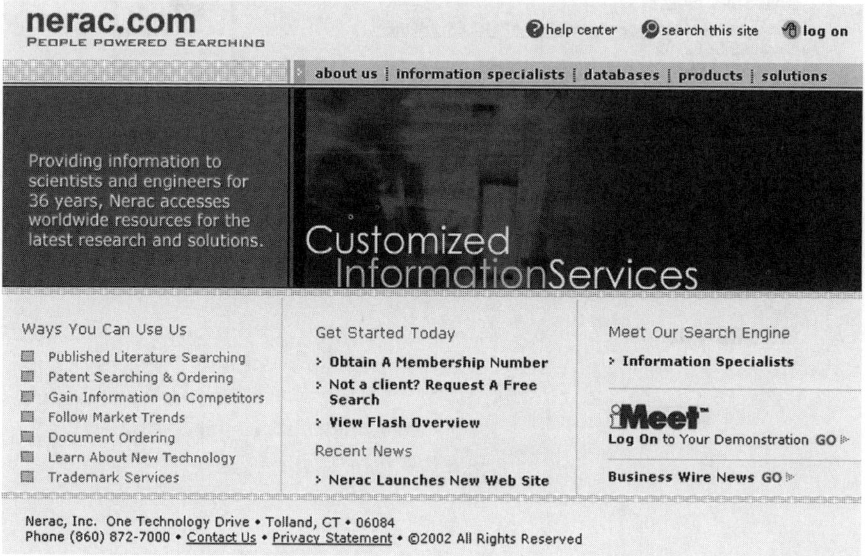

FIGURE 3.34

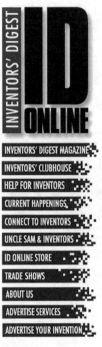

This site is designed for anyone who has ever said, "I've got a great idea. .
.Now what do I do?" It's also THE spot for anyone who's searching for the
next HOT product! Check out our magazine site and then follow our links to
the wonderful world of invention! SITE SCHEMATIC

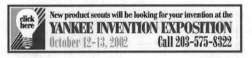

INVENTORS' DIGEST MAGAZINE

INVENTORS' CLUBHOUSE

HELP FOR INVENTORS

CURRENT HAPPENINGS

CONNECT TO INVENTORS

UNCLE SAM & INVENTORS

ID ONLINE STORE

TRADE SHOWS

ABOUT US

ADVERTISE SERVICES

ADVERTISE YOUR INVENTION

Search our Site:

[   ] [GO]

sitemap

INVENTORS' DIGEST
30-31 Union Wharf
Boston, MA 02109
(617) 367-4540

1-(800)-838-8808
(Subscriptions/Back
Issues)
CONTACT US

YOU ARE VISITOR
3 4 6 6 9 7

FIGURE 3.35

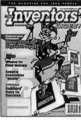

September/October
2002

Cover Story:
Proposed
Changes at the
USPTO: A Raw
Deal or a
Square Deal?

Complete Table
of Contents

■ Co-Founder
National Inventors' Month® - August
Help kids get inventive!

■ **GET THE LATEST ISSUE!**

■ **PAST ARTICLES ONLINE**

■ **WHAT OUR READERS SAY**

■ **HOT NEWS**

■ **INVENTOR'S CLUBHOUSE**
Avoid Scams... The Inventing Process...
Inventors Who Did It! (Success Stories)...
Answers to Common Questions...
Inventor Organizations...Product Seekers...
Invention Professionals

Patent Office
proposes huge
increases to patent
fees! (click here)

A PEEK INTO THE
FUTURE

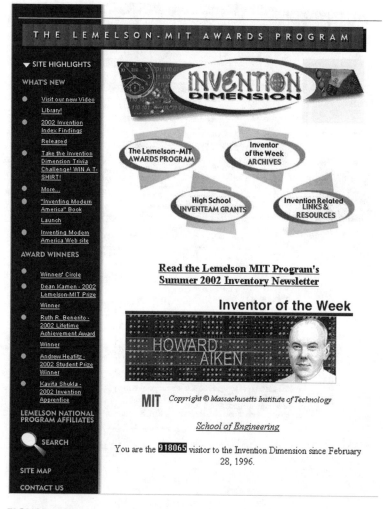

FIGURE 3.36

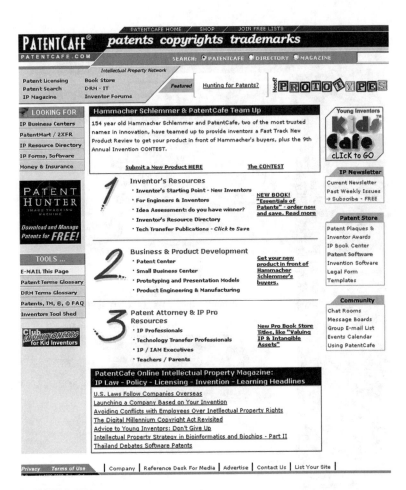

FIGURE 3.37

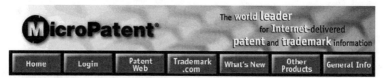

PatentWeb®

◎ Order Digital Patents

Why wait? Download patent documents from the world's largest digital collection of 33+ million patents to your PC or printer.

◎ Patent Research

Conduct **full-text** and **front-page** research using our databases of the **United States**, **Europe**, **PCT(WIPO)**, and **Japan**. UNLIMITED daily and annual subscriptions available.

Open a new **account today!**

CLICK HERE

◎ File Histories

Get your file histories fast and directly from MicroPatent with our file history order service. They're accurately organized, economically priced, and you can check the status of your order at any time. Click here for pricing or click above to go to the login page, type your login name and password, then click on the "Order/Download" button to place your request.

◎ TOPS™ - Corporate Patent Solution

TOPS (Total On-Demand Patent Solution) unites the best of our PatentWeb services, in **one unlimited** corporate account. Subscribe today and give *all* of your users access to a wealth of US and international patent information on MicroPatent.

◎ PatentImages® Viewer

Designed by our experts, our software (Free) helps you view, print, and file your downloaded patent documents in MicroPatent's own .mpz format.

◎ OG Notices (FREE)

Review front matter of the USPTO *Official Gazette*. To use it, simply login and select OG.

Home | Login | PatentWeb™ | Trademark.com™
What's New | Other Products | General Info

FIGURE 3.38

4   Online Filing Basics

INTRODUCTION

The major issues in online filing of patents arise in the security of transmission and authentication of the filer. These issues have kept the patent offices busy designing secure systems. The U.S. Patent and Trademark Office (USPTO) is ahead of the rest of the world in implementing an almost-complete system of online filing of patents; the European Patent Office (EPO) started accepting online filings in mid-2002, and in mid-2003 the World Intellectual Property Organization (WIPO) will begin accepting online PCT applications at first to the International Bureau only and then gradually to other receiving offices. Sufficient details of the operations of the online filing systems of the three organizations are provided in this book to prepare you for acquiring the hardware and software needed to benefit from this remarkable change in the way patents are developed and filed.

The online filing of patents is generally a four-step process:

1. Identification: This is the step where the applicant or filer establishes his identity in a manner that is certifiable; it is important to know that individuals, not firms, are identified even if they are part of an organization. Patent offices assign security keys either as software (USPTO and WIPO) or as hardware (EPO).
2. Proprietary software setup: The patent offices have developed their own proprietary software systems; restrictions apply to download eligibility. WIPO does not require use of any specific software, as long as the application meets the standards specified. Recently, the USPTO has awarded contracts to five private vendors to further develop its proprietary software and to offer other services for filing online applications through these vendors.
3. Preparation of specification: The body of patent applications is prepared using word-processing and scanning software as needed, and then brought into the environment of the authoring software provided by the patent office to convert the files to an appropriate form (XML for USPTO and WIPO). If your files are already in the form specified, such as PDF or XML, you may use them directly in the submission software.
4. Bundling, conversion, and submission of application: The software provided by the patent office pools all the required components of the application, does a validation check to make sure all parts are complete, converts the files to an appropriate form (e.g., XML; in the U.S. it is done in Step 3), encrypts and compresses the files (ZIP files), and transports them to patent office servers using a secure socket layer with identification system. An electronic receipt is generated.

USPTO

To become eligible to file a U.S. patent application online, the following steps should be followed exactly as described.

OBTAIN A CUSTOMER NUMBER

All those who do business with the USPTO, including *pro se* applicants, attorneys, and agents, need first to register. This step requires securing a Customer Number, which will be used to identify the name and address of the applicant and his agent or attorney. The Customer Number gives you exclusive access to your application information through the PAIR (Patent Application Information Retrieval) system described in Chapter 11. There is no special requirement or qualification needed to secure a Customer Number. If you are an attorney or an agent qualified to practice before the USPTO, you will identify yourself as such so that the USPTO will know where to send your mail. (*Note:* A Customer Number can be obtained for a firm or individual; however, a firm is not qualified to act as an agent or attorney.) To obtain your unique Customer Number, you should use form PTO/SB/125A (http://www.uspto.gov/web/forms/sb0125.pdf); the second page of this form is for continuation of attorney/agent registration number information); after filling it out you may fax it to the USPTO Electronic Business Center at (703) 308-2840; or you can mail it to U.S. Patent and Trademark Office, Box CN, Washington, D.C. 20231. This step is not related only to electronic or online filing of patents but common to all applications; therefore the correspondence is not sent to the EFS (Electronic Filing System) division of the USPTO. The Customer Number should not be disseminated frivolously (Figure 4.1).

A few weeks after filing the request, you will receive in the mail a Customer Number and a sheet of imprinted barcode labels, courtesy of the USPTO. At this point it is a good idea to generate more barcode labels, as you will be placing these on your future correspondence. You may choose to use barcode-generating software or simply make a high-resolution photocopy of the sheet received from the USPTO on self-sticking labels. Another practical approach is to scan the barcode in GIF format at 300 dpi and insert this graphics file on your correspondence where necessary (recommended method).

Corrections to the Customer Number database may be required from time to time; to do so, use form PTO/SB/124A (http://www.uspto.gov/web/forms/sb0124.pdf) to make a change. This may be more important to attorneys changing firms or when reorganizing the management of a group of patents. You can fax or mail this form to the Electronic Business Center using the contact information given earlier.

ASSOCIATE CUSTOMER NUMBER WITH PATENT APPLICATION(S)

Once you have your Customer Number, you must now associate your currently filed patent applications with it. You should now download the Microsoft® Excel spreadsheet template by logging on to http://www.uspto.gov/ebc/documents/cust_req _instructions.xls. An example of a completed spreadsheet is given in Figure 4.2.

Please type a plus sign (+) inside this box →☐

PTO/SB/125A (08-00)
Approved for use through 10/31/2002. OMB 0651-0035
U.S. Patent and Trademark Office; U.S. DEPARTMENT OF COMMERCE
Under the Paperwork Reduction Act of 1995, no persons are required to respond to a collection of information unless it displays a valid OMB control number.

**Request for
Customer Number**

Address to:

Assistant Commissioner for Patents
Box CN
Washington, DC   20231

To the Commissioner of Patents and Trademarks:
Please assign a Customer Number to the Correspondence Address indicated below.

Firm *or* Individual Name	
Address	
Address	
City	State ZIP
Country	
Telephone	Fax

Please associate the following practitioner registration number(s)with the Customer Number assigned to the Correspondence Address cited above.

☐ Additional practitioner registration numbers are listed on supplemental sheet(s) attached hereto

Request Submitted by:

Firm Name (if applicable)	
Name of person submitting request	
Signature	
Telephone Number	Date

Burden Hour Statement: This form is estimated to take 0.2 hours to complete. Time will vary depending upon the needs of the individual case. Any comments on the amount of time you are required to complete this form should be sent to the Chief Information Officer, U.S. Patent and Trademark Office, Washington, DC 20231.   DO NOT SEND FEES OR COMPLETED FORMS TO THIS ADDRESS. SEND TO: Assistant Commissioner for Patents, Box CN, Washington, DC 20231.

FIGURE 4.1

After completing the Microsoft Excel spreadsheet, you will need to copy it to a floppy disk and send the disk to USPTO, Box CN, Washington, D.C. 20231. If you do not have pending applications on file, then skip to Step 3. After your first application is filed, you must return to the filing the diskette step. (*Note:* This needs to be done only once.) The purpose of this filing is to associate your Customer Number to different permanent addresses required for communicating with you. The instructions at the USPTO are not clear. (*Note:* You must send the file in .xls format only and return the entire spreadsheet without removing any information footnotes that were meant for you.) The USPTO computer reads only the fields that are marked by capital Xs; changing this feature of the file will misalign the data and cause

	A	B	C	D	E	F	G
1	Customer:	XXXXXX	<----	(Six digit Customer Number)			
2					NOTE: Bold X's indicate where data is entered.		
3	Sarfaraz K. Niazi			<---- Enter Correspondence Address.			
4	Niazi Consultants Inc.				Line 3 firm name		
5	20 Riverside Drive				Line 4 street address		
6	Deerfield, Illinois 60015				Line 5 street address or city, state zip		
7	XXXXXXXXXXXXXXXXXXXXXXXXX				Line 6 street address or city, state zip		
8	XXXXXXXXXXXXXXXXXXXXXXXXX				Line 7 street address or city, state zip		
9	XXXXXXXXXXXXXXXXXXXXXXXXX				Line 8 street address or city, state zip		
10					Line 9 street address or city, state zip		
11	Rows 10 through 15 are blank, data entry begins in row 16 and is continous until all application and/or						
12	patent information is entered. No headers or titles are used on subsequent pages.						
13	Patent	Application	Patent	Filing	Correspondence	Practioner of	Fee
14	Number	Number	Date	Date	Address	Record	Address
15	(7 Digits w/o ",")	(8 digit w/o "/" or ",")	mm/dd/yy	mm/dd/yy	yes/no	yes/no	yes/no
16	XXXXXXX	9681119	XX/XX/XX	1/10/2001	yes	yes	yes
17	Left or Ctr algn	Left or Ctr algn	mo/da/yr	mo/da/yr	l, r or c algn	l, r, or c algn	right align

FIGURE 4.2

misreading. The rationale for this rather cumbersome step is to update the USPTO computer database by associating correspondence address with Customer Number in the preinspection section of the Patent Office; when the Customer Number is established, this information is not automatically communicated to the patent processing system. (One may have different addresses for correspondence regarding a patent application and regarding the Customer Number database.)

REQUEST A DIGITAL CERTIFICATE

The USPTO needs to establish your digital identity on the Internet. To do so, the USPTO has developed an elaborate system of obtaining a digital signature and confidentiality certificate. Before making this request, you should read the PKI (Public Key Infrastructure) Subscriber Agreement (PTO-2042; Certificate Action Form or PAIR Access Form, see Figure 4.3) carefully as it describes your legal obligations to the USPTO. You should now fill out the form, which allows you to access the Patent Application Information Retrieval system (http://www.uspto.gov/ebc/documents/certificateactionform.pdf).

Note that this is an "action" form, which is used for the initial request for a number, or to replace or cancel it. You should know that the key assigned by USPTO is not like the password on your Internet applications and is not recoverable; a new key is always issued to replace the old key. Also note that you need to identify that you are a registered attorney/agent or a *pro se* applicant. This is one of the rare forms submitted to the USPTO that requires notarization (or certification by a designated USPTO officer, if you want to walk it to the Office); therefore, it cannot be faxed. The original form (no copies) should be mailed to USPTO, Box EBC, Washington, D.C. 20231.

OBTAIN ACCESS CODES

After your application for a digital certificate has been approved you will receive two codes: (1) an Authorization Code, which will be sent by mail and (2) a Reference Number, which likely will be sent via e-mail. Some of the biggest goof-ups happen

UNITED STATES PATENT AND TRADEMARK OFFICE CERTIFICATE ACTION FORM

(Block 1) REQUESTOR STATUS	PTO USE ONLY
☐ Registered Attorney, Registration Number [ ] ☐ ProSe Inventor	

(Block 2) REQUESTOR INFORMATION - (PRINT INFORMATION ABOVE GREY LINE)

Given Name	Middle name	Family Name

Street Address		APT

City	State Code	Postal Code	Country Name

Telephone Number	Facsimile Number	Email Address

Customer Number [   ]   Additional Customer Numbers Attached ☐

(Block 3) ACTION

Certificate Application ☐   I request a Certificate be issued to me by the USPTO.

Certificate Revocation ☐ I request that my Certificate be revoked.	Reason (Select One): New Certificate ☐ No Longer Needed ☐ Issued Legal Name Change ☐ Other ☐ Key Compromise [ ] Date Last Known to be Un-compromised [ ]

Key Recovery: ☐ I request that my encryption key be recovered.	Reason (Select One): Forgotten or Lost Password ☐ Entrust Profile Corrupted or Lost ☐ Other [ ] Describe [ ]

(Block 4) SIGNATURE

I have read and understand the Subscriber Agreement (Version 1, December 1999) and my signature on this document, by hand, is my agreement to abide by the agreement and the rules and policies of the USPTO regarding the agreement.

I certify that the information, statements and representations provided by me on this form are true and accurate to the best of my knowledge. I understand that a willfully false certification is a criminal offense and is punishable by law (18 U.S.C. 1001).

_____   _____
(Requestor signature required from block 1)   Date (mm/dd/yyyy)

(Block 5) IDENTIFICATION

SUBSCRIBED and SWORN to before me by _____
this ____day of _____, _____. _____ of _____
(county)
Notary Public _____
MY COMMISSION EXPIRES: _____

(Notarial seal)

PRIVACY ACT AND PAPERWORK REDUCTION ACT STATEMENTS ATTACHED

US PTO Form PTO-2042   Approved for use through 3/31/03   OMB Control Number 0651-0045
Patent and Trademark Office: U.S. DEPARTMENT OF COMMERCE

FIGURE 4.3

at this stage. Many times the USPTO will send you the two codes in separate e-mails as they come from two different departments; oftentimes an applicant may have to call to get a number.

The Authorization Code comes from the Office of Information System Security. The key codes are case sensitive and require entering spaces and dashes as listed. Save these e-mails.

For the Reference Number contact the USPTO at 800-786-9199 (in the United States and Canada) or 703-308-4357 or by email at usptoinfo@uspto.gov. The reason we are giving you such detailed information is in case you make mistakes in entering the access code numbers. You get only one chance to enter them; if you make a mistake, the file will become corrupt and you have to request a new set of numbers.

At this point, you are ready to download software for EFS or PAIR and to take advantage of electronic filing of patent applications or patent application status checks via the Internet.

SET UP THE SOFTWARE

Before starting the setup of software needed to communicate with the USPTO, you must check the hardware and software requirements (Table 4.1).

TABLE 4.1
System Requirements

	Minimum	Recommended for Best Results
Pentium processor	233 MHz	266 MHz or higher
Memory	64 Mb RAM	128 Mb RAM
Screen display	800 × 600	1024 × 768 or higher
Browser	Internet Explorer 5.0	Internet Explorer 5.5
Plug-in TIFF viewer	AlternaTIFF plug-in v1.3.5 or higher[a]	
Free hard disk space	42 Mb	
Internet connection	56 kbps or faster modem	
Operating system	Windows 95/98 (Service Release 2 or higher)/2000/NT 4.0 (Service Pack 3 or later)	
Applications	Microsoft® Word 97/2000 including Office Assistant for PASAT or Corel® WordPerfect 9 (Service Pack 2 or higher) for the Template for Specification Authoring	
	Graphics package (for TIFF image formatting) such as Imaging for Windows	
Printer driver(s)	MDAC 2.1	
Scanner	Capable of producing black-and-white TIFF images at 300 dpi; CCITT Group 4 compression	

[a] AlternaTIFF plug-in is freeware available at http://www.alternatiff.com.

Do not install the software until you have received your Customer Number and the two codes; you may download the software, however. Because the USPTO is continuously updating its software to add newer features, the program itself includes a "current-version" check, which is a very useful feature; I will later advise you on how to keep it flagged all the time. The software that you will download is

- ePAVE (electronic Packaging and Verification Engine) compiles the patent application and transmits it to the USPTO; it can be downloaded at http://www.uspto.gov/ebc/efs/downloads/epave.htm.
- PAIR (Patent Application Information Retrieval) system allows you to log on to the USPTO server through a secure system; it can be downloaded at http://www.uspto.gov/ebc/efs/downloads/ptodirect.htm.
- PASAT (Patent Application Specification Authoring Tool) is a plug-in for Microsoft® Word (default; can be downloaded at http://www.uspto.gov/ebc/efs/downloads/pasat.htm) or Corel® WordPerfect (requires installation of a specific program and can be downloaded at http://www.uspto.gov/ebc/efs/downloads/wptempl.htm).
- PatentIn is a computer program designed to expedite the preparation of USPTO patent applications containing nucleic acid and polypeptide sequences; the software can be downloaded at http://www.uspto.gov/web/offices/pac/patin/patentinv3.htm.
- TSA (http://www.uspto.gov/ebc/efs/downloads/wptempl.htm) if you are using WordPerfect instead of Microsoft Word. Whereas the USPTO provides support to WordPerfect, it should be noted that the default is Word; also, the use of WordPerfect is more cumbersome. Unless there is a special licensing reason (such as WordPerfect being a corporate licensed software), I recommend that you switch to Word.

Install all software (choose between Word and WordPerfect, and PatentIn if needed) at this time. Please pay attention to the following statement of restriction:

Notice: Cryptographic Software Notice and Acknowledgment. The USPTO Direct software includes cryptographic software subject to export controls under the Export Administration Regulations and anyone receiving the software by downloading or otherwise may not export the software without a license. Acknowledgment: I acknowledge that I understand that the cryptographic software that I receive or download is subject to export controls under the Export Administration Regulations and that I may not export the software without a license. References to the Export Administration Regulations are references to 15 CFR 7(c). The software is issued by the U.S. Department of Commerce, Bureau of Export Administration (BXA) under laws relating to the control of certain exports, reexports, and activities.

WIPO

The World Intellectual Property Organization administers the Patent Cooperative Treaty (PCT) filings worldwide. PCT-EASY (Electronic Application System) is the software designed to facilitate the preparation of PCT international patent applications in electronic form and, ultimately, the transfer of such applications by electronic means. It is anticipated that by late 2003, you will be able to file PCT applications online using the PCT-SAFE software that is under development; in the meantime, the online filing functions remain limited. You can download the current software at the WIPO Web site (http://www.wipo.org/pct-safe/en/pct_easy/welcome.htm); from the same URL, you can request the software on CD. PCT-EASY is updated periodically using a small executable file, called a patch, which modifies the software to reflect any new designations, fee amounts, or other changes. In the future, if you are a registered user of PCT-EASY, you will be notified and will receive patches via e-mail if you desire. You will be able also to periodically check the PCT-EASY Web site to download new patches. You can check when the software was last updated on the user registration screen (see PCT-EASY Registration below).

Currently the use of PCT-EASY software is limited to:

- A request form module that provides for the input and validation of data typically included in the PCT Request Form and the attachment of the abstract in electronic form
- Option to print out a PCT computer-generated request form, replacing the existing PCT/RO/101 form, for the purposes of PCT-EASY filing
- Option to copy to diskette the PCT-EASY Request Form data file, and an attached abstract template and electronic address book, both of which facilitate data entry in the request form module for submission with the complete paper filing
- Preparing an abstract and attaching to the file, and a module for import and export of file for records management

PCT-EASY REGISTRATION

The PCT-EASY registration screen is accessed from the Options command of the Tools menu in the EASY File Manager (Figure 4.4). It contains important registration information that is used by the software in many different ways; select the PCT-EASY application bar to view these details. Please ensure that your name and address details are current. If you have not yet registered or in the event of a change in details, update directly on this screen, print out a registration sheet by selecting the print icon, and forward this information to the PCT-EASY Help Desk at World Intellectual Property Organization, 34 Chemin des Colombettes, CH-1211 Geneva 20, Switzerland; phone +41 22 338 9523, fax +41 22 338 8040, and e-mail (scan and attach) pcteasy.help@wipo.int. Soon it will be possible to upload this information online. The applications are not submitted to the Help Desk.

PCT-EASY INSTALLATION

Routine procedures for installation of new software are followed using either the CD-ROM or the downloaded .exe file:

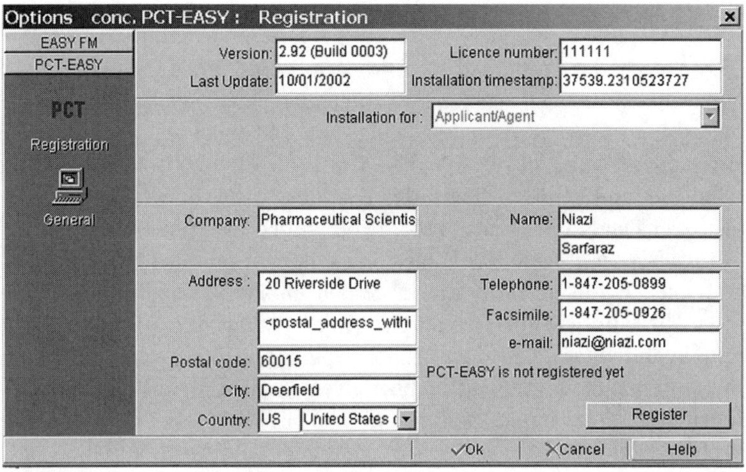

FIGURE 4.4

1. Select your language for installation.
2. Indicate the license number provided with your registration; if you do not have one, enter 111111.
3. Click OK.
4. You will be prompted to create a password, if you desire. To do so, check the password protection check box, type in the password and then confirm it by typing it a second time. Please make careful note of this password, as it will be needed for accessing PCT-EASY.

There should never be more than one version of PCT-EASY software installed on a machine. If an earlier version has already been installed, simply follow the instructions for installing PCT-EASY, making sure that the same installation path has been chosen. Existing files will be updated as required and user templates will be updated accordingly. The Uninstall facility included in this version of PCT-EASY assists the user when removing the software from the hard disk. In the EASY Applications Group in the Program Manager, double-click on Uninstall.

PCT-SAFE

WIPO is developing electronic filing software, PCT-SAFE, which will enable users to file PCT international applications in completely electronic form, either online over the Internet or using physical media (e.g., diskettes, CD-ROMs, DVDs). In order to facilitate the transition to E-filing, this new system is based on the present PCT-EASY software, currently used in some 40% of all PCT applications. The technical details about the structure of PCT-SAFE have been made available.

EPO

The online patent filing system of the European Patent Office is called the *epoline®*.
This online filing product enables you to submit patent applications to the EPO
electronically. To use *epoline* online filing, you first must register and receive the
software and validating device by mail from the EPO (http://www.epoline.org).
Unlike the U.S. and WIPO systems, this is a rather long, drawn-out procedure that
may take weeks and even months before you will be ready to use the system. EPO
handles requests on a batch basis, meaning they will produce the software copies
and the related hardware only after a certain number of applications have been
received. The application for registration is available at http://www.epo-
line.org/onlinefilingdocs/enrolmentEN.doc. You can mail the form to EPO or send
it by fax (preferred method) to the number given on the form; also you have a choice
of completing the form online, adding a bitmap or JPEG signature, and sending the
document to *epoline* Customer Service, using the Send function; your application
will then be processed by the EPO. Once it has been accepted, you will be sent the
following items free of charge:

1. CD-ROM containing Online Filing software
2. Smart card reader
3. Smart card (separate mailing)
4. Pin code (separate mailing)
5. Documentation

These items will enable you to use not only *epoline* Online Filing, but other
secure *epoline* services also as they become available.

5 USPTO EFS Overview

EFS PURPOSE

The purpose of the Electronic Filing System (EFS) of the U.S. Patent and Trademark Office (USPTO) is to electronically file specific types of patent application-related submissions via the Internet. An EFS user must be identified as one of the following authorized patent application filers:

- Applicant
- Assignee
- Assignee undivided part as set forth in 37 CFR 1.33(b)
- Registered Attorney or Agent

EFS is a system for submitting new utility patent applications, provisional patent applications, assignment documents, publication-ready application information for pre-grant publications, Information Disclosure Statements, and computer readable format (CRF) sequence listings for pending biotechnology patent applications as described in MPEP (*Manual of Patent Examining Procedure*) and 37 CFR 1.821–1.825.

EFS use is based on patent business rules and statutes. A new utility patent application is originally filed electronically. All applications filed after November 29, 2000 are subject to the pre-grant publication rules (see 37 CFR 1.211 to 1.221). The electronic filer will indicate how the application will be published (i.e., early, at 18 months, or not at all) during submission of the electronic application. EFS applications are assigned a filing date and an application number, and entered into the normal paper-based flow of examination after being printed in a standard format.

A pre-grant submission is a submission of a copy (possibly amended or redacted) of an application specification already filed at the USPTO, together with patent application information that will be published along with the specification. The pre-grant submissions will be published but will not be entered into the examination process.

To file a pre-grant publication submission electronically the applicant should already have a filing date, an application number, and a confirmation number. The amendments or modifications that appear in these submissions are not made automatically in the corresponding application file at the USPTO. These amendments must be submitted to the USPTO on paper according to conventional procedure. Please refer to the American Inventors Protection Act of 1999 (http://www.uspto.gov/web/offices/dcom/olia/aipa/index.htm).

EFS SOFTWARE OVERVIEW

The Electronic Filing System provides patent applicants and practitioners with software capabilities and technical guidance to author patent application information for electronic submission to the USPTO via the Internet. EFS is comprised of two software components: (1) authoring software that complies with the USPTO business rules and electronic data capture standards; and (2) submission software that creates forms, validates, bundles, compresses, and submits secure application files and information. The USPTO makes the EFS authoring and submission software available at no cost.

EFS implements patent business rules and practices using Internet technologies; XML (Extensible Markup Language) is one of the technical standards that it implements. XML is a nonproprietary standard approved by the World Wide Web Consortium (W3C); it is a format used for exchange of information between different automated applications. Because the data is tagged, it can be passed intelligently from one system to another. XML allows the USPTO to publish pre-grant publication submissions without having to rekey the information.

Applicants author their patent application specifications offline as intelligent, tagged, electronic documents using the EFS software, which automatically tags the patent application specification and other related application information in XML.

The authoring tool allows patent applicants to code (tag) the various parts of their application in XML, while operating in a commercially available word processing program environment. The USPTO provides two authoring tools as part of EFS; you may author a patent application specification as an XML-tagged document by using (1) PASAT (Patent Application Specification Authoring Tool) for Microsoft® Word or (2) TSA (Template for Specification Authoring) for Corel® WordPerfect.

The submission software is called ePAVE (electronic Packaging and Validation Engine). It is used to create forms and submit the electronic application information. Using ePAVE, applicants author other patent application information, including fee transmittal, transmittal information, bibliographic application information, and assignment information, as XML forms. After successful transmission, the software returns an acknowledgment that includes the date of receipt at the USPTO and an assigned patent application number.

A USPTO Customer Number and digital certificate must be obtained prior to using the EFS software. When you file electronically, you can pay fees using either a USPTO deposit account or a bankcard (i.e., credit card).

WHAT EFS SUPPORTS

1. Electronic filing of the following new utility patent application parts: specification, CRF biosequence listing text files, computer program listing text file appendices, large table text file appendices, declaration, power of attorney, application transmittal, fee transmittal, application data sheet, small entity statement, invention disclosure statement (IDS), and assignment recordation.

2. Electronic filing of publication-ready patent application information as a subsequent filing for pre-grant publication. Pre-grant publication submissions can include utility or plant specification, patent application information for publication on the front page of the publication, submission transmittal, and fee transmittal.
3. Electronic filing of information disclosure statements with new utility applications and as subsequent submissions for previously filed applications.
4. Electronic filing of sequence listing(s) in CRF for pending applications. The CRF sequence listing is submitted according to patent business rules in ASCII (text) file format.
5. Electronic filing of assignment recordation documents for previously filed patent applications and patents.
6. Windows® 95/98/2000/NT 4.0. You will need an Internet service provider or Internet connection also to use EFS.
7. Accepts images, including figures and declarations, as TIFF (Tagged Image File Format) files only.
8. Requires a scanner capable of producing black and white TIFF images at 300 dpi using CCITT Group 4 compression.
9. Requires a CD recorder for submissions larger than 10 MB in size. CD submissions should be CD-ROM or CD-R.

WHAT EFS DOES NOT SUPPORT

1. EFS does not allow you to electronically file international (PCT), design, plant, reissue, reexam, or secrecy order patent applications.
2. You cannot electronically submit all documents to be matched with the paper file wrapper during the prosecution of an application, including amendments.
3. EFS does not support electronic filing of submissions larger than 10 MB via the Internet.
4. EFS does not support electronic filing of color images.

BASIC STEPS TO USING EFS

Getting Started

Before you can file electronically, you must obtain your Customer Number and digital certificate from the USPTO. These items are used to confirm your identity and to ensure the security of your electronic transmission. Procedures for obtaining these numbers were provided in the previous chapter.

WORD PROCESSING AND IMAGING PROGRAMS

Install or upgrade to a word processing application that permits XML authoring (Microsoft Word 97 or 2000, or Corel WordPerfect 9.0). Note that later versions of these software applications offer some distinct advantages; it is recommended that you use the latest versions available.

Acquire software to create and view image files in the TIFF format. Create image files, e.g., drawings, declaration, assignment conveyance documents, small entity statements (no longer required). Images can be drawings, figures, tables, complex chemical formulae, complex math equations, and custom characters. Scan or convert all images (using the specified settings for drawings and forms).

FILE PREPARATION

Prepare your files using the recommended software with specific precautions for the images and text formatting:

- **Preparing images:** Before you can attach images to your electronic submission, they must meet the specifications established by the USPTO for electronic filing. Scan or convert all images using the following settings: 300×300 dpi, black-and-white only, Group 4 compression, maximum size $8\,1/2 \times 11$ in. for drawings and forms. These specifications apply to the following items: inline graphics (including complex chemical structures, math equations, tables, and custom characters), drawings (figures), declaration forms, assignment documents, and small entity statements
- **Naming your files:** File names are limited to 25 characters and must be alphanumeric. You can also use the hyphen and period characters in file names. The USPTO recommends that you use the 8.3 file-naming convention when you name folders and files that will be used with ePAVE. This convention specifies up to eight characters for the name of the file and three characters for the file extension, with the two components separated by a period — for example, newfile1.doc. It is important that you do not use special characters or spaces in your file names, as this will cause errors when you attempt to submit to the USPTO. Do not use any characters other than letters, numbers, hyphens (-), and periods (.). When you name your ePAVE submission folder, the folder name must differ from the names of any files or figures that are included in your submission.
- **Working with source documents:** If you are authoring from a source document, convert the document text to Arial, CG Times, or Times New Roman. Create a working or source document folder on a local or shared drive to store all files relating to the submission, making sure you follow the file-naming conventions specified in this document. Copy all specification-related files into this folder: all images, source document(s), the specification that you authored using PASAT (*.s4w and *.s4t). Once you have begun authoring your specification, do not move any files from this folder. Images inserted into a PASAT document are not embedded in the document. There is a hyperlink created to the file path of the image. If the image is moved from the folder once it has been inserted into the PASAT document, the hyperlink will no longer point to the image.

OBTAIN SPECIFICATION AUTHORING TOOLS

EFS offers of a choice of two authoring tools for preparing submissions in XML format (PASAT and TSA). The primary difference between the two programs is the level of automation available during the authoring process. Both tools produce the required EFS submission files. Tag the specification text using an XML word-processing application. If necessary, attach images to the specification document while authoring the XML document. View the authored XML tagged specification document using a Web browser (e.g., Internet Explorer 5.5 with TIFF viewer plug-in) and the USPTO standard style sheet that is provided as part of the EFS authoring software).

OBTAIN SUBMISSION SOFTWARE

The EFS submission software (ePAVE) uses the Entrust Direct™ Public Key Infra-structure (PKI) architecture to ensure that your transmission is protected against unauthorized viewing.

EFS software must be installed on your local computer drive and not a network drive; however, you may load EFS software on the network for software distribution purposes. For best results, EFS files (XML and TIFF) should be placed on the local drive during authoring and submission. While authoring, these may be backed up on the network (such as the ePAVE submission folder).

The specification document created by the authoring tools, as well as the fee, transmittal, and application data sheet documents created by ePAVE, are formatted in XML. The USPTO uses Internet Explorer (IE) 5.5 in conjunction with style sheets to render the XML in human-readable form. XML rendering is not supported in versions of IE prior to version 5.

Use the ePAVE application to create the submission package, view and print your submission, validate it, and send it to the USPTO. You can file patent applications electronically almost 24 hours a day, 7 days a week. You immediately receive an electronic acknowledgment receipt that includes a USPTO-assigned application serial number and a date. The electronic submission is automatically validated for com-pleteness against the USPTO business rules, reducing the chances of an incomplete application being filed, particularly in the case of pre-grant publications because the data that the applicant submits electronically is the data that the USPTO publishes.

The use of EFS reduces processing costs as well as cycle time and provides accurately tagged data for both publication and search purposes. Electronic Infor-mation Disclosure Statements eliminate the requirement for mailing paper copies of U.S. patents and published applications. Author-tagged patent application transmit-tal, fee transmittal, application data sheet, and assignment cover sheet are done using ePAVE as follows.

- Create a submission package by attaching the tagged specification XML document, the TIFF images containing scanned pages of the oath, decla-ration, or power of attorney using ePAVE. ePAVE will automatically attach the transmittal, fee transmittal, application data sheet, assignment cover sheet, and associated assignment conveyance forms.

- Digitally sign the submission package using ePAVE and your digital certificate.
- Submit the submission package to USPTO via the Internet using ePAVE.
- Receive the electronic acknowledgment receipt that the USPTO sends you upon successful completion of the transmission.

The following limitations apply to the actual file that you submit to the USPTO:

- EFS maximum file size is 10 MB for electronic transmission, one CD for mailed submission.
- New utility assignment maximum number of cover sheets is five.
- Provisional application assignment maximum number of cover sheets is five.
- Subsequent filing assignment maximum number of cover sheets is 15.
- Each assignment cover sheet must have a minimum of one TIFF per cover sheet, but there is no limit on the number of TIFFs that can be referenced except for the ePAVE 10 MB file size restriction.

OBTAIN PTO DIRECT SECURITY™

PTO Direct Security software allows applicants to view the status of their application as it appears on the USPTO server. The use of PTO Direct is not required as it is only used to create a digital certificate allowing the applicant to view their proprietary information. PTO Direct is a USPTO-branded version of the Entrust™ product suite, which is used to protect data from unauthorized disclosure and to ensure patent application security, integrity, and authenticity. Patent business customers who obtain a digital certificate from the USPTO will be provided with PTO Direct to create a digital certificate that is used to access the PAIR system via the Internet and to use ePAVE. The Entrust/Direct certificate is assigned to a practitioner or inventor and is associated with a USPTO-assigned Customer Number for correspondence so access to patent application data is protected.

TECHNICAL ISSUES

SETUP

EFS Software on Multiple Computers

The installation of EFS software components, ePAVE, PASAT, and TSA are subject to terms noted in the individual licenses. In order for ePAVE to upload an electronic submission properly, a user must transfer a digital certificate file. The digital certificate is created using the USPTO Direct Security software after receiving reference information from the USPTO. There is no need to reinstall this software on multiple machines once you have created a profile. Users can simply transfer the digital certificate file to the computer of their choice.

Use of EFS Software on a Network

EFS software components are client applications. ePAVE can be used with network Internet connections and with networked machines. In order to install ePAVE or some of its components, you must have local administrator privileges. If you are unsure if you have these privileges, contact your IT staff. The ePAVE installation program will prompt you if local administrator privileges are required for installation (refer to the ePAVE user manual for more details.)

The most important consideration in effective use of EFS in a network environment is file management. The application files created with the authoring tool (PASAT or TSA) or with ePAVE must reside in network storage that is commonly mapped to all machines working with the application. For example, a network drive where files will be stored should be referred to by the same relative path for all machines that will be working with the application. All EFS files are best stored in a dedicated folder. This allows common access to the files from any PC in the network and allows EFS to locate and attach/bundle all the files constituting the application in assembling the submission. Because EFS software associates an application's files based on path name, their location should not be changed once the files have been stored.

FILE MANAGEMENT

1. File names are limited to 25 characters and must be alphanumeric.
2. The 8.3 file naming convention is recommended.
3. Do not use special characters in your file name, i.e., &, -, [spaceband], #. To enable electronic filing of patent applications that contain special characters or symbols EFS supports the Lucida Sans Unicode font, which covers the most commonly used characters. The EFS authoring tool, PASAT, will translate symbols to the correct Unicode characters. In addition, the filer may create custom characters and save them as TIFF images. These images can be inserted into the application specification document. ePAVE does not accommodate use of special characters during form creation. Use only ASCII text when creating forms in ePAVE.
4. When creating your ePAVE submission folder, its name must differ from the names of any submission files and figures that will be included in the submission.
5. If authoring from a source document, convert the source document text to Arial, CG Times, or Times New Roman. Special characters, such as certain math or chemical symbols, may need to be scanned as TIFF images
6. Create a working or "source" document folder on a local or shared drive to store all files relating to the submission. Save the authored specification to this folder using the file naming convention mentioned earlier. Copy all specification-related image and source files into this folder.

Web Browser

The Web browser enables the filer to connect to the EFS Web site and to file a submission electronically. Internet Explorer 5.5 allows for Internet access, provides faster ways to complete work, supports portable computers and USPTO standard style sheets.*

The USPTO standard style sheets determine how the XML files (specification, transmittal, fee transmittal, and application data sheet) created by the EFS software tools are rendered or displayed in the browser for viewing and printing. For example, the headings of sections in the specification are bolded and paragraphs are double-spaced.

OPERATIONAL ISSUES

Following are the most pertinent and frequently raised points of clarification about the use of EFS; these are arranged in grouping of topics and offer an excellent learning opportunity.

General

- The number of cover sheets per submission and properties per cover sheet is limited based on the submission type. Each of these can have a minimum of one TIFF per cover sheet, but per cover sheet we have no limitation except the ePAVE 10 MB restriction.
  - 5 cover sheets per new utility application and only that property may be referenced in the cover sheet
  - 5 cover sheets per provisional application and only that property may be referenced in the cover sheet
  - 15 cover sheets per submission for subsequently filed assignment submissions; each cover sheet may reference up to 999 properties
- Applications that have been amended during prosecution can be substituted for the originally filed application if they are submitted in compliance with the electronic filing system technical specifications and timely filed. Refer to 37 CFR 1.215(c). *Note:* EFS submission of patent application information to be published is a separate filing from the paper filing of the amendment in the course of prosecution.
- An electronic request for non-publication of a previously filed patent application cannot be made. 37 CFR 1.213 states that requests for non-publication must be made at the time the patent application is filed at the USPTO. You may abandon your application by filing a paper request to

---

* There is a known issue with printing documents in Internet Explorer 5.0. Text or images, which print near the end of a page, are occasionally split horizontally with the lower portion of the text or image printing on the next page. The pages can sometimes be made to print correctly by adjusting the printer margins using the browser's Page Setup. IE 5.5 has better support for page layout and does not split text or images.

avoid publication. *Note:* Any express abandonment must be received more than 4 weeks prior to the projected publication date.

- EFS submissions must be smaller than 10 MB (approximately 2000 type-written pages) in order to be filed via the internet. You can submit a new utility patent application document authored as an EFS submission on CD-ROM or CD-R to the USPTO for larger submissions. Very large files (over 10 MB) are inappropriate for the Electronic Filing System via the Internet. Part 4 of the Legal Framework for Use of the EFS describes in detail the EFS filing scenario for large submissions using compact discs. The process described requires the workstation to be connected to a CD recorder. If you attempt to file a utility patent application or pre-grant publication submission that exceeds the EFS system limit of 10 MB, the system will generate a message and advise you to submit the large application on CD or CD-R. If a specification with drawings or a biosequence listing (or both) attached causes the large application size, submit the EFS application on CD as instructed in the Legal Framework for Use of the EFS. If large tables or computer program listing caused the large application size, you may submit the application according to the requirements of 37 CFR 1.52(e) with the large section on CD and the rest in paper. The filing date of any EFS new utility application sent in on CD will be based on the date the CD is received at the USPTO, if delivered by hand or regular U.S. mail. The date will be indicated in an acknowledgment. If the CD package was sent to the USPTO via Express Mail under 37 CFR 1.10, then the date of deposit with the U.S. Postal Service will be used. Pre-grant publication patent application filings can also be submitted to the USPTO on CD-ROM or CD-R. One page of text is about 3 kb; one image is generally less than 50 kb in CCITT Group 4 compression and is about 960 kb when uncompressed (users should submit files that are compressed). The actual limit in terms of page count and number of images will vary with the amount of formatting of the text and the complexity of the drawings. As an approximation, these are the limits of the system for electronic submission via the Internet.

3000 pages text	0 drawings	9000 k text
2000 pages text	60 drawings	6000 k text, 3000 k figures
1000 pages text	120 drawings	3000 k text, 6000 k figures
100 pages text	170 drawings	300 k text, 8500 k figures

- You may electronically file a patent application that contains a computer listing over 300 lines long. Include the computer program listing file as a text attachment in ePAVE.
- An electronically filed patent application that contains a biosequence listing can be submitted. You may author an XML-tagged patent application specification that contains biosequence listing information and references. In addition, you may attach a text file containing a computer

readable form sequence listing as part of the electronically filed submission package. See 37 CFR 1.52, 1.96, and 1.821–1.825 for the rules and limitations covering these submissions. The biosequence listing is authored using a sequence-listing editor (e.g., PatentIn; Chapter 9) that produces a valid computer readable form sequence listing in compliance with stated format rules.

- You should not file your application in paper and electronically on the same day just to ensure that you will get the filing date. Duplicate filings will result in duplicate applications with different serial numbers. You will also be charged two filing fees.
- To publish an application pending at the USPTO and filed before November 29, 2000, consult 37 CFR 1.221, which provides for such publications. Applicants must file a request for voluntary publication and a copy of the application via EFS, with a processing fee of $130 and a publication fee of $300.
- You need not be an attorney or patent agent to use EFS. Independent inventors may file their own applications. However, such *pro se* inventors must obtain digital certificates and Customer Numbers from the USPTO prior to using the EFS software.
- When a user submits a request for a multiple assignment transfer, multiple cover sheets are completed with either one legal document (if the transfer is documented in one assignment) or multiple legal documents attached in ePAVE.
- You may use ePAVE to author and print an application data sheet that satisfies the requirements of 37 CFR 1.76 for a paper new utility patent application filing. To begin authoring the application data sheet, select the Forms tab on the ePAVE screen, then select Application data in the Available Forms box. Enter text in each data entry field as appropriate to your new utility patent application filing and then view and print the application data sheet you have authored. The USPTO encourages you to consider electronically filing your new utility patent application documents, including the application data sheet.
- Preliminary amendment or other amendments are not being accepted. EFS only accepts new utility patent applications, CRF biosequence listings, pre-grant publication, provisional applications, assignments for previously filed patent applications, and Information Disclosure Statements. *Note:* The USPTO is continuously updating its submission interface; please check with the USPTO at http://www.uspto.gov/ebc/efs/index.html for the current status of allowed submissions online. Substitute specifications cannot be filed by EFS currently.
- For applications involving federal support, the authoring tool used to create the specification document will prompt you for information such as a federal grant number, a federal contract number, and the granting agency so that this information can be properly tagged. *Note:* A patent application that may contain national security-related material or a patent application associated with a patent application under secrecy order must

not be filed electronically. Refer to the applicable MPEP rules related to proper submission of this sensitive technical content (37 CFR 5).

- A continuation of an earlier filed application may be filed using EFS. The specification authoring tools will allow you to reference parent applications. The EFS submission software (ePAVE) will guide you through the process of authoring the parent application information as XML-tagged data. You will enter this information on the screens provided to create a patent application data form. The USPTO will accept regular domestic utility applications (except Continuing Prosecution Applications and Requests for Continuing Examination). Refer to the EFS Legal Framework for more details.
- EFS is used to electronically author and submit publication ready text publication submissions. Pre-grant publications can be submitted using EFS.
- The use of EFS is mandatory for the following publication submissions:
  - Voluntary publication of an application filed before but pending on November 29, 2000, per 37 CFR 1.221
  - Republication of a previously published application per 37 CFR 1.221
  - Publication of the application as it has been amended during prosecution per 37 CFR 1.215(c)
  - Publication of the application in redacted form per 37 CFR 1.217(b)
- The use of EFS is optional for early publication of a new utility application filed on or after November 29, 2000, per 37 CFR 1.219
- If the USPTO publishes your application with errors that were your fault, you may submit a correction request; however, republication requests must be submitted using EFS. There is a $130 processing fee and a $300 publication fee to have a corrected version published. If the errors were created by the USPTO, you must request a corrected publication within 2 months of the publication date. There is no fee when it is the USPTO's fault.

SPECIFICATION AUTHORING

- The authoring tool allows patent applicants to code (tag) the various parts of their application in XML while still operating in the environment of a commercially available word processing program. The USPTO provides two authoring tools as part of EFS: PASAT for Microsoft Word users or TSA for WordPerfect users. Any other related application information will be authored using the EFS submission software (ePAVE). Examples of related application information include fee transmittal, transmittal information, bibliographic application information, and assignment information.
- The difference between the PASAT and TSA authoring tools is the level of automation available during the authoring process. Currently, PASAT for Word offers additional automation capability over the TSA Tool for WordPerfect. However, both tools produce the required EFS submission files.

- The original specification document can be reformatted to comply with the USPTO technical specifications (e.g., XML tagged) after the inventor(s) has read and signed the declaration, as long as the content of the original specification document is not modified in any way. In addition the individual submitting the new utility patent application (e.g., attorney, agent, or inventor) via the electronic filing system must certify that the attached specification and related patent application documents have been viewed using the USPTO style sheet or software, and that this is the document the filer intends for initiation or further prosecution of a patent application noted in the submission. The USPTO does not consider the minor rearranging of the parts of the application as a change in the content of the application (see 37 CFR 1.63(b)(2)). The applicant will be careful to avoid adding any new matter to the application in the process, except headings and other organizational indicia needed to fit the EFS requirements for submission.
- It is preferable to cut and paste a document; opening a file written in a different application does not allow detailed XML tagging and is not a preferred method. The tools for auto-tagging the specifications document may become available as technology progresses, likely through third-party software vendors. *Note:* USPTO has recently awarded contracts to five private vendors to do so.
- If you are working with foreign associates and receive specification on paper, this can be retyped into the authoring tools; if clients are transferring files back and forth with their associates, the EFS can be used, as long as they are using the same path names and file names on both machines if storing files on a network drive. For best results, all EFS files (XML and TIFF) should be placed in one folder on the local (C:) drive during authoring. This entire folder can be sent to other users for viewing or editing.
- The sections of specification that the authoring tools provide for in accordance with MPEP include:
  - Title
  - Copyright Statement
  - Cross Reference to Related Applications
  - Federal Research Statement
  - Compact Disc Appendix
  - Background of the Invention
  - Summary of the Invention
  - Detailed Description of the Drawings
  - Detailed Description of the Invention
  - Program Listing, Claims
  - Abstract of the Disclosure
  - Figures
- Applicants may include other subsections such as Field of the Invention or Examples within Background of Invention, Summary of Invention, and Detailed Description. The section heading presented in the EFS authoring

tools comes from the 37 CFR 1.77. These are just recommendations; the headings of these sections may be changed. To change the heading of a section, just click in the heading (e.g., Background of the Invention) and type over the heading text. You may rename the heading of a section (e.g., change Background of the Invention to Field of the Invention) or add a subsection by inserting the section tag. *Note:* You should keep information in the appropriate section. For example, you should not put detailed description information in the Summary section.

- Before you delete a section from the specification document, note that each application is required to include a Title, a Detailed Description of the Invention, at least one Claim, and an Abstract. These sections cannot be deleted. Other preferred sections may be deleted by deleting the associated section tags and content.

- If you want your application published as amended during prosecution, you should not underline inserted text and bracket deletions in your authored specification. Instead, submit a clean copy (without brackets and underlining) of the specification and claims with the same content as the application currently pending before the USPTO via EFS. Integrate the amendments into your submission. For example, delete and insert text per amendment instructions.

- If you want your application published in redacted form, you should not bracket what is to be deleted in your authored specification. Instead, submit a clean copy (without brackets and underlining) via EFS. You are submitting a publication-ready specification text via EFS. If you bracket deletions, the bracketed information will be published in that form and it will no longer be confidential, as the public will see the text. However, you must submit a bracketed paper copy and a clean copy in paper for inclusion in the paper file wrapper. See 37 CFR 1.217 for more information.

- Type the title inside of the provided brackets; the brackets are provided as placeholders for the title. You should delete the brackets after entering the title.

- It is recommended that you convert the source document to Word or WordPerfect before copying it to the Specification section of TSA.

- TSA allows you to add sections to or delete sections from the specification at any time during the editing process. To add a section to the specification document, select the appropriate section from the Template>Add menu; to delete a section, select the appropriate section from the Template>Delete menu. If you delete a section, the content within the tags will also be deleted. To restore a mistakenly deleted section, immediately press Ctrl+Z or select Undo from the Edit menu. *Note:* Required sections cannot be deleted and will not be listed on the Template>Delete menu.

- To insert a subheading or subsection in TSA (Examples, etc.), position your cursor at the desired insertion point before or after a paragraph element. Click on the Valid Elements box (usually a long blank box on the toolbar) to select Section. This will insert tags for the heading and first paragraph of your subsection and allow you to insert the additional paragraphs you want associated with this subsection. Replace the default text "Heading" with your subheading title. If the authoring tool splits a paragraph in two, you can change them to a single paragraph by copying the text from the "second" paragraph and pasting it into the first, then delete the undesired paragraph tags and text. In PASAT, you can click once on the paragraph label in the left margin which reads, for example, [ ] or [0006], to highlight the paragraph and press delete.

- PASAT allows you to add sections to or delete sections from the specification at any time during the editing process. To edit the specification sections: Select the Edit Sections option from the Tools menu. The Edit Sections dialog box appears. Its layout and functions are identical to those of the Create New Specification dialog box, which you use while creating a new specification. Check or clear the check boxes adjacent to the section names to add or delete the corresponding sections. Click the OK button. If you have requested that one or more sections be deleted from the specification, a confirmation box appears. To confirm the section deletion request, click the OK button. The dialog box closes. The sections are added to or deleted from the specification per your definition. PASAT will adjust the structure by adding or removing the appropriate tags.

- To delete an optional section in PASAT, select Edit Sections from the Tool menu, then clear the unneeded section. The section tags and content will be deleted. To add a subheading or subsection, position your cursor at the desired insertion point. Use the Office Assistant, right click, or click on the Valid Elements box (usually a long blank box on the toolbar) to select Section. This will insert heading tags for your subsection and allow you to insert the paragraphs you want associated with this subsection. Replace the default text with your subheading title.

- Tables may be inserted into the specification document as TIFF images. Also, PASAT provides a capability to create a table within the XML specification document or to insert the table by highlighting the table in a Microsoft Word document and selecting Paste Table from the Edit menu. Using the current EFS software to submit tables more than 50 pages long is not appropriate. At this time only the submission of listings in biotech applications are to be filed as attachments using EFS. According to patent business rules only three items may be submitted on CDs for paper applications (37 CFR 1.52(e)): (1) sequence listings in biotech applications, (2) tables more than 50 pages long, and (3) computer program listings more than 300 lines long.

- EFS currently accommodates only sequence listings in biotech applications. Future releases of EFS software will accommodate filing of large tables and computer program listings more than 300 lines long.

- The PASAT Office Assistant can be turned off by selecting an option on the View menu or by clicking the X in the upper right corner of the Assistant. However, for right-click shortcuts to work you must turn the Office Assistant off in the View menu.

- The.s4w and .s4t files contain your specification document contents and tags in PASAT format. The .err and .log files are used for debugging purposes; the .err file is created upon loading an .s4w specification and upon importing or exporting an XML specification from PASAT whether or not errors exist. The .log file is created during authoring to log certain events, such as misplaced tags. If there are errors that should be corrected, you will be warned upon validating the specification in PASAT. The .s4w, .s4t, .err, and .log files should not be sent to the USPTO.
- If you paste bolded or italicized text into PASAT, the text appears bold. When you view the specification in Internet Explorer, the bold text from PASAT appears italicized because bold and italicized text pasted into PASAT is tagged as <emphasis>. The style sheet for PASAT displays the text in emphasis tags as bold. The style sheet for Internet Explorer displays the text in emphasis text in italics. The USPTO views and prints the specification using the style sheet for Internet Explorer.
- You may get the following error when validating the specification: "Element 'emphasis' not allowed in the current position. Possible missing tag before illegal element." It happens when text that is both bold and italicized is pasted into PASAT; the text is tagged with double <emphasis> tags. This will cause a validation error.
- Mistranslations and formatting changes occur when you copy from a Microsoft Word source document and paste into PASAT. If the user authors a Word document with AutoCorrect (Tools menu), the following formatting goes in.
  - Smart quotes (quotation marks that are curly instead of straight) do not translate at all. Therefore the quotes are lost. Apostrophes are translated to quotes. Thus Bill's becomes Bills. This behavior is a little different between Word 97 and 2000 (in Word 2000, the smart quotes translate).
  - Fractions become one character instead of three ($\frac{1}{2}$ versus 1/2). Single space fractions lose space after the fraction.
  - Double hyphen (--) becomes a single dash (—), which is lost in translations.
- When you paste a special character from a source document, PASAT inserts an <unknown symbol> tag. Although the character is available in the PASAT symbol manager, PASAT does not paste it. Fonts are represented in the computer as numeric codes, usually from 1 to 127. Different fonts may use different codes to represent the same character. Many fonts use codes that are not Unicode compliant. When pasting text, PASAT is not able to translate these codes to character entity references. For best results do not use symbol fonts such as Symbol or Wing Dings in the source document; instead use the Times New Roman, Arial, Lucida Sans Unicode, or Courier fonts when creating the source document or convert the source document by selecting the entire document and changing to one of these fonts.

- When copying text from your source document and pasting it into PASAT, some words may be deleted. Currently, PASAT is unable to translate nonbreaking spaces and smart quotes. In addition, when you copy from a source document to PASAT with a nonbreaking character, the string of text following the character is lost. So the text string created in Word "Carbon[non-breaking space]fibers are strong" is pasted into PASAT as "Carbon are strong." The nonbreaking space should be translated as a space in PASAT. Users are advised to carefully review the content pasted into the XML template to identify any space problem or missing text string. Developers expect to fix the problem in the next release.
- Currently, PASAT is unable to translate en and em dashes. These dashes must be converted to normal dashes before pasting.
- PASAT users have reported difficulty in using the PASAT Managing Claim Dependencies features. Unfortunately at this time there is not an alternative PASAT capability to manage claim dependencies. Steps are being taken to evaluate the current implementation of this editing capability to determine what program fixes may be needed and how the user interface can be simplified to better support management operations for the claim dependencies.

FIGURES, DRAWINGS, CHEMICAL STRUCTURES, AND MATHEMATICAL EQUATIONS

- The same drawing standards apply to EFS submissions as with paper submissions. The new utility patent applications submitted through EFS must have scanned TIFF images of the drawings. These drawings will be printed and drawing standards under 37 CFR 1.84 will be applied. With respect to pre-grant publication submissions, the TIFF images of the figures will be reviewed. The applicant will be notified if the figures are not suitable for publication.
- By cropping your images, you avoid double margins being applied to the images (one margin from the scan and another margin from your Web browser) and cropping eliminates white space between the image and other contents in your specification.
- EFS accepts only specific file formats: TIFF image files; ASCII text file biosequence listings, computer program listings, and large tables; and XML documents.
- TIFF image files must be 300 dpi, black-and-white TIFF images with CCITT Group 4 compression. EFS also accepts uncompressed TIFF images, but this is not recommended. Many graphics programs produce TIFF output; the Windows® Imaging accessory program will produce TIFF files with CCITT Group 4 compression. The image files should be on a local disk drive; ePAVE may have difficulty locating image files on a different drive, especially a network drive. The USPTO is investigating

accepting a wider range of file formats, including ChemDraw® and Mathematica® files in future releases.

- The drawing requirements as set forth in 37 CFR 1.84 for TIFF images will allow the applicant to submit images that will satisfy all the quality requirements under 37 CFR 1.84. The USPTO will print images using the following margins on $8\frac{1}{2} \times 11$ paper: top 1, left 1, right 0.75, bottom 0.75. These margins satisfy 37 CFR 1.84(g). The margins that will be applied to both the specification and the drawings on $8\frac{1}{2} \times 11$ paper are the same as described here. You may set up your Web browser for these margins by choosing the Page Setup option from the File menu so that your printed copy of the specification and drawing will have the same margins as the USPTO copy.

- If your invention can only be illustrated using micrographs, they must be converted to black-and-white TIFF files. In addition, you must submit three copies of the photographs and the appropriate petition and fees, via mail, according to the current standard U.S. practice.

- The reason you must use TIFF images is that the patent applications must be archivable. For this reason, only nonproprietary and stable formats may be used for electronic PATENT files. TIFF is both nonproprietary and retains integrity when compressed (for transmission and storage) or archived. This format is also viewable in a wide variety of software packages. As noted in a third party vendor's online sales documentation "TIFF is compatible with a wide range of scanners and image-processing applications. It is device independent and is used in most operating environments, including Windows, Macintosh, and UNIX. Most scanner manufacturers and desktop publishing applications have implemented this nonproprietary industry standard for data communication." Another reason for use of the TIFF file format is that use of proprietary file formats in the development of products requires obtaining licenses for the technology. An example of such technology is LZW compression technology used in GIF images that requires a license from Unisys. JPEG files may cause a loss of data when compressed or archived. Some compression algorithms simplify images to compress them, which results in an image that has lost some data.

- Color images or different image file types (JPEG, GIF, etc.) are not acceptable. EFS only accepts images in black-and-white TIFF format. In the future, EFS technical standards will be updated as needed to accommodate filing color images and use of other standard file formats. Two issues that limit the file types that are accepted are proprietary file types and loss of data during compression. The native output of some programs is not readable without the program itself. Some compression algorithms (such as JPEG) simplify images to compress them, which results in an image that has lost some data.

- In PASAT, the Figure Manager assists you with adding, removing, and moving figures. A thumbnail of each figure appears as the figure is added. Clicking on the thumbnail will show the file name at the top of the Figure

Manager window. To add another figure, select the figure that you would like your next figure to follow. Select the Add Below button and attach the new figure file. To delete a figure attached twice, use the Figure Manager, click on the thumbnail of the second occurrence, and then click the Remove button. In TSA, use the XML Tree. Double-click the Figure tag of the second occurrence, and press the Delete key. You must also remove the image reference from the Insert/File References list. See the authoring tool user manuals for detailed instructions.

- The TIFF files should ideally reside on a local drive rather than a network. For best results, TIFF files should be placed on your local drive during authoring and submission, in the same folder as your XML specification. While authoring, you may wish to keep a backup copy on your network. When submission is completed, we recommend copying the ePAVE Submission Folder, which includes all your submission files, to your network for archival purposes.

- AutoCAD® may be used to prepare drawings; save these drawings as TIFF images with Group 4 compression. TIFF images have a file extension of .tif. You may use any software package capable of producing 300 dpi, black-and-white Group 4 TIFF images. Imaging for Windows can be used to save TIFF images. Other software packages you may use are Microsoft Visio®, AutoCAD, CorelDraw®, Adobe Photoshop®, and Adobe Illustrator®.

- Tables may be inserted into the specification document as TIFF images. Also, PASAT provides a capability to create a table within the XML specification document or to insert the table by highlighting the table in a Microsoft Word document and selecting Paste Table from the Edit menu.

- Complex work units such as chemical formulas, mathematical equations, and some tables should be saved as TIFF images and inserted into the submission document. The EFS ePAVE software will bundle these files with the specification for submission to the USPTO. ChemDraw® Ultra 6.0 and Pro 6.0 allow you to save your structures in TIFF format. The TIFF image files created from ChemDraw are suitable for submission via EFS.

- The number of figures submitted by EFS is limited by memory size. A TIFF image in Group 4 compression takes from about 3 to 300 kb, depending on the level of detail in the figure. The number of drawings that you can submit will depend on the length of your specification text and the electronic size of your TIFF files.

- EFS requires one figure per image. The specification will be authored using an XML authoring capability. The image file for each drawing/figure will be tagged within the specification document.

- If your application contains many superscripts and subscripts, the following applies regarding their tagging: If you type your application directly into the templates or paste text into TSA, then each superscript and subscript must be tagged in the same manner that these characters were formatted in the word processing environment. If you have a previously prepared document, when you copy text from that document into PASAT, it will recognize the special formatting and insert the appropriate tags.

- If your application contains many special characters such as Greek letters, you may insert these by typing directly into PASAT, and using the Insert/Symbol menu item to insert identified special characters. If you are copying and pasting from a previously prepared document, PASAT will attempt to recognize the special character and paste it into the template. If PASAT does not recognize the character, it will be replaced with an unknown symbol tag in large red text. PASAT will prompt you to replace these occurrences. If you are typing into TSA, use the Insert/Text References... menu item to insert the special characters. If you are copying and pasting from a previously prepared document, TSA will attempt to recognize the special character and convert it to the Unicode character equivalent. If TSA does not recognize the character, a warning message will appear upon validating the document. The EFS approach to special characters is to use character entity references (codes), which will display and print correctly in the authoring tools and the browser. Details about special characters can be found in the EFS authoring manuals. The EFS supports the Lucida Sans Unicode font, which covers most commonly used characters.

ADDITIONAL APPLICATION DATA

- You do not have to submit a declaration with an EFS filing. A declaration is not mandatory for electronic filing of a new utility patent application as based on current filing rules. However, it is required to complete the application. The application will not be forwarded for examination until the executed declaration is received by the USPTO.
- The Oath or Declaration is submitted scanned with each page saved as a single TIFF file. ePAVE will prompt you to attach the Declaration to the patent application submission package during the submission process. Each page of the Declaration is scanned as a single TIFF file. Affidavits must be filed on paper.
- The priority information associated with your application submission is done by placing the information in the appropriate tab in ePAVE (continuity data or foreign priority). The domestic priority data should be placed in the Cross Reference to Related Applications section of your specification document. Refer to the EFS user manual for specific details.
- The assignment recordation associated with your new patent application submission is authored in ePAVE, which will author tagged assignment recordation information.
- To author any additional instructions or comments about the condition of the electronic new utility patent application or pre-grant publication submission, ePAVE provides a Comments data entry screen. The information entered on this screen will appear on the transmittal forwarded to the USPTO along with the attached documents and other forms completed

using ePAVE. The transmittal can be viewed and printed by both the applicant and the USPTO using the standard style sheet. For instance, in the Comments section you can enter a general description of the changes made in the corrected publication text. These comments will facilitate viewing of the published patent application. For example, you can include correction information: Correction of US 00/000000 A2 Mar 1 2001; see Claim 7; see Drawing Figures 3 and 4; see paragraphs 27, 42, 98, and 103.

- A small entity statement is an optional submission for a new utility patent application. Submission of a small entity statement is not necessary for a pre-grant publication filing. However, you may create a TIFF image of your small entity document and attach it as directed in ePAVE.

VIEW/PRINT

- The EFS software provides viewing and printing capabilities for each application document submission. Highlight the submission document and select View from the ePAVE Attachment tab to view the documents created by ePAVE. The USPTO standard style sheets provide the format in which the attorney or administrative staff will view and print the documents. Because the style sheet is usable in an Internet browser, the specification document can be viewed on a desktop with access to Internet Explorer 5.5. In ePAVE the applicant and attorney also may view the other submission components (transmittal, fee transmittal, and application data sheet) before sending the package by choosing the View button on the Attachments tab in ePAVE.

- To view the specification without installing EFS, you must have Internet Explorer 5 or 5.5 and a TIFF plug-in on the computer. Next, move the following files from the creator's PC to the viewer's hard drive (place all files in the same folder): specification (XML file); u-specif.dtd (validation rules document); specif.xsl (style sheet); and all TIFF files. On the viewer's computer, use My Computer or Explorer to locate and double-click on the XML specification file. The browser will launch, apply the style sheet, and display the specification. Any subsequent editing must be done in the EFS authoring tool. For best results, all EFS files (XML and TIFF) should be placed in one folder on the local (C:) drive during authoring. This entire folder can be sent to other users for viewing or editing. The built-in TIFF editor in PASAT can be used to view the USPTO patent database images. However, AlternaTIFF v.1.3.5, the freeware recommended for use with Internet Explorer 5.5 can be used to view the USPTO patent database images.

- Style sheets of the USPTO determine how the authored XML files (specification, transmittal, fee transmittal and application data sheet) created by ePAVE, PASAT, and TSA are rendered in the browser for viewing and printing the content of the submission. For example, the headings of the recommended sections in the specification are bolded, and the paragraphs of the specification are double-spaced. The style sheet formats the XML tagged information. To render your submission for viewing and printing as it is received at the USPTO, you must use the USPTO standard style sheets. The USPTO uses these style sheets to print out the legal record of your new submission including the specification, transmittal, fee transmittal, application data sheet, assignment recordation, and biosequence transmittal.

- To print out the transmittal, fee sheet, or the application data sheet, ePAVE allows the user to render these sheets in an Internet browser for viewing and printing. To view the fee sheet, application data sheet or specification, select the Attachments tab, select the attachment you wish to print, and click the View button. To view the transmittal, click the Print button, which opens up the file that you are working on in Internet Explorer 5.5 with the USPTO standard style sheet; from there you can print that file. For more information, refer to the EFS user manual.
- If you cannot view your TIFF images in the authoring tool but can view them after selecting the View option on the ePAVE Attachments tab, verify that the files are located on your local drive, not a network drive. Next, check the settings of each TIFF image (300 dpi, black-and-white Group 4 compression). If any of these requirements are not met, make the correction, delete and reattach the image(s) in the authoring tool, then remove and reattach the XML specification on the ePAVE Attachments tab.
- The ability to view and print XML documents depends on your Web browser's capability. Currently, Netscape does not support use of XML with XSL style sheets, therefore you cannot use Netscape to preview or view your specification.

TRANSMITTING TO THE USPTO

- An electronic signature can be whatever you designate; it can be as simple as /s/ or a typed name.
- If you get an error (e.g., missing signature) on the Validation tab before you proceed to the Submit tab, you must enter an electronic signature prior to submission of the patent application electronic package. The signature identifies you as the electronic filer. The electronic signature you enter will be viewed and printed at the USPTO as part of the electronic filing process.
- The red and white Xs beside the TIFF files listed on the ePAVE Attachments tab are there to verify that your TIFF images are located on your local drive, not a network drive. ePAVE may not be able to locate files on a network drive. Next, check the settings of each TIFF image; if any of these requirements are not met, make the correction, delete and reattach the image(s) in the authoring tool, then remove and reattach the XML specification on the ePAVE Attachments tab.
- Compressing your files ensures that they do not exceed the acceptable 10 MB limit.

- Do not file a paper copy of your patent application after filing your new utility patent application electronically. As noted in the Legal Framework, the official copies of all application documents filed via EFS are the paper versions printed from the electronic files received by the USPTO. If the print version of any document is unreadable and cannot be recovered from the USPTO stored EFS files, you will be notified promptly. In this unlikely scenario, you would present (1) the acknowledgment receipt, (2) a paper version and an electronic version (on floppy disk or CD-R) of the files as submitted, and (3) a petition indicating that the files are the same as those mentioned in the acknowledgment receipt for that application number.
- The USPTO will accept electronic filings from 6 a.m. Sunday to 11 p.m. Saturday (Eastern Time), 52 weeks per year. For the purpose of determining the filing date of a new utility patent application, the receipt date for new utility patent application filings on Saturdays, Sundays, and holidays is handled in the same manner as Express Mail submissions to the Post Office. The Office of Initial Patent Examination will execute the formalities review and send out the official filing receipt. Notices about any planned EFS server outages (e.g., for maintenance) will be given in advance on the EFS Web site.
- The USPTO establishes the date of receipt on the day that the application is completely and successfully received at the USPTO, as shown on the acknowledgment receipt. The date at the USPTO is used for the purpose of the date-of-filing original patent applications. If an application is received on Saturdays, Sundays, or holidays, the USPTO will apply that date to the submission, similar to the Express Mail practice of 37 CFR 1.10. The filing date of any EFS new utility application sent in on CD will be based on the date the CD package is received at the USPTO, if delivered by hand or regular U.S. mail. The delivery date will be indicated in an acknowledgment. If the CD package was sent to the USPTO by Express Mail under 37 CFR Section 1.10, then the date stamped by the U.S. Postal Service will be used. Part 3 of the Legal Framework describes in detail the EFS filing scenario for large submissions using compact discs. The process described requires the workstation to be connected to a compact disc recorder.
- The acknowledgments and notifications to the applicant indicated above in this EFS process do not constitute the granting of an official filing date for the application. That official date will be noted on the paper filing receipt (37 CFR 1.54), PTO Form-103X, which is sent after printing the application, and reviewing the submitted application parts for compliance with 35 USC 111 filing date requirements. However, the acknowledgment receipt establishes the date of successful submission of the associated documents, and is thus a crucial part of the application process.
- If the printed version of any document received by the USPTO is unreadable, and if it cannot be recovered from the stored files received by electronic submission, then the applicant will be promptly notified by phone, fax, or e-mail as indicated in the EFS instruction. Even with prompt

processing, if EFS receipts are high the review may take place a few days or a week later. If an error occurs and the application cannot be reconstructed, the applicant may have to resubmit the application and petition for the original filing date. Such events are expected to be rare. Under this scenario, the applicant would present (1) the acknowledgment receipt, (2) a paper version and an electronic version (on floppy disk or CD-R) of the files as submitted, and (3) a petition verifying that the attached files are exactly the same as mentioned in the acknowledgment receipt for that application number. The acknowledgment receipt will establish that the resubmitted documents were exactly those submitted on the date of receipt. However, the acknowledgment receipt is of no value if an applicant submits the wrong data files under EFS, just as a postcard receipt has no value if an applicant submits a wrong application in paper filings. Applicants are responsible for ensuring that a filing contains the correct application files.

- The application's date of receipt is the date that it is fully and successfully received at the USPTO, as shown on the acknowledgment receipt. The date at the USPTO is controlling for the purposes of original patent applications. There is no certificate of transmission practice for new application or provisional application e-filings (37 CFR 1.8).

- Hours of operation will be clearly expressed in the EFS instructions. If a transmission is attempted during a down time, the Office cannot accept it and will, if possible, respond with a notice that the Office is closed. No acknowledgment receipt will be sent. The "closed" notice will advise the applicant to use alternative filing methods, such as hand delivery of paper to the USPTO or Express Mail (under 37 CFR 1.10), to establish the filing date. Note that new applications filed under 37 CFR 1.53 cannot be submitted by fax (37 CFR 1.6(d)(3)), and that normal certificate of mailing procedures do not apply to new applications (37 CFR 1.8(a)(2)(i)(A) and (D)). Applicants are strongly advised to transmit their electronic filings sufficiently early in the day to allow time for alternative paper filing when transmission cannot be initiated or correctly completed.

- If an application is successfully received on a Saturday, a Sunday, or a federal holiday within the District of Columbia, the Office will assign that receipt date at the USPTO to the submission. The USPTO will be open for receiving applications in electronic form during scheduled hours every day of the week. Electronic filing with EFS will provide applicants with the opportunity to receive a filing date on any day of the week, including Saturdays, Sundays, and federal holidays within the District of Columbia. In addition, consistent with 35 USC 21(b), when the last day for taking any action or paying any fee in the USPTO falls on a Saturday, a Sunday, or a federal holiday within the District of Columbia, the action may be taken or fee paid on the next business day. Thus, under U.S. law, applicants will still be permitted to take action on the next business day when the last day for taking action falls on a weekend or federal holiday, regardless of the mode or form of filing.

- Because the conditions for priority rights are governed by the national law in the country of filing, applicants are cautioned to consider possible adverse consequences regarding the determination of priority periods under Article 4(c)(3) of the Paris Convention when filing international applications in the U.S. Specifically, the ability to file applications electronically on weekends may result in loss of priority rights in foreign jurisdictions designated in international applications filed with the USPTO, if applicants elect to take advantage of sections 21(b) or 119(e)(3) of Title 35. In such circumstances, other patent offices may deny the priority claim on the basis that the international application was not timely filed according to their national law. For this reason, applicants may prefer not to rely upon the "next business day" provisions of sections 21(b) and 119(e)(3) of Title 35 when filing applications with the USPTO, and instead file the application before the Convention year has expired.
- The length of time it takes to transmit your EFS submission depends on the speed of your modem speed or Internet connection, server usage, and the size of your submission. Note that ePAVE will compress your submission, reducing the size of the original files.
- If you cannot log on and file your submission and it is a mandatory e-file submission, then know that submissions of more than 10 MB can be submitted on CD-R. If your submission is smaller than 10 MB, you should resubmit your electronic submission at a later time and check the USPTO Electronic Business Center Web site for notices about system status. Part 3 of the Legal Framework for Use of the Electronic Filing System describes in detail the EFS filing scenario for large submissions using compact discs. The process described requires the workstation to be connected to a compact disc recorder.
- Your EFS application is processed once the submission is successfully received at the USPTO. An acknowledgment receipt is then transmitted to the filer. The receipt contains information describing the transmission. It includes an application serial number, the names and sizes of all electronic files received, and the time and date of receipt by the USPTO. Once the electronic filing submission is received at the USPTO, the files are printed on paper. The receipt of the electronically filed papers are entered into the pre-exam system. After formalities review processing, the official paper filing receipt is mailed to the applicant or attorney of record. Because the EFS application is associated with a Customer Number, the applicant or attorney can use the digital certificate and Customer Number to access the PAIR system to view the status of the electronically processed application. The status of the EFS filed application becomes available via PAIR upon the completion of data entry into the pre-exam system.
- You may not request a specific publication date in the EFS submission. Requests for a specific publication date are treated as a request to publish as soon as possible (see 37 CFR 1.219).
- Your electronic patent application documents should be viewed using the appropriate USPTO standard style sheet prior to submission. Both EFS

XML authoring software programs provide a view capability for the patent application specification using the USPTO standard specification style sheet. The EFS submission software also provides a view capability for patent application documents on the Attachments tab. The USPTO uses the same standard style sheets to view and print electronically filed patent application submission documents.

- The package sent to the USPTO is stored in a .zip file, which contains a copy of all XML, TIFF, ASCII text, style sheets, and DTD files that were submitted. This bundle can be unzipped and viewed. If the files are unzipped, they should be stored with the acknowledgment receipt so you can identify what was submitted.

- The USPTO will print a confirmation number on your official filing receipt starting with the implementation of pre-grant publication. The confirmation number is an additional four-digit identifier assigned to your application. It can be found in the upper left-hand corner of the official filing receipt. If your application is associated with a Customer Number, you may obtain the confirmation number in the PAIR system. When you file a pre-grant publication or an electronic information disclosure statement (eIDS) submission using EFS, you will need to enter both the application serial number that is associated with the submission as well as the confirmation number. Upon transmission of the submission, EFS will verify that the application serial number with the associated confirmation number is in a valid status for the submission.

- The use of a Certificate of Transmittal does not apply when filing an application submission electronically. The Certificate of Transmittal is the Internet equivalent to the existing Certificate of Mailing and Certificate of Facsimile practice (see 37 CFR 1.8; MPEP 502, 502.01), and it is designed to accord Internet filed submissions the same significance as submissions filed by facsimile. This certificate can only be used for subsequent filings. The certificate does not apply to new utility patent filings. EFS submission software will allow use of the Certificate of Transmittal when you elect to electronically submit either a CRF biosequence listing or certain pre-grant publication submissions. The use of the Certificate of Transmittal applies to "as-amended," previously published publications or early publication EFS pre-grant publication submission types. As with all certificate practice, the local date at the place of submission as indicated on the Certificate of Electronic Transmission will be considered for the purpose of determining if the documents were submitted in a timely manner. This practice does not apply to redacted publication application submissions because that type of subsequent submission must be received by the USPTO at a specified date.

RECEIPT OF FILING

- Knowing what happens after you click the Send button will help you to know if your application has been received completely. The application files (e.g., X, Y, and Z) that you can print out and view on your computer are sent to the USPTO (wrapped, encrypted, and digitally signed). When the USPTO receives them, they are unwrapped, decrypted, and stored. If the files are successfully received, an acknowledgment receipt containing the name and size (in bytes) of every file is sent within seconds. This information about the files is the same information that you can view on your computer. You can view the byte size of a file by right-clicking the file name in the Windows File Manager and selecting Properties from the pop-up menu. If the acknowledgment receipt lists X, Y, and Z with the same size as on your computer, you know the USPTO received the files intact. The USPTO also includes a security software produced message digest code on the acknowledgment receipt, which indicates that the files were received by the USPTO in the original condition. If a question arises as to when the documents were submitted, the acknowledgment receipt and message digest will be considered strong evidence of what you submitted. Simply print out the files listed in the acknowledgment receipt. Submit these printouts, an electronic version of the files, and the acknowledgment receipt in a petition to the USPTO. In addition, ePAVE creates a .zip file in your submission folder, which contains all of the electronic files you sent to the USPTO. You should save this .zip file as evidence of your submission along with the electronic copy of the acknowledgment receipt (.rsp file). The .rsp file is automatically saved in your submission folder.

- Once the electronic file is received by the USPTO, new utility and provisional applications are printed to paper for standard processing. Pregrant publication submissions are stored and tracked electronically for timely forwarding to the USPTO publication database contractor. If an assignment is submitted, the assignment and attachments will be processed electronically into the Office of Public Records workflow system (Patent and Trademark Assignment System). The eIDS submissions are printed to paper and a search string is created so that examiners can review the references electronically.

- Upon completion of submission, a filing date will be displayed. The time and date are assigned after the EFS server receives all the contents of the submission. The EFS acknowledgment receipt will be sent immediately to the applicant's computer with the date/time, a message of successful transmission, and other pertinent information. Part 3 of the Legal Framework for Use of the Electronic Filing System describes in detail the EFS filing scenario for large submissions using compact discs. The process described requires the workstation to be connected to a compact disc recorder.

- The USPTO establishes the date of receipt on the day that the application is completely and successfully received, as shown on the acknowledgment receipt. The date at the USPTO is used for the purpose of the date-of-filing original patent applications. If an application is received on a Saturday, a Sunday or a holiday, the USPTO will apply that date to the submission, similar to the Express Mail practice of 37 CFR 1.10. The filing date of any EFS new utility application sent in by CD will be based on the date the CD package is received at USPTO, if delivered by hand or regular U.S. mail. That date will be indicated in an acknowledgment. If the CD package was sent to the USPTO by Express Mail under 37 CFR Section 1.10, then the date of deposit with the U.S. Postal Service will be used. Part 3 of the Legal Framework for Use of the Electronic Filing System describes in detail the EFS filing scenario for large submissions using compact discs. The process described requires the workstation to be connected to a compact disc recorder.

- The USPTO retains electronic files as long as there is a legal or business reason for use of the patent application information.
- You need not submit a paper copy of the same biosequence listing electronically filed to the USPTO.

FEES/PAYMENT

- Payment methods for EFS include deposit account and bank (credit) card payments; however, payment of filing fee is not necessary, as in paper application, to get a filing date; however, until the fee is paid, the applications remains incomplete.
- If you are paying the fee for a new utility patent application submission, you should not include the fee transmittal form with the submission package. If you have mistakenly saved the fee XML transmittal document (which attaches the file to the submission package), you should go to the Attachments tab of ePAVE, click on the XML file labeled "fee-transmittal," then click the Remove button.
- If you request early publication for a new application (or for a voluntary, redacted, or amended submission), you must pay the $300 publication fee when you make the request. If you do not request early publication, the $300 publication fee will be due when the issue fee is due.
- You must pay a publication fee for the publication of patent applications that are published early upon request, for voluntary publication of applications which are pending on November 29, 2000, and republication of previously published applications. For all other utility application publications, the publication fee is paid with the issue fee. Unless a request for nonpublication is made at filing, a publication fee of $300 is required for each application that the USPTO publishes.
- A processing fee is required when an applicant requests voluntary publication of an application pending on November 29, 2000, and when applicant requests republication of an application that has been previously published.
- You need not pay the assignment fee when filing a new application with an assignment recordation form along with assignment documents; however, nonpayment will result in a notice of nonrecordation of the submitted assignment.

- ePAVE will validate the payment information you enter on the screen to ensure that all required fee information is present prior to sending your electronic application submission package to the USPTO. If a credit card problem is identified, USPTO will notify you about the problem using the correspondence information you provide as part of the application submission.
- Include statements that pre-grant publication submissions do not contain any "new matter" in the Comments screen of the ePAVE software program. The comment then will appear on the transmittal document.

TROUBLESHOOTING/ERRORS

- Notices are posted on the Electronic Business Center (EBC) and EFS Web sites explaining any scheduled system outages. The electronic filer should also receive error messages when the system is not responding. If your new application filing is time sensitive and EFS is not available, file your new utility application in paper. Otherwise, try to file electronically at a later time. Contact the EBC Customer Support Center at 703.305.3028 or 866.217.9197 (toll-free) to find out when system operations will be restored.
- If the Print Preview screen in IE 5.5 gives you a printout with one word in the specification document not visible (a rare problem), adjust the margin settings in your browser by choosing the Page Setup option from the File menu bar, then decreasing the values for the left and right margins. Go back to the Print Preview window and determine if the new margin values resolved the problem. The source of the problem may be the combination of different browser versions, with printer types, margin settings, and font versions and sizes.
- Double-clicking on error lines on the Validation tab brings up details on the error messages. The "bibd-transmittal" error is to be corrected in the Application Data form. The application data sheet is where bibliographic information is captured.
- If you enter partial fee information on the screen, a validation error related to fee transmittal appears. To avoid this error, fill in all other text fields for Deposit Account or click on the Credit Card button. Then click the Deposit Account button to clear the default date from the Date Signed field. The signing date for the deposit account is filled with current date by default, to encourage the user to complete other data in the deposit account block. If no other data is entered, a parsing error occurs.
- A credit card expiration date error appears even though you leave the credit card number blank because the ePAVE validation program detected that a default date in the credit card expiration date was entered. The error message appears to indicate that some fee payment information is missing even though the expiration date is not necessarily the specific fee information missing. When a validation error occurs, return to the Forms tab.

Reopen the fee form and complete payment information or override the error and submit for new utility filings.

- The * 1234 * notation on your application data sheet form and fee transmittal facilitates correct database entry of the Customer Number and deposit account number. Once your application is printed at the USPTO, this notation appears on the fee and application data sheet as a bar code, which can be scanned by the USPTO's Office of Initial Patent Examination.

- The specification documents or any XML forms authored using ePAVE contain the following words in the header notation Electronic Version #.#.# and Stylesheet Version #.#, which are a version control naming convention that USPTO is implementing with the use of the Electronic Filing System. The USPTO will know what version of the technical standard and USPTO standard style sheet was used to create the electronically filed patent application document.

- There is an inconsistency in the way the cursor tabs through text fields on different screens in ePAVE; this inconsistency will be corrected in a future release.

- To enter the First Named Inventor (first and last names) when authoring an electronic submission transmittal document, enter the first and last name of the first-named inventor on the ePAVE Application Data form Inventor Tab screen. The first name displayed on the Inventor Tab screen will be the name that appears on the transmittal document. You only need to enter the First Named Inventor once.

- To select the U.S. as the country associated with your residence or an application document, use the ePAVE screens that have a country text field which provides a list box for you to select the appropriate country. United States is the default entry for some country text fields. If you type in the first few letters of the country name, the program takes you to a position in the list near the selected country name.

- If you downloaded TSA from the EFS Web site but could not find the template after it was unzipped, you will find it using the following path: C:\Program Files\USPTO\WordPerfect Authoring Tool.

- A Visual Basic runtime error "Invalid Entity Name" occurs and PASAT becomes inoperative when an unknown symbol was identified in your specification text and you clicked Yes in the Symbol Manager dialog box to insert the missing symbol and you highlighted the TIFF image thumbnail, located on the Custom Character tab. To avoid this error when prompted by PASAT to use the Symbol Manager, after PASAT displays the Unknown Symbol tag click the No button. Next place the cursor either directly in front of the Unknown Symbol tag or directly after it, and select the Symbol option from the Insert menu. The custom character selected will be successfully inserted into the specification text using the workaround. After successfully inserting the symbol, you should then highlight the Unknown Symbol tag and delete it.

6 USPTO EFS Scenarios

INTRODUCTION

A full understanding of how the Electronic Filing System (EFS) of the U.S. Patent and Trademark Office (USPTO) works requires familiarization with its terminology, the process of patent application publication, and the submission process, which can vary with the type of application filed. This chapter reviews the common elements of different applications, as well as their peculiarities.

TERMINOLOGY

A new application is one that is being originally filed electronically. These applications are subject to the pre-grant publication rules, and they contain some information that dictates how they will be published (i.e., early, at 18 months, or not at all). These applications are assigned a filing date and an application number, then entered into the normal flow of examination, and published according to the same rules as new paper filings.

A pre-grant submission is a copy (possibly amended or redacted) of a specification already filed at the USPTO, together with some information that dictates how it will be published. These submissions are published but not entered into the examination process; they already have a filing date, an application number, and a confirmation number. The amendments or modifications that appear in these submissions are not automatically made in the corresponding application file at the USPTO; they must be made according to conventional procedure.

PATENT APPLICATION PUBLICATION PROCESS AND EFS SUBMISSIONS

As required by the American Inventors Protection Act and the 1999 amendments to 35 USC 122(b), the USPTO began publishing applications filed on or after November, 29, 2000, at 18 months after their earliest claimed priority date. As each paper application is filed, it is electronically scanned and assigned a projected publication date. If the applicant requests nonpublication at the time of filing and makes the appropriate certification, then no publication date is assigned.

The application enters the publication queue14 weeks prior to the publication date. If the applicant requests early publication and pays the publication fee, the application immediately enters the 14-week publication queue. The publication queue includes the following EFS submissions:

- New utility applications filed via EFS after November 29, 2000, are added in the same manner as new applications filed in paper.

- Original redacted and amended submissions filed before the original application enters the 14-week publication cycle are used to replace the data captured at the time of filing; their publication dates are not changed unless applicant requests early publication when making the EFS submission.
- Republication amended and corrected publications enter the publication cycle immediately.
- Voluntary publications of applications pending on November 29, 2000, which would otherwise not be published until they were patented, enter the publication cycle immediately.

Once each week, application management software creates a list of cases to be published 14 weeks later. This list includes applications due for publication on their 18-month date and immediate publication requests. This schedule is synchronized with the time frame used for printing issued patents; it is important to applicants submitting amended or redacted applications for publication, for the following reasons:

- If the amended or redacted submission is made before the application enters the publication queue, the newly submitted data will replace the initially filed data. The publication fee is due at the same time as the issue fee (provided no request for early publication was filed).
- If the submission is made after the initial data is already in the publication queue, the new submission will be added to the next-available publication cycle as a republication. The fees in this instance are $130 for processing and $300 for publication in addition to the $300 publication fee associated with the earlier publication.

The USPTO delivers the data to a printing contractor using the following schedule:

- **14 weeks prior to publication:** Applications due for publication at 18 months enter the publication queue along with requests for immediate publication. This is the applicant's last chance to submit an amended or redacted copy before first publication.
- **12 weeks prior to publication:** Data gathered and validated at the USPTO.
- **64 weeks** from **earliest filing:** Applicant's last chance to submit a redacted copy to replace the originally filed copy.
- **4 weeks prior to publication:** Applicant's last chance to abandon application and avoid publication. Please do not wait this long. This date represents the last opportunity for the USPTO to remove the application from the publication queue. Applicant may submit a letter of abandonment after this point; however, there is no guarantee that the USPTO will be able to pull the application from the publication queue.

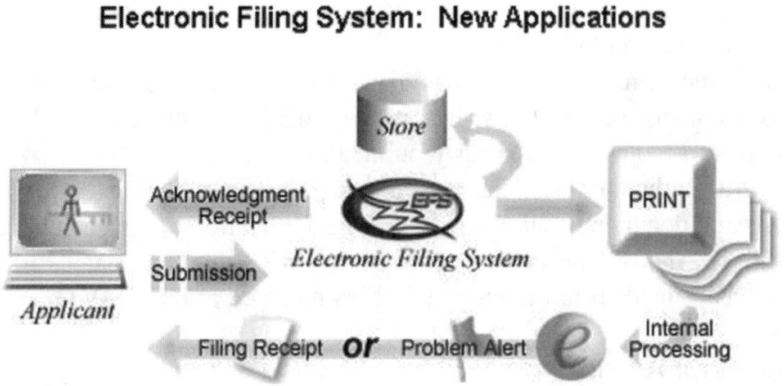

Electronic Filing System: New Applications

FIGURE 6.1 Electronic Filing System: New Applications

NEW UTILITY APPLICATION (FIGURE 6.1)

THE APPLICANT

1. Qualifies for PKI (public key infrastructure) security key pairs and receives a digital certificate from the USPTO.
2. Receives authoring and submission software from the USPTO.
3. Authors application specification following USPTO technical guidelines and template to produce structured document and compliant image files.
4. Uses submission software supplied by the USPTO to validate and transmit application via the Internet.

THE USPTO

1. Receives electronic submission in EFS, unwraps and decrypts files.
2. Stores files in secure repository under Electronic Records Management control.
3. Checks file attributes for file integrity and successful transmission; alerts applicant if a problem is encountered.
4. Sends an electronic acknowledgment receipt to applicant with date, file names and sizes, and a message digest.
5. Prints documents to paper and reviews pages to determine readability.
6. Paper files become the official submission and enter the normal workflow. They are inserted into the file wrapper. The paper copy is used for publication of the patent application.
7. In due course, a filing receipt is issued when all the necessary elements are received.
8. If a problem occurs with the printed application, the USPTO first checks the electronic version in EFS. If a new copy is needed, the applicant will be able to resubmit files upon presentation of the acknowledgment receipt.

Rule bases: 35 USC 111–113, 122; applicable 37 CFR sections, including 1.76 "Application Data Sheet"

When: Same as for paper filings under applicable individual sections.

Fee: Same as for paper filings; fees may be paid by bank card (credit card) or deposit account. Fee for early publication is $300.

Comment: Voluntary use. See previous section in this chapter for types of applications and documents permitted. For large application files, use compact discs (37 CFR 1.52). The official copies of all documents submitted using EFS are the paper versions printed from the electronic files received at the USPTO.

PREPARATION FOR AUTHORING

The description here is specific to filing a utility application but the method is common to all other applications and other document filing except where differences are noted.

Prior to using the EFS software, assemble the patent application information. Obtain a TIFF image of each drawing figure, including complex chemical formulae or mathematical equations, that will be included in the text of your specification. Obtain a scanned image of the declaration with the signature(s) of the inventor(s). A scanned image of a small entity statement may be included even though these statements are no longer required.

Application-related information such as fee information, small entity status, type of publication, nonpublication request, and information equivalent to that on a typical transmittal letter will be created using ePAVE (see Chapter 10). Image files (equivalent to these patent application papers) are not required because these forms are created using ePAVE.

The text of the application specification may be typed directly into either the EFS specification authoring tool, or it may be copied and pasted from a source document. If an electronic copy of a source document exists, it should be accessible.

SPECIFICATION

Specific use of the Patent Application Specification Authoring Tool (PASAT) and the Template for Specification Authoring (TSA) is described in Chapters 7 and 8. Using either authoring tool you will create an electronic copy of the specification as required by 35 USC 112 and 113, including the claims and associated drawing figures. The output of this authoring process will be a structured electronic document with links to the image files containing figures, chemical formulae, or mathematical equations.

VIEWING

When the specification is formatted, it can be viewed using the USPTO standard style sheet in Internet Explorer (5.0 or higher). During the submission process you must certify that the documents you intend to submit have been reviewed. You will be able to view and print the specification, including drawings, declaration, and forms (e.g., fee transmittal, application transmittal) created using ePAVE.

SUBMISSION FOLDER

ePAVE, the EFS submission application, allows you to create a submission folder that will contain all the electronic files to be sent to the USPTO as part of the electronic filing. For a new utility patent application filing, the authored XML-tagged specification document, along with any linked image files, are attached. ePAVE prompts you to attach the scanned declaration file and will automatically include the other XML document files you have created, such as the application data sheet, fee transmittal, and transmittal document, in the submission folder.

SUBMISSION

After the specification and declaration are attached and other appropriate information has been entered, ePAVE will validate the contents to ensure that you have included the necessary items. For a new application submission, you can override certain validation errors. While this is not recommended, under current patent business rules a new patent application may be filed with fewer than all of the required parts. However, follow-up action will be necessary to complete the application and correct any deficiencies; an additional fee may be required.

The Submit screen requires you to certify that the content of the submission has been reviewed.

The last two steps prior to submission allow you to electronically sign the application transmittal and authenticate the digital certificate. Authentication is accomplished by providing the computer directory location of your certificate profile and entering a password. An individual authorized to file the application (e.g., attorney or agent) must make the electronic signature. A support staff member under direction of the attorney or agent may apply the signature using the digital certificate.

ePAVE will submit the patent application package via your Internet connection in encrypted and compressed form to ensure the security and integrity of the submission. Upon receipt of the application, the USPTO will decrypt and decompress the file and send you an electronic receipt. This receipt includes the application number, date and time of receipt, names and sizes of files submitted, and some patent application identifying information, such as the first-named inventor, the title of the invention, and the attorney docket number. You can print this electronic postcard and maintain it as evidence of the time, date, and content of the filing. ePAVE automatically saves the electronic receipt in the submission folder on your computer. After the electronic files have been printed to paper and have undergone a formalities review, the USPTO will mail the official patent application filing receipt (on paper).

NOTES

For submission of a new utility patent application you will be given three options for pre-grant publication:

1. Early publication will result in publication at 14 to 15 weeks from filing; a $300 publication fee along with the standard filing fee is due.
2. Normal publication will result in publication at 18 months from the earliest claimed priority date; the publication fee is due at the time of payment of the issue fee.
3. A request not to publish has no fee associated with it because publication will not occur. A request for nonpublication requires the filer to certify that the application has not been and will not be the subject of a patent application in a foreign country or an international authority that publishes such filings after 18 months.

Ordinarily, the application as filed in paper or via EFS is used for the production of the patent publication. For more information regarding pre-grant publication, see 37 CFR 1.211–1.221 for a full description of the process.

Electronic Filing System:
EFS Filing Scenario with Compact Discs:

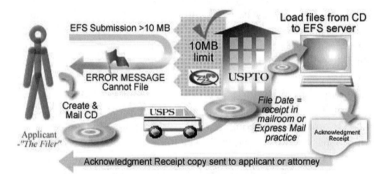

FIGURE 6.2 Electronic Filing System: Compact Disc Scenario

EFS FILING SCENARIO WITH COMPACT DISC (CD-R) (FIGURE 6.2)

THE APPLICANT

1. Receives an ePAVE error message indicating that the package is larger than 10 MB.
2. Prints the transmittal form from ePAVE.
3. As instructed by the error message, applicant copies the indicated encrypted header.enc and submissiondoc.zip.enc files to CD-R.
4. Applicant mails the CD-R(s), transmittal form, and a cover letter to the USPTO or sends the items via Express Mail.

The USPTO

1. Uploads encrypted CD-R files to EFS server.
2. Acknowledgment receipt is produced by the EFS server and printed by the Office of Initial Patent Examination (OIPE); date adjusted by hand.
3. A copy of the acknowledgment receipt is inserted to the application paper file wrapper.
4. A copy of the acknowledgment receipt is sent to the applicant or to the applicant's attorney.

If an applicant or attorney attempts to file a patent application or an 18-month publication submission that exceeds the EFS system limit of 10 MB, the system will generate an error message and advise the applicant to submit the application on CD-R. The submission cannot be forwarded to the USPTO via the Internet using ePAVE. If a biotechnology sequence listing, a computer program listing, or tables caused the large file size, the applicant has the option of submitting the application according to the requirements of 37 CFR 1.52(e) with the large section on CD-R and the rest in paper. However, regardless of the cause of the large size of the submission, EFS can be used also to file the application in the following manner (the process requires the workstation to have a compact disc recorder). Applicant, upon creating a large application (> 10 MB) will be instructed by ePAVE to:

1. Print out the transmittal form.
2. Copy the two files indicated by ePAVE to CD-R. These files contain the entire application. Do not include other files. Do not use floppy or zip disks or other media.
3. Place the CD-R and the transmittal form in a jewel case made for CDs and insert into a padded mailing envelope. Enclose a cover letter explaining that the submission contains an application that was too large to be submitted via ePAVE.
4. Hand deliver or send the envelope via Express Mail (37 CFR 1.10).

You are advised to keep a copy of the CD-R and transmittal form for your records. If you have concerns about readability you may make a backup copy of the CD-R and send both copies to the USPTO. Label the CD-Rs "Copy 1" and "Copy 2," and include a signed statement that the two copies are identical. Copy 1 will be used for processing, unless it is unreadable. You are advised to electronically "compare" the file on the CD-R with the files on the computer to be sure of accuracy. You are advised also to compare the file size of the encrypted files copied to CD-R and the files residing on your workstation.

When the USPTO receives the application package in its mailroom, the date of receipt is recorded. In due course, the CD-R will be uploaded to the EFS server, where the files are unsigned, decrypted, and unzipped. The application files are then processed as EFS submissions.

If the submission is a new application (as opposed to a resubmission of an application under 18-month publication), an acknowledgment receipt is printed. However, the acknowledgment receipt will be modified to indicate that the USPTO mailroom date of receipt or the Express Mail date is the official date of receipt (the date of uploading to the server will not be used). The acknowledgment receipt is placed in the file with the printed application, and a copy is sent to the applicant.

If the files contain large tables, sequence listings, or computer program listings, the Office has the option of not printing the large files, instead creating two CD-Rs of such data and treating them as outlined in 37 CFR 1.52(e). If the file is an amino acid/nucleotide sequence listing, then one additional copy will be created and used as the computer readable file. In any case, one CD is placed in the file, and one is put in the Office's CD repository.

In other respects, processing will continue as if the application had been submitted by the standard EFS channels.

For applications that are originally filed using EFS, the paper copy of the specification that is printed from the EFS submission and placed in the file wrapper is the official copy, with one exception. Sequence listings, large tables, and computer program listings may be submitted on CD-R only, in accordance with 37 CFR 1.52(e). If the Office decides in a particular instance to copy one of these files onto a CD-R instead of printing it to paper, the CD-R becomes the official copy, the active authoritative copy. The decision of media, paper or CD, is determined by the length of the submission and the feasibility of printing it to paper. The Office will follow the procedures of 37 CFR 1.821.

NEW UTILITY APPLICATION WITH ASSIGNMENT

Patent assignment: 35 USC 261; 37 CFR 1.21, 3. Include with your new utility patent application an assignment recordation form and an assignment conveyance document. Other rule bases are the same as for a new utility application.

The patent assignment documents are electronically stored and processed through the Patent and Trademark Assignment System (PTAS). An assignment cover sheet and assignment conveyance documents may be included with new utility applications. The conveyance documents should be scanned as TIFF images (black-and-white, 300 dpi, CCITT Group 4 compression). In ePAVE you will create the cover sheet. Each new filing may include from 0 to 5 cover sheets and their associated conveyance images.

PROVISIONAL APPLICATION

Rule bases: 35 USC 111(b), 112 T 1, 113, 122. Provisional applications under 35 USC 111(b) can be electronically filed using EFS.

The process for handling EFS provisional patent applications is the same as for new utility patent application EFS filings except for the following features:

1. Provisional application must include the application data sheet (37 CFR 1.76) as the cover sheet and the bibliographic information required by 37 CFR 1.51(c)(1). The entry of a Customer Number for a correspondence address will assign to the provisional application the correspondence address associated with the Customer Number and will enable information about the application to be obtained using the private side of the Patent Application Information Retrieval (PAIR) system. The ePAVE system can be used to create the required application data sheet.

2. The EFS transmittal form will automatically include information identifying the electronic submission as a provisional application.

3. If the provisional application submission to be electronically filed is subject to U.S. government property interest, an explanation should be entered in the EFS transmittal form Comments section. Provisional applications containing national security-related matter cannot be electronically filed.

4. Payment of the basic provisional filing fee is required. As for paper filings, fees must be paid by bank card (credit card) or deposit account: $80 for small entity, $160 for large entity.

5. The acknowledgment receipt returned after a successful electronic filing of a provisional application will contain the USPTO assigned provisional application number.

6. Provisional application submissions under EFS will be printed to paper, reviewed for completeness, and a paper filing receipt will be mailed to the applicant. The paper file wrapper containing the electronically filed documents (i.e., the provisional application) will not be examined or published. *Note:* The provisional application does not require the inclusion of a claim, oath, or declaration.

7. Provisional applications submitted under EFS must be in the English language only. The USPTO permits paper applications to be filed in a language other than English (37 CFR 1.52(d)), but applications submitted through the EFS must currently be in the English language.

8. Allows filing under 35 USC 111(b) without a formal patent claim, oath, or declaration, or any information disclosure statement and provides the means to establish an early effective filing date in a nonprovisional patent application filed under 35 USC 111(a). Provisional applications are not published and do not require claim text to be part of the specification; however, the XML template needs one claim tag entered with or without place-holding text to be valid. The output of this authoring process will be a structured electronic document with links to the image files containing figures, chemical formulae, or mathematical equations.

You can override certain validation errors. While this is not recommended, under current patent business rules a new patent application may be filed with fewer than all of the required parts. However, follow-up action will be necessary to complete the application and correct any deficiencies; an additional fee may be required.

Electronic Filing System: Pre-Grant Publication Submissions

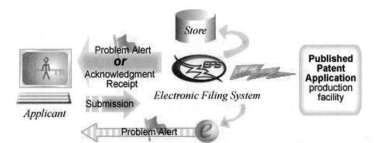

FIGURE 6.3 Electronic Filing System: Pre-Grant Publication Submission

18-MONTH PUBLICATION (FIGURE 6.3)

THE APPLICANT

1. Qualifies for PKI (public key infrastructure) security key pairs and receives a digital certificate from the USPTO.
2. Receives authoring and submission software from the USPTO.
3. Authors an as-amended, redacted, voluntary, previously published, or early application specification following the USPTO technical guidelines and template to produce structured document and compliant image files. Includes statement of "no new matter."
4. Uses submission software supplied by USPTO to create and validate XML documents, and transmit application via the Internet.

THE USPTO

1. Receives electronic submission in EFS, unwraps and decrypts files.
2. Stores files in secure repository under Electronic Records Management control.
3. Checks file attributes for file integrity and successful transmission; alerts applicant if a problem is encountered.
4. Sends an electronic acknowledgment receipt to applicant with date, file names and sizes, and a message digest. Determines if applicant complied with timeliness and other formal matters associated with certain submissions.
5. Documents are sent in electronic form to the facility that produces the published patent application document.
6. If a problem occurs with the published application, the USPTO first checks the electronic version in EFS. If a new copy is needed, the applicant will be able to resubmit files.

The same ePAVE software that is used for filing new patent applications is used also for the resubmission of patent applications for the purposes of 18-month publication. See 37 CFR 1.211–1.221 for the relevant rules.

Ordinarily, a paper copy of a patent application is used for the production of the patent application publication; however, the following can be used as well:

- The publication of a redacted copy of an application (37 CFR 1.217)
- The publication of the application as amended (37 CFR 1.215)
- The voluntary publication of an application filed before but pending on November 29, 2000, under 37 CFR 1. 221
- A republication under 37 CFR 1.221 of an application previously published under 37 CFR 1.211

Then the application must be submitted in electronic form using the EFS. If the applicant requests early publication of the application under 37 CFR 1.219 he may submit an electronic copy using EFS, but EFS submissions are currently only able to be used for publication purposes if the application was already on file in the USPTO. Accordingly, to obtain early publication either file the application on paper or through EFS, and once a confirmation number is obtained (on the filing receipt) resubmit the application using EFS with a request for early publication. Alternatively, the second EFS submission may be eliminated, but publication will be based on a paper version of the application. Requests for early and voluntary publication and republication require payment of publication and processing fees (see 37 CFR 1.217–221).

The following statement is automatically entered and printed on the completed EFS application data sheet for every 18-month publication electronic submission:

I state that this resubmission of the application contains no new matter. If this resubmission is a redacted copy of an application submitted under CFR 1.217, the applicant hereby certifies that the redacted copy of the application eliminates only the part of description of the invention that is not contained in any application filed in a foreign country, directly or through a multilateral international agreement, that corresponds to the application filed in the Office and otherwise does not introduce any new matter. Additionally, if this submission is a redacted copy of an application submitted under 37 CFR 1.217, the applicant further certifies that the documents and certification required by 37 CFR 1.217(c) will be filed in paper.

In accordance with 37 CFR 10.18(b), by presenting to the Office (whether by signing, filing, submitting, or later advocating) any paper, the party presenting such paper, whether a practitioner or nonpractitioner, is certifying that:

All statements made therein of the party's own knowledge are true, all statements made therein on information and belief are believed to be true, and all statements made therein are made with the knowledge that whoever, in any matter within the jurisdiction of the Patent and Trademark Office, knowingly and willfully falsifies, conceals, or covers up by any trick, scheme, or device a material fact, or makes any false, fictitious or fraudulent statements or representations, makes or uses any false writing or document knowing the same to contain any false, fictitious or fraudulent statement or entry, shall be subject to the penalties set forth under 18 USC 1001, and that violations of this paragraph may jeopardize the validity of the application or document.

Entry of one electronic signature appearing on the EFS submission transmittal will acknowledge all the certification statements contained in the EFS submission.

Electronic submissions for 18-month publication under EFS of as-amended applications, voluntary or previously published publications, or early publications may be made with a certificate of transmission. Consistent with the certificate practice of 37 CFR 1.8, the local date at the place of submission as indicated on the certificate of transmission will be considered for the purposes of determining if the electronic application was submitted in a timely manner. This does not apply to redacted applications submitted under 37 CFR 1.217 that must be received on the specified date at the USPTO.

VOLUNTARY PRE-GRANT PUBLICATION

Rule basis: 37 CFR 1.221(a).

When: On or after November 29, 2000, for cases pending on November 29, 2000.

Fee: $300 for publication plus $130 for processing.

Comment: Applications are published 14 to 15 weeks from submission through EFS. Eighteen-month publication applies only to applications filed on or after November 29, 2000; however, applications filed prior to this date and pending at USPTO may be published under 37 CFR 1.221(a). If you have made amendments to the claims during prosecution, you may file the application with the amended claims. For more information regarding pre-grant publication, see 37 CFR 1.211–1.221 for a full description of the process.

Note: In order to prevent replacement of the wrong specification with an EFS pre-grant publication submission, the USPTO is issuing confirmation numbers for each application number. Once an application is perfected (i.e., in condition for publication), a four-digit confirmation number is generated and transmitted to the applicant. This confirmation number is used in conjunction with the application number to identify pending applications. Be sure to enter the correct application filing date as failure to do so will prevent publication. In EFS, when an applicant is submitting an application for publication or republication, the applicant must enter both the application number and the confirmation number in order to submit the application. This procedure is necessary because many applications will have identical filing dates and similar application numbers; thus a typographic error in the application number could result in failure to publish an application or improper publication of an application. The combination of the application number and the randomly generated confirmation number will prevent this.

Publication-ready applications are prepared following the same process used to create a new utility patent application.

AMENDED PUBLICATION AS FIRST PRE-GRANT PUBLICATION BY THE USPTO

Rule basis: 37 CFR 215(c).

When: For an application that has been amended during prosecution with no claim to priority and no request for early publication, the last date for submission is 14 months from the filing date or at least 1 month from filing, whichever is later. For example, if an application with no claim to priority was filed January 2, 2001, an applicant must submit the EFS copy of the application as amended no later than March 2, 2002.

For an amended application with foreign priority dating back an extra year, less time is provided for filing an amended application. For example, if there is foreign priority dating to January 2, 2000, and a filing date in the U.S. of January 2, 2001, 14 months from earliest priority under 35 USC is March 2, 2001. An applicant must submit an EFS copy of his application by March 2, 2001 (2 months after the filing date) for the submission to be timely.

For an application claiming priority to a PCT application with 2 years of priority claim, applicants would have 1 month from filing in the U.S. to file the amended pre-grant publication submission.

Fee: No fee is charged via EFS if applicant does not submit request for early publication. A $300 publication fee will be collected at the time of payment of the patent issue fee. If, however, an early publication request is indicated, then a $300 application fee will be collected via EFS when the submission is filed.

Comment: If an amended publication is submitted after the initial application enters the publication queue (or after it has been published), it is considered a republication request. A $300 publication fee and a $130 processing fee for the republication are due, in addition to the $300 publication fee for the first publication. For more information regarding pre-grant publication, see 37 CFR 1.211–1.221 for a full description of the process.

Note: In order to prevent replacement of the wrong specification with an EFS pre-grant publication submission, the USPTO is issuing confirmation numbers for each application number. Once an application is perfected (i.e., in condition for publication), a four-digit confirmation number is generated and transmitted to the applicant. This confirmation number will be used in conjunction with the application number to identify pending applications. Be sure to enter the correct application filing date as failure to do so will prevent publication.

REDACTED PUBLICATION SUBMISSION AS FIRST PRE-GRANT PUBLICATION BY THE USPTO

Rule basis: 35 USC 122(b)(2)(B)(v); 37 CFR 1.217.

When: Applicants have 16 months from the earliest claimed priority under 35 USC to submit a redacted application for publication. See 37 CFR 1.217 and 35 USC 122(b).

Fee: No fees are collected through EFS. A publication fee of $300 is due at the time of payment of the issue fee. If early publication of a redacted publication is requested, the $300 publication fee is due on filing.

Comment: Redacted publication is available only when an applicant has filed an application outside of the U.S. with less content than was filed in the U.S.

To prevent publication of the full content as filed in the U.S. by limiting publication to what will be published abroad, the applicant will file a redacted application (see 37 CFR 1.217(a)). In addition to electronically filing the redacted publication information, applicant must submit, in paper, a copy of the application with the redacted information in brackets to indicate changes in the application on record. Applicant is also required to file, in paper, an unmarked copy of the redacted specification document for distribution to the public (see 37 CFR 1.217(c)). A $130 fee and a certification that a less-extensive foreign filing is the basis for foreign priority are associated with the paper copies rather than the EFS submission (see 37 CFR 1.217(d)(3)). For more information regarding pre-grant publication, see 37 CFR 1.211–1.221 for a full description of the process.

Note: In order to prevent replacement of the wrong specification with an EFS pre-grant publication submission, the USPTO is issuing confirmation numbers for each application number. Once an application is perfected (i.e., in condition for publication), a four-digit confirmation number is generated and transmitted to the applicant. This confirmation number will be used in conjunction with the application number to identify pending applications. Be sure to enter the correct application filing date as failure to do so will prevent publication.

REDACTED PUBLICATION SUBMISSION AFTER INITIAL PUBLICATION

Rule basis: As for amended republication, 37 CFR 1.221(a).

When: Must be filed no later than 16 months from the filing date.

Fee: $300 for publication plus $130 for processing.

Comment: This scenario arises when applicant wants to republish a redacted application that has been amended. Applicant may want to publish some of the pending claims. A standard redacted publication will not be possible after the as-filed application has been published. For more information regarding pre-grant publication, see 37 CFR 1.211–1.221 for a full description of the process.

Note: In order to prevent replacement of the wrong specification with an EFS pre-grant publication submission, the USPTO is issuing confirmation numbers for each application number. Once an application is perfected (i.e., in condition for publication), a four-digit confirmation number is generated and transmitted to the applicant. This confirmation number will be used in conjunction with the application number to identify pending applications. Be sure to enter the correct application filing date, as failure to do so will prevent publication. The same tool will create the patent specification for 18-month publication as required by 35 USC 122(b).

CORRECTED PUBLICATION DUE TO ERROR

Rule basis: 37 CFR 1.221(a).
When: After initial publication.
Fee: $300 for publication plus $130 for processing if the error arose through action by applicant. No fee if the error arose at USPTO.
Comment: This is a republication. Applicant may submit the most-recent version of the pending claims with this publication. If the correction is necessary because of a serious error on the part of the USPTO (i.e., affecting the scope of the claims), applicant must submit a paper copy to the USPTO within 2 months of the date of the error and provide an explanation about the error. No fee will be charged for this republication if it is necessitated by a material mistake on the part of the USPTO. See 37 CFR 1.221(b). For more information regarding pre-grant publication, see 37 CFR 1.211–1.221 for a full description of the process.
Note: In order to prevent replacement of the wrong specification with an EFS pre-grant publication submission, the USPTO is issuing confirmation numbers for each application number. Once an application is perfected (i.e., in condition for publication), a four-digit confirmation number is generated and transmitted to the applicant. This confirmation number will be used in conjunction with the application number to identify pending applications. The same tool will create the patent specification for 18-month publication as required by 35 USC 122(b).

COMPUTER READABLE FORMAT BIOTECHNOLOGY SEQUENCE LISTING FOR PENDING PAPER APPLICATION

Rule basis: 37 CFR 1.821–1.825.
When: For a pending application that requires a computer readable format (CRF) sequence listing copy. 37 CFR 1.821(e) requires nucleotide and/or amino acid sequence disclosures in patent applications to include a copy of the sequence listing to be submitted in CRF in accordance with the

requirements of 37 CFR 1.824. The CRF is a copy of the sequence listing and will not necessarily be retained as part of the patent application file.

Fee: Pay fees due by submitting a fee transmittal in paper to the USPTO.

Comment: Voluntary use for pending paper applications. CRF biosequence listing can be created using the USPTO sequence listing authoring tool, PatentIn, or any other biosequence creation tool or editor. You can obtain a free copy of the PatentIn software and its instruction manual at http://www.uspto.gov/web/offices/pac/patin/patentinv31.htm.

The authoring tool used must produce an acceptable text file as defined in MPEP (*Manual of Patent Examining Procedure*). Use of the PatentIn program is not required for compliance with the sequence rules, but its use is highly recommended as experience has shown that submissions developed with PatentIn are far less likely to include errors than those developed in other programs. The PatentIn file format can be submitted using ePAVE.

In ePAVE a sequence transmittal is prepared and accompanies the electronically filed sequence listing. Upon receipt at the USPTO the sequence listings are automatically forwarded to the automated biosequence search system.

Note: In order to prevent replacement of the wrong specification with an EFS pre-grant publication submission, the USPTO is issuing confirmation numbers for each application number. Once an application is perfected (i.e., in condition for publication), a four-digit confirmation number is generated and transmitted to the applicant. This confirmation number will be used in conjunction with the application number to identify pending applications. Be sure to enter the correct application filing date as failure to do so can create problems. For a CRF biosequence filing, ePAVE will automatically include the other XML document files you created, such as the biosequence transmittal and the transmittal document, in the submission folder. You will attach the text file containing the biosequence listing as part of the submission folder at the ePAVE Attachment tab.

FILING AN ASSIGNMENT RECORDATION FOR A PREVIOUSLY FILED PATENT APPLICATION USING EFS

Rule basis: 35 USC 261; 37 CFR 1.21, 3.
When: For previously filed patent applications and patents.
Fee: $40 per cover sheet per property.
Comment: Voluntary use for previously filed applications and patents.

37 CFR 3.1 defines an assignment as "a transfer by a party of all or part of its right, title, and interest in a patent or patent application, or a transfer of its entire right, title, and interest in a registered mark or a mark for which an application to register has been filed." EFS only accepts assignments for patents, patent applications, and PCT applications at this time.

For an assignment for a patent or patent application to be recorded at the USPTO it must include a completed cover sheet per 37 CFR 3.28 and 3.31 and an assignment conveyance document.

To file a new assignment document using EFS you will need to scan the assignment conveyance documents and save them as TIFF images (300 dpi, black-and-white, CCITT Group 4 compression). Using ePAVE, you will create XML-tagged cover sheet(s). An EFS submission of assignment for previously filed patent applications, patents, and PCT applications will include a transmittal, a fee form, at least one assignment cover sheet, and the assignment TIFF images. The cover sheet may refer to up to 999 properties. Up to 15 cover sheets may be included in each submission. Each cover sheet will refer to from 1 to 5 conveyance document TIFF images. If the method of delivery selected is fax and the submission is proper for recordation, a notice of recordation and a copy of the cover sheet will automatically be faxed to the filer.

APPLICATION DATA SHEET

An application data sheet can be authored and printed using EFS software. ePAVE is used to author and print an application data sheet that will satisfy the format requirements of 37 CFR 1.76. As cited in MPEP, an application data sheet may be voluntarily submitted in either provisional or nonprovisional applications, and contains bibliographic data arranged in a format specified by the Office. The use of this optional submission of an application data sheet is beneficial to the applicant as it improves accuracy of filing receipt and of recorded data. You may submit the printed application data sheet you produce using EFS software to the USPTO as part of a paper new utility patent application filing. However, the USPTO encourages you to consider electronically filing your entire new utility patent application including the application data sheet. If you prefer to create a customized application data sheet, you may do so; however, the suggested format is designed to more effectively turn a customer's paper document into an electronic USPTO data record. For further information on the layout and required information for application data sheets, go to http://www.uspto.gov/web/offices/pac/dapp/sir/doc/patappde.html.

CASE STUDY FOR A NEW UTILITY APPLICATION

OVERVIEW

The following is a detailed look at the process behind filing a new utility application. Details on the use of PASAT, TSA, or ePAVE are provided in Chapter 10. This case study is intended to demonstrate the steps taken prior to and during the authoring of the patent application specification document, creating the necessary transmittal forms and cover sheets, and transmitting all developed documents electronically. *Note:* The details provided here and the related documents were actually filed with the USPTO and resulted in the allowance of a patented invention.

BACKGROUND

The author of this book (the inventor) has discovered that the effectiveness of sildenafil citrate (Viagra®) can be substantially improved if it is administered concomitantly with a group of nutritional products, which are needed in eliciting the action of Viagra. The author, who is an agent himself, sought to file this application as a *pro se* inventor.

PREPARATION FOR AUTHORING THE PATENT APPLICATION SPECIFICATION DOCUMENT

Before authoring the patent application specification document, the filer has already installed the necessary software, and obtained a Customer Number and a digital certificate from the USPTO.

The necessary documents have been reformatted to Arial font because he will cut and paste information into the specification document he will create in PASAT. The necessary scans have been saved as TIFF files (300 dpi, black-and-white, with CCITT Group 4 compression). For this document, the filer has scanned in pages of declaration. There were no figures or complex chemical equations; otherwise, these would have had to be scanned as well.

AUTHORING THE PATENT APPLICATION SPECIFICATION DOCUMENT

With the source document open, the filer launches PASAT and opens a new utility application template. To do so, choose the New Specification option from the File menu. (If you choose the Open option, you will go to your Microsoft® Word files instead.)

Warning

PASAT is a Microsoft Visual Basic template that Word views as a macro. If you have Word set with a high level of security, you will see the message "Macros and Disable" and you will be unable to load PASAT. Be sure you change the security setting of macros to "low." To do so, quit the application and launch Word. Choose the Macros option from the Tools menu, then choose Security and set it to "low."

Changing this security setting to low means that you must have a virus-scanning program installed to protect your computer from malicious macros that are sometimes embedded in Word attachments to e-mails.

Prior to the template appearing, a window displays the various sections that will need to be filled out for this specification (Figure 6.4). The sections in bold (Title of Invention, Detailed Description, Claims, and Abstract of Disclosure) are required for this specification, whereas the other sections are optional. From the list, the filer

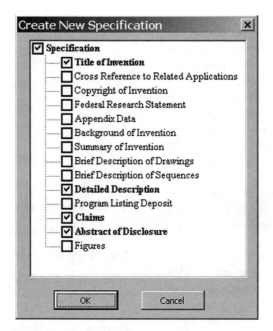

FIGURE 6.4 Create New Specification Window

selects the required sections and the optional Figures section he needs and clicks OK.* A blank template appears along with the Office Assistant that will help him in preparing the specification. The filer copies the title from the source document and, after placing the cursor at the appropriate spot, pastes it into the specification. The filer does this for each of the required sections, as well as for those optional sections he chooses to include (Figure 6.5).

At various points in the process of creating the patent application specification, the filer saves the document-in-progress as an .s4w file in the same folder as the source documents and scanned images. The file location is important for knowing where to find it if he has to put it aside and come back to it later (if he realized after he started that he was missing a piece of information or a scan, he could save his work and not have to start all over again later). The.s4w format facilitates the easy translation of the document into the final .xml format that will be transmitted to the USPTO.

---

* The author has experienced difficulties in selecting only the needed sections, as recommended by the EFS. Some examiners are accustomed to seeing paper applications that contain all the sections, with optional sections marked "Not Applicable." In several instances, the examiners have required the author to resubmit an electronic specification with all sections included and indicating "Not Applicable" in the sections that were not required. The official position of the USPTO is that it is not necessary to do so; however, if you want to save time in the event that your application ends up in the hands of an examiner who requires the entire application, it is better, at least until the EFS becomes the norm, to choose all sections and indicate "Not Applicable" as needed.

While entering data in the Detailed Description section, the filer sees a special scientific character. After placing the cursor in the specification document where he wants the symbol to appear, the filer uses the Office Assistant* to select the symbol from a reference table. The Insert Symbol option opens a window from which he selects the symbol (in this case a right arrow). He clicks Insert at the bottom of the window, then clicks Close. The Insert Symbol window closes and the symbol now appears in the specification document (Figure 6.6).

Later, while copying another paragraph into the specification document, the filer tries to copy and paste a special character that could not be converted. After pasting the paragraph into the specification, he sees in large red type: Unknown Symbol. These large red call-outs make it easy to see that he is not missing any valuable data in the specification document, and save him the time of having to look at every character. The Office Assistant

SPECIFICATION

[Electronic Version 1.2.8]

[Insert title of invention]

Cross Reference to Related Applications

Copyright Statement

Federal Research Statement

Appendix Data

Background of Invention

Summary of Invention

Brief Description of Drawings

Brief Description of Sequences

Detailed Description

Program Listing Deposit

|Beginning of Program|
|Insert Program Here|
|End of Program|

Claims

FIGURE 6.5

will take him to a reference table to enter arrows and standard characters such as ® or ™. He highlights the Unknown Symbol text and again uses the Office Assistant to place the proper character into the specification document.

If the Detailed Description had included a complex mathematical equation or chemical structure that is too cumbersome for copying and pasting, a scan should be made of the object. This scanned object would then be inserted at an appropriate place (corresponding to where it existed in the original write-up). Placing his cursor where the object is to appear, the filer uses the Office Assistant to pull the object into the document. The Office Assistant opens a dialog box for him to select the object file; after selecting the correct file and clicking the OK button, the image is placed in the specification document.

Notice that an Electronic Version number appears below Specification (Figure 6.7); do not delete it as USPTO uses this to make sure that the conversion tools used

---

* The Office Assistant feature in Microsoft Word is very useful; make sure it always visible. If you are using your Word program with this feature hidden (some people find it annoying), make sure you activate it from the Help menu when you begin using PASAT.]

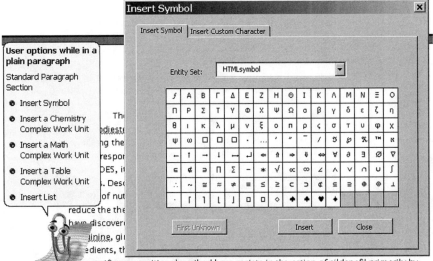

FIGURE 6.6 Using the Office Assistant to Insert a Symbol

SPECIFICATION

[Electronic Version 1.2.8]

[Composition and method of use in treating sexual dysfunction using cGMP-specific phosphodiesterase type 5 inhibitors]

Detailed Description

[0001]   Adequate sexual function is a complex interaction of hormonal events and psychosocial relationships. The term "sexual dysfunction" generally includes any sexual dysfunction in an animal, preferably a mammal, more preferably a human. The animal can be male or female. Sexual dysfunction may include, for example, sexual desire.

FIGURE 6.7

are appropriate to that version. Note also that the spell-check feature has indicated words that are not found in its dictionary.

The Claims section, although more complex, works like the others, with the filer copying and pasting information from the source document into the specification. One addition to the usual procedure is that he uses the Office Assistant to distinguish between claims, e.g., dependent and independent claims (see detailed instructions for working with PASAT in Chapter 7). He also types some new claims directly into the document. After typing the first claim text or section of the first claim, the filer uses

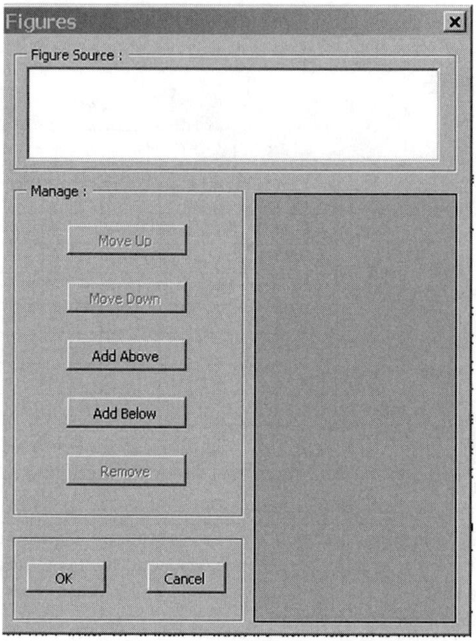

FIGURE 6.8   Figure Manager Window

the Office Assistant to create a new claim text for the second section of the claim. After typing the second section, he uses the Office Assistant to create another claim.

The last section to be completed for the purpose of this case study is Figures. With the Office Assistant, the filer opens the Figure Manager window to link the scans to this document. The Figures window allows him to add (and remove) images, arrange the order, and even see a preview of the image, which aids in verifying the image file name to the image itself* (Figure 6.8).

Once all the sections are complete, the filer saves the document and then exports it as an .xml file by clicking on File and Export XML Specification. The authoring tool does all the converting work, resulting in the .xml file that will be sent to the USPTO. After saving the converted file, the filer views the .xml file in PASAT. This launches Internet Explorer 5.0 and displays the file as it will be seen at the USPTO. He can now view his work and verify the attached scans at actual size.

The last step is to use the Save As option to save the application specification as a .doc file.** This version of the file can be archived or sent to other individuals who do not have the PASAT software installed.

---

* Figures to be added would be indicated in the Create New Specification window (shown in Figure 6.4). The Figure Manager (shown in Figure 6.8) opens when you place the cursor under the Figure listing in the main text and select Figure Manager from the Insert menu.

** It was earlier advised not to alter the name of the directory containing the documents created by PASAT or ePAVE; the reason for this advice was that each of these programs creates other program files, which must be presented in the path recorded in the document in order to open it, as well for reading and sharing.

CREATING NECESSARY TRANSMITTALS AND THE COVER SHEET

With the specification document complete, the filer works on the other necessary forms, such as the fee transmittal, application data sheet, and assignment cover sheet. All of these forms are developed using ePAVE.

The filer launches the application and chooses the New option from the File menu, then selects New Utility Patent Application (Figure 6.9). Then the filer picks a location and creates a folder where the files developed in ePAVE will be stored. ePAVE then displays a window with a series of tabs for the filer to use to enter information (Figure 6.10).

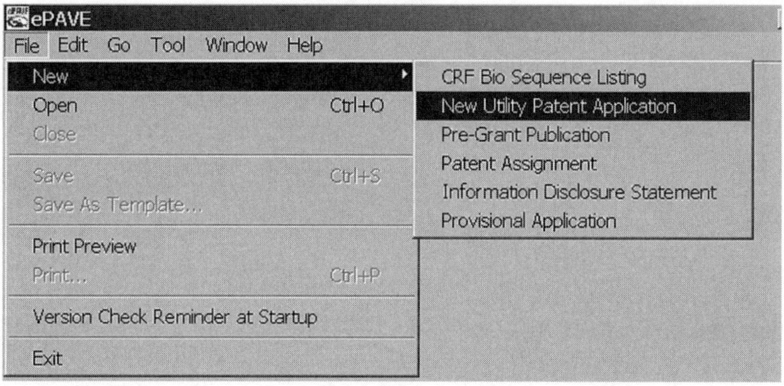

FIGURE 6.9   New Utility Patent Application Path in ePAVE

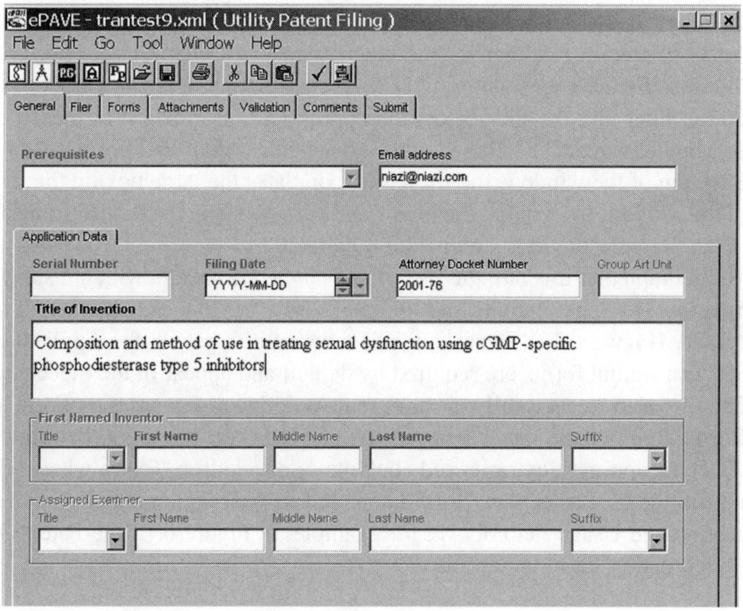

FIGURE 6.10   ePAVE General Tab

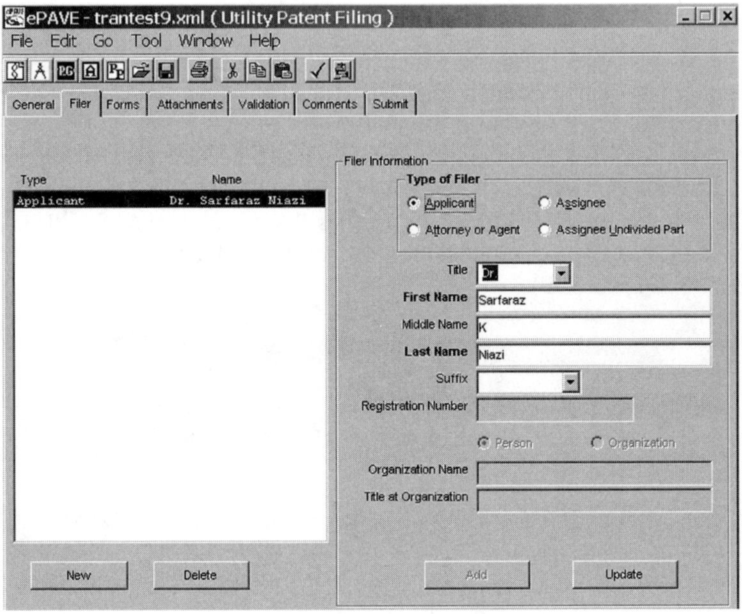

FIGURE 6.11 ePAVE Filer Tab

As the applicant goes through the various tabs, some of the fields are not available ("grayed") because they do not apply to a new utility filing (Prerequisites field, Figure 6.10) or they are not to be filled in by you (Filing Date field). On the General tab, the only available fields for the filer to enter information are the Email address and Attorney Docket Number.* After entering that information, the filer clicks on the Filer tab (Figure 6.11).

On the Filer tab, the filer enters the appropriate information in the Title, First Name, Middle Name, Last Name, and Suffix fields. After clicking the Add button at the bottom of the window, the formation populates the large box on the left-hand side of the window. Note that if the filer is an attorney/agent, the Registration Number field would require the filer's registration number.

After completing this tab, the filer clicks on the Forms tab, which displays a list of forms the filer must include and optional forms the filer may choose to include if necessary (Figure 6.12). Because this is a new utility patent, the Application data and Fee Transmittal forms are required by default and appear in the Selected Forms list. The filer also elects to fill out the Patent Assignment Recordation Form and the IDS Form. To move the forms from the Available Forms list to the Selected Forms list, select the appropriate forms and click the Add>> button. To see what each form is used for, the filer selects the form name and its description appears in the Form Description and Usage field above; for example, in Figure 6.12 the Patent Assignment Recordation Form is described.

---

* Assigned by attorneys and agents for their internal recordkeeping.

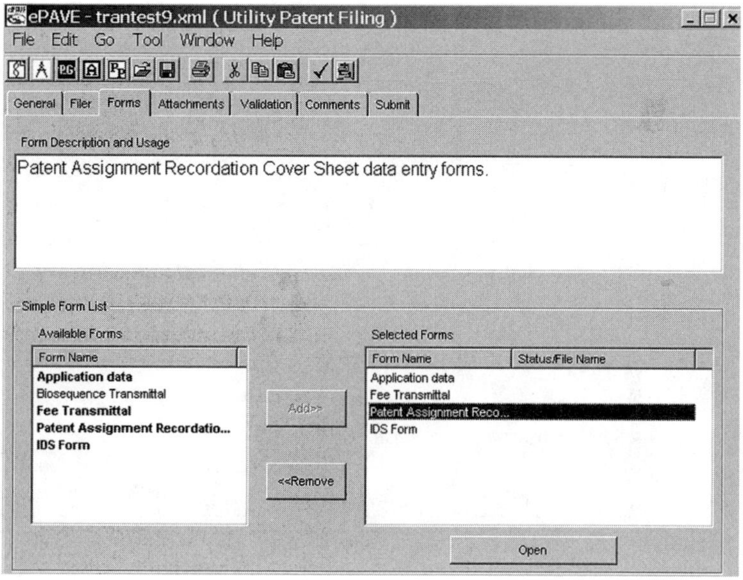

FIGURE 6.12 ePAVE Forms Tab Showing Description of Patent Assignment Recordation Form

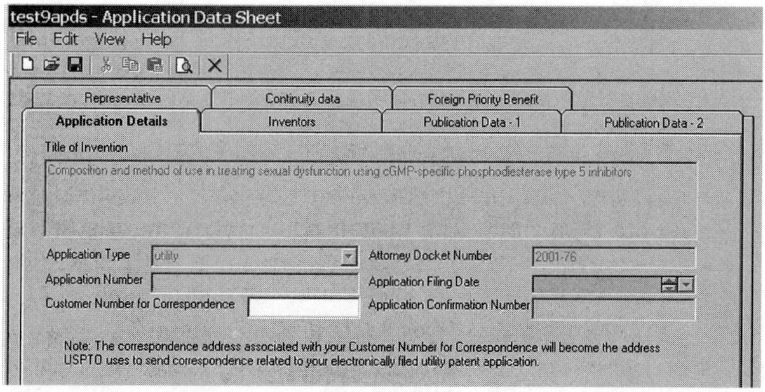

FIGURE 6.13 Application Data Sheet Tabs

The filer double-clicks the Application data form and a window appears, showing a series of tabs for the various parts of that form (Figure 6.13). The filer enters information into fields of the various tabs; for example, the Application Details tab for the type of application, the Inventors tab for listing the names of all the inventors, the Publication Data-1 tab for publication information. He then saves the Application data sheet, and returns to the Forms tab.

The filer then opens the Fee Transmittal form (Figure 6.14) to indicate the filing status, determine the fees due, and enter the method of payment. There are three tabs on the Fee Transmittal form. The process is the same as what was described in

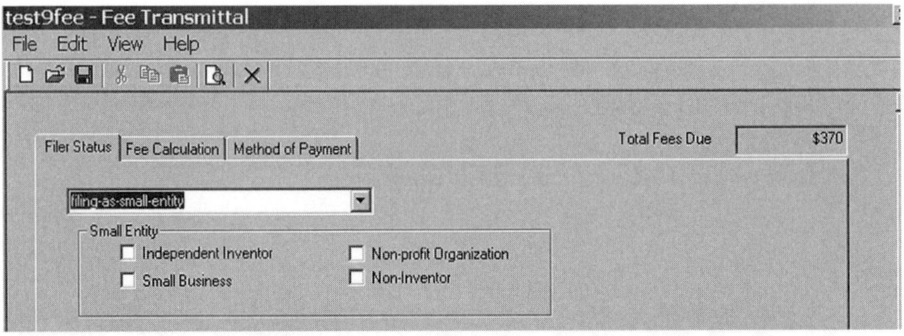

test9fee - Fee Transmittal

File   Edit   View   Help

Filer Status | Fee Calculation | Method of Payment | Total Fees Due $370

[filing-as-small-entity   ▼]

Small Entity
   ☐ Independent Inventor   ☐ Non-profit Organization
   ☐ Small Business   ☐ Non-Inventor

FIGURE 6.14   Fee Transmittal Tabs

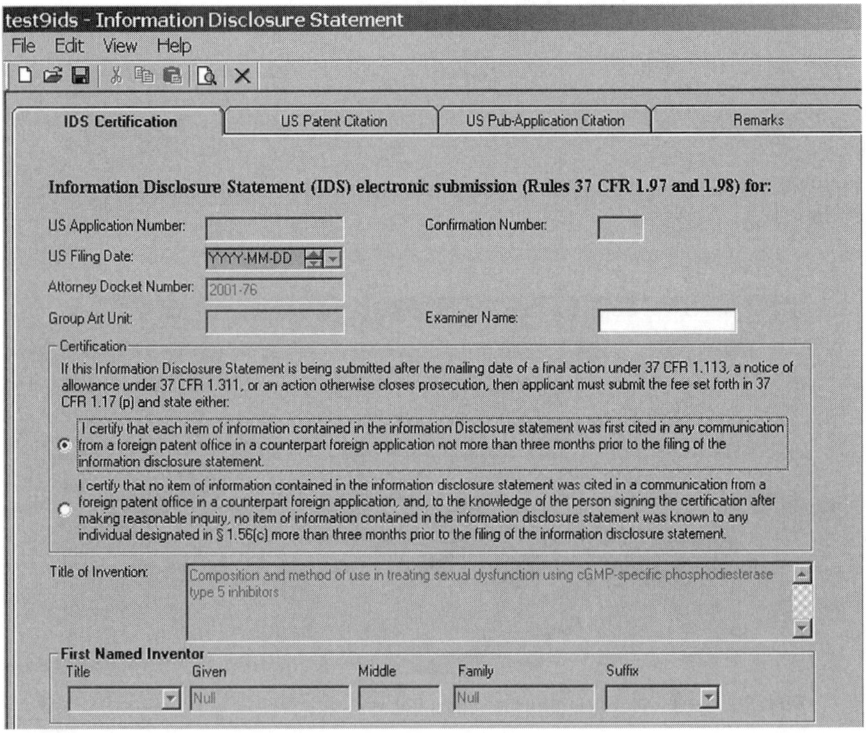

test9ids - Information Disclosure Statement

File   Edit   View   Help

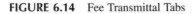

IDS Certification | US Patent Citation | US Pub-Application Citation | Remarks

Information Disclosure Statement (IDS) electronic submission (Rules 37 CFR 1.97 and 1.98) for:

US Application Number: [   ]   Confirmation Number: [   ]

US Filing Date: [YYYY-MM-DD ▲▼]

Attorney Docket Number: [2001-76]

Group Art Unit: [   ]   Examiner Name: [   ]

Certification
If this Information Disclosure Statement is being submitted after the mailing date of a final action under 37 CFR 1.113, a notice of allowance under 37 CFR 1.311, or an action otherwise closes prosecution, then applicant must submit the fee set forth in 37 CFR 1.17 (p) and state either:

⦿ I certify that each item of information contained in the information Disclosure statement was first cited in any communication from a foreign patent office in a counterpart foreign application not more than three months prior to the filing of the information disclosure statement.

○ I certify that no item of information contained in the information disclosure statement was cited in a communication from a foreign patent office in a counterpart foreign application, and, to the knowledge of the person signing the certification after making reasonable inquiry, no item of information contained in the information disclosure statement was known to any individual designated in § 1.56(c) more than three months prior to the filing of the information disclosure statement.

Title of Invention: Composition and method of use in treating sexual dysfunction using cGMP-specific phosphodiesterase type 5 inhibitors

First Named Inventor
Title   Given   Middle   Family   Suffix
[▼] [Null]   [   ] [Null]   [▼]

FIGURE 6.15   Information Disclosure Statement Form

working with the Application data tabs. Here, the filer fills out the Filer Status, Fee Calculation, and Method of Payment tabs to determine the cost of filing and select how the fees will be paid. The Total Fees Due field (on the right-hand side of the window) displays the cost of filing and calculates as the filer adds or alters information in relevant fields. The filer then saves the Fee form and returns to the Forms tab.

As in the other tabs described, the filer opens the IDS (Information Disclosure Statement) Form (Figure 6.15) if this is planned (it is an optional element although

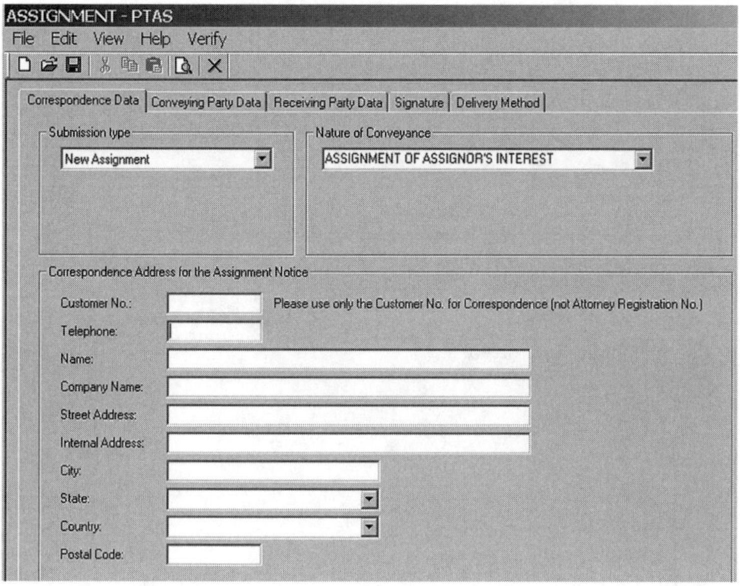

FIGURE 6.16   Assignment PTAS (Patent and Trademark Assignment System)

highly recommended for various legal reasons, not discussed here) and fills out the required information under all tabs. The Remarks tab allows the filer to share information with the examiner. Notice that there is a provision for filing IDS after the application has been submitted and thus the Certification is required, details of which are part of patent practice issues.

Finally, the filer selects the Patent Assignment Recordation form and the window displays tabs for the parts of that form (Figure 6.16). Shown here is Assignment of Assignor's Interest, the other two allowed options are Lien and Mortgage. Working through the tabs, the filer fills out the necessary information for the Correspondence Data, Conveying Party Data, Receiving Party Data, Signature, and Delivery Method tabs. After saving the Assignment Recordation form, the filer returns to the Forms tab. Because the filer has filled out the two required forms and the optional form, the filer continues by clicking the Attachments tab (Figure 6.17).

The Attachments tab is where the filer attaches the .xml specification document that was exported from the .s4w file created in PASAT. The filer clicks the Attach... button on the right-hand side of the window, and then from the dialog box that appears, navigates to the location of the .xml specification file. Notice that the default for clicking the Attach... button is specification. After adding specification, a prompt asks the filer about attaching the declaration. The filer had stored all scanned pages in the same directory where the .xml file is stored; to see other documents, the filer will have to select from the drop list of the dialog box; when declaration is selected, *TIFF files become visible; only one file can be attached at a time. This tab also allows him to view and remove any of the attachments listed, useful if the filer accidentally attached the wrong specification file.

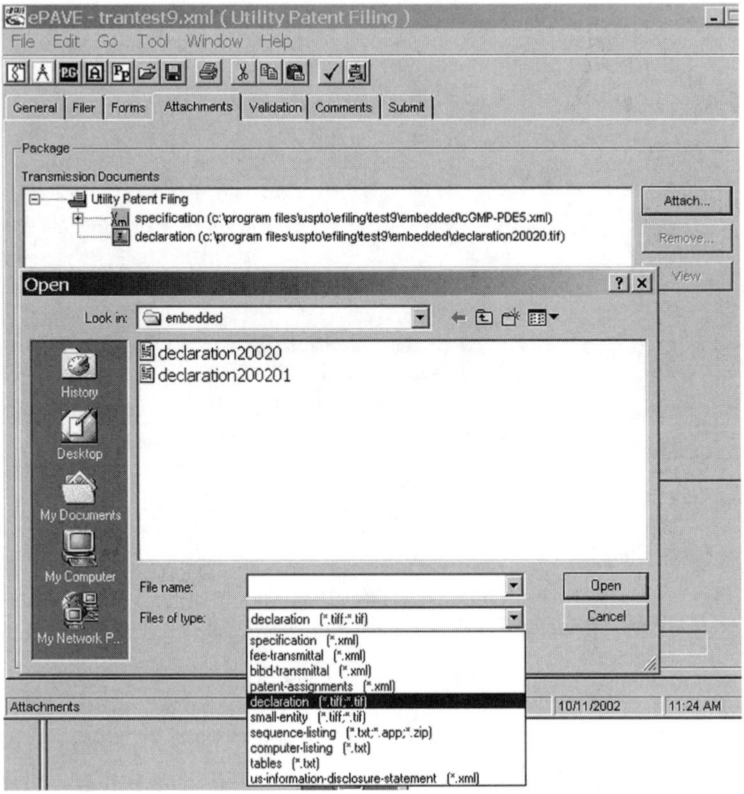

FIGURE 6.17   ePAVE Attachments Tab

The Validation tab allows the filer to check his forms for completeness prior to transmitting to the USPTO system (Figure 6.18). Any possible errors or warnings are listed and can be printed or selected and viewed in greater detail. After looking over the results of the Validation tab, the filer amends key fields and revalidates his work. The second time the field is blank, indicating an error-free submission. The example in the figure shows how various errors are flagged.

Because the filer has no additional comments to add to this submission, he skips the Comments tab and proceeds to the Submit tab (Figure 6.19) to transmit the forms created in ePAVE and the specification exported from PASAT. On the Submit tab, the filer selects the two required check boxes as a sign of agreement to the two statements. The filer then electronically signs and dates the submission with the dialog box that appears after clicking on the Sign & Date button. Here the filer enters his name as signature. Once that is done, the filer clicks the Send to USPTO button to begin transmitting his files. Before transmission begins, the Entrust Profile Login window appears where the filer enters his log-in name and password (the PKI signature).

This window facilitates the encryption of the submission as it is transmitted to the USPTO system. It is based on the Entrust profile and password designated when

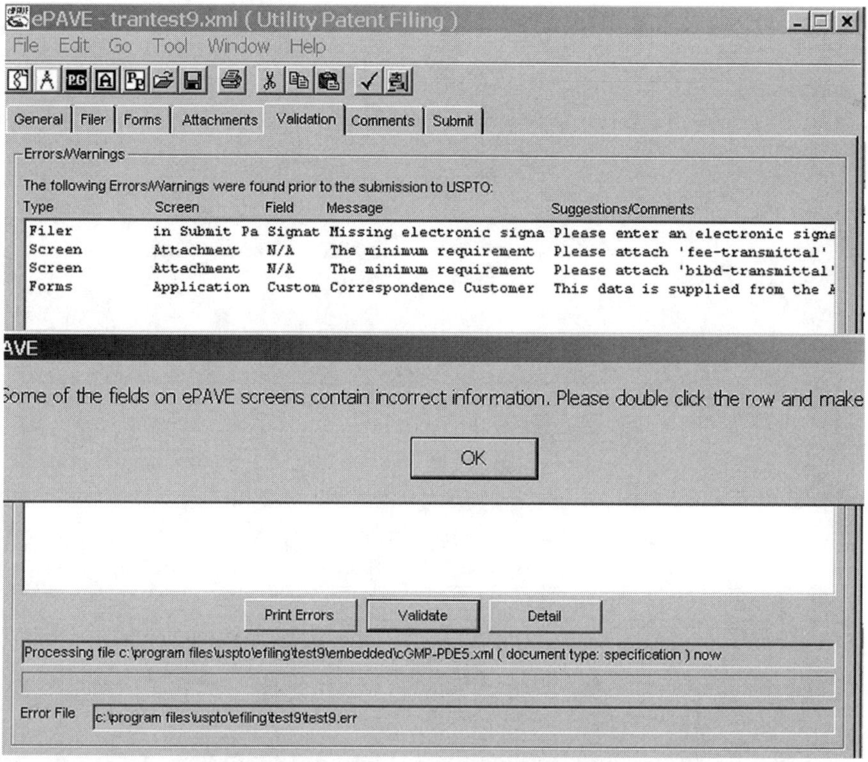

FIGURE 6.18 ePAVE Validation Tab Showing Errors/Warnings

the filer created his digital certificate using the USPTO Direct security software. After clicking OK, the files are transmitted. When transmission is complete, the server returns an acknowledgment receipt to the filer (Figure 6.20). The receipt is saved in the same folder that was created for this particular submission. The receipt includes, among other things, a unique EFS ID number, a timestamp of the date and time of receipt at the USPTO, and the Upload Status, which confirms that the submission was successfully uploaded to the USPTO server. The filer prints out the receipt for his records.

TRACKING DOWN THE APPLICATION

The USPTO Direct software allows applicants to review the status of their application online. To do so, the applicant loads the USPTO Direct application, which will ask for a password. If you enter the wrong password (it is case sensitive), the configuration file will automatically be corrupted and you will have start all over again with getting the key (Figure 6.21).

From the main menu, the applicant clicks Patent Application Information Retrieval, which takes the applicant to a menu where he can seek information on patents and patent applications. The default Customer Number is already in the drop list; for law firms having several Customer Numbers, the selection can be made from

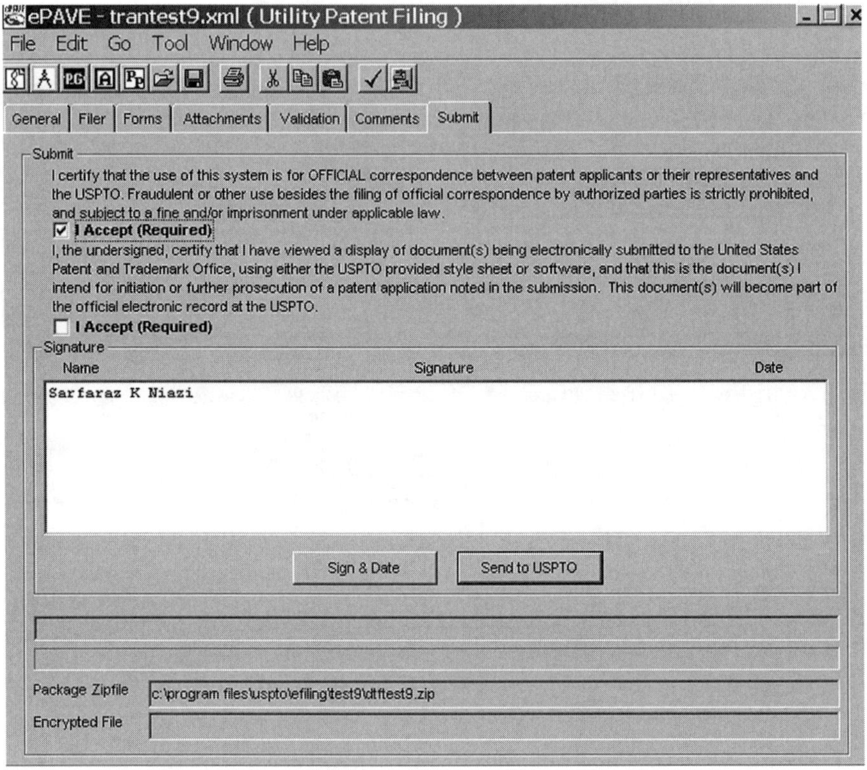

FIGURE 6.19 ePAVE Submit Tab

this drop list. The easiest way to look at all of your pending and approved applications at the USPTO is to use the search button for your Customer Number.

Notice that you get to the menu in Figure 6.22 by clicking on the Patent Application Information Retrieval link; this menu is different from what you would get if you were to connect to PAIR from the public USPTO Web site. The screen in Figure 6.23 shows the details of author's pending and issued patents. Here the applicant can sort the information by clicking on the various headings; the most frequently used is Status Date. To see details about the history of prosecution, the applicant clicks on the Application No. (not the Patent No.); following is what appears in the prosecution history of the patent application discussed above (Figure 6.24):

From 03-26-2001 filing date to 09-28-2001 date of allowance (6 months) and recordation of patent on 01-15-2002 is one of the faster records of achievement made possible by careful writing of the application to avoid formal matter rejections, prompt response to office actions, and continuous monitoring of the status of application. Details of various drop lists and other means of following up on the pending application are described in detail in the chapter on USPTO Direct (Chapter 11).

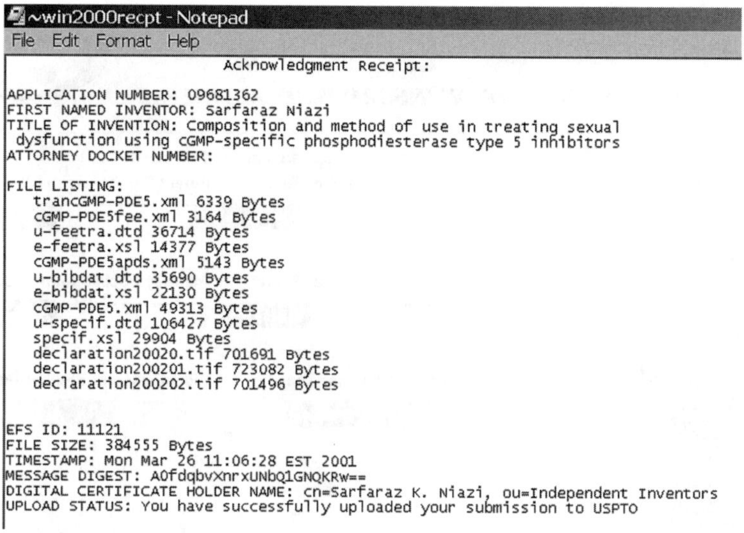

```
~win2000recpt - Notepad
File   Edit   Format   Help
                        Acknowledgment Receipt:

APPLICATION NUMBER: 09681362
FIRST NAMED INVENTOR: Sarfaraz Niazi
TITLE OF INVENTION: Composition and method of use in treating sexual
 dysfunction using cGMP-specific phosphodiesterase type 5 inhibitors
ATTORNEY DOCKET NUMBER:

FILE LISTING:
    trancGMP-PDE5.xml 6339 Bytes
    cGMP-PDE5fee.xml 3164 Bytes
    u-feetra.dtd 36714 Bytes
    e-feetra.xsl 14377 Bytes
    cGMP-PDE5apds.xml 5143 Bytes
    u-bibdat.dtd 35690 Bytes
    e-bibdat.xsl 22130 Bytes
    cGMP-PDE5.xml 49313 Bytes
    u-specif.dtd 106427 Bytes
    specif.xsl 29904 Bytes
    declaration20020.tif 701691 Bytes
    declaration200201.tif 723082 Bytes
    declaration200202.tif 701496 Bytes


EFS ID: 11121
FILE SIZE: 384555 Bytes
TIMESTAMP: Mon Mar 26 11:06:28 EST 2001
MESSAGE DIGEST: AOfdqbvXnrxUNbQlGNQKRw==
DIGITAL CERTIFICATE HOLDER NAME: cn=Sarfaraz K. Niazi, ou=Independent Inventors
UPLOAD STATUS: You have successfully uploaded your submission to USPTO
```

FIGURE 6.20 Acknowledgment Receipt

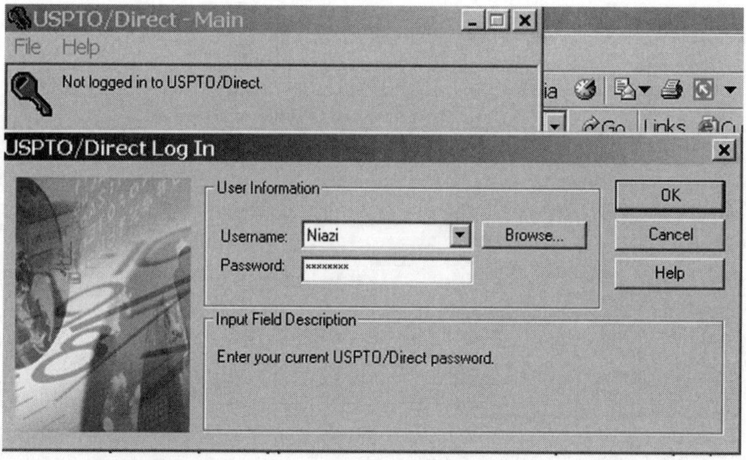

FIGURE 6.21 USPTO/Direct Log In Window

Once you are inside the secure web of the Patent Office, you can look at another applicant's or attorney's information database and, conversely, they can view yours. For example, if you enter any attorney docket number in the screen prompting you to choose the search method, you will be able to see all records with that particular attorney docket number, which may belong to several Customer Numbers. The patent issues as shown in Figure 6.25.

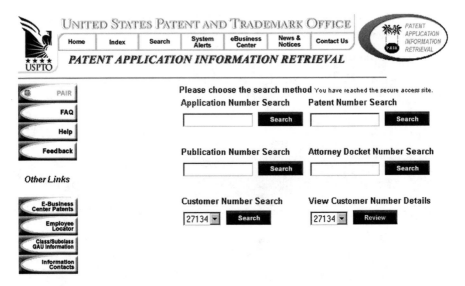

FIGURE 6.22 Acknowledgment Receipt

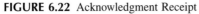

FIGURE 6.23 Detail of Pending and Issued Patents

Search results for application number: 09/681,362

Application Filing Date:	03-26-2001	Class / Sub-Class:	424/728.000
Issue Date of Patent:	01-15-2002	Location:	FILE REPOSITORY (FRANCONIA)
Examiner Name:	WINSTON, RANDALL O	Status:	Patented Case
Group Art Unit:	1651	Attorney Docket Number:	20020
Earliest Publication No:	-	Patent Number:	6,338,862
Earliest Publication Date:	-	Customer Number:	27134
Confirmation Number:	5294		

PTA History	Continuity Data	Web Patent Database

Retrieve Maint.Fees to Pay	View Maint. Payment Windows	Payment Window: 4 ▾	View Maint. Statement

Maintenance Fees Available: Mon-Fri 5:30 AM to Midnight, Sat-Sun-Hol. 7:30 AM to 8:00 PM E.T.

File Contents History

Number	Date	Contents Description
27	01-15-2002	Recordation of Patent Grant Mailed
26	10-02-2001	Workflow - File Sent to Contractor
25	12-28-2001	Weekly Patent Issue Receipt
23	12-13-2001	Receipt into Pubs
22	12-11-2001	Application Is Considered Ready for Issue
21	10-09-2001	Mailroom Date of Issue Fee Payment
20	12-11-2001	Receipt into Pubs
19	11-19-2001	Receipt into Pubs
18	09-28-2001	Receipt into Pubs
17	09-28-2001	Receipt into Pubs
16	09-28-2001	Mail Notice of Allowance
15	09-28-2001	Notice of Allowance Data Verification Completed
14	09-28-2001	Notice of Allowability
13	07-30-2001	Case Docketed to Examiner in GAU
12	08-10-2001	Date Forwarded to Examiner
11	08-07-2001	Supplemental Response
10	08-10-2001	Date Forwarded to Examiner
9	08-07-2001	Response after Non-Final Action
8	07-31-2001	Mail Non-Final Rejection
7	07-30-2001	Non-Final Rejection
6	06-18-2001	Case Docketed to Examiner in GAU
5	05-22-2001	Case Docketed to Examiner in GAU
4	05-17-2001	Application Dispatched from OIPE
3	05-15-2001	Correspondence Address Change
2	04-04-2001	Application Scanned
1	03-26-2001	Initial Exam Team nn

FIGURE 6.24 Prosecution History of Patent Application

‖‖‖‖‖‖‖‖‖‖‖‖‖‖‖‖‖‖‖‖‖‖‖‖‖‖‖‖‖‖‖‖‖‖‖
US006338862B1

(12) **United States Patent**
     Niazi

(10) Patent No.:   **US 6,338,862 B1**
(45) Date of Patent: **Jan. 15, 2002**

(54) **COMPOSITION AND METHOD OF USE IN TREATING SEXUAL DYSFUNCTION USING CGMP-SPECIFIC PHOSPHODIESTERASE TYPE 5 INHIBITORS**

(76) Inventor: **Sarfaraz K Niazi**, 20 Riverside Dr., Deerfield, IL (US) 60015

(*) Notice: Subject to any disclaimer, the term of this patent is extended or adjusted under 35 U.S.C. 154(b) by 0 days.

(21) Appl. No.: **09/681,362**

(22) Filed: **Mar. 26, 2001**

(51) Int. Cl.^{7} A61K 35/78
(52) U.S. Cl. 424/728; 424/725; 514/565
(58) Field of Search 424/728, 725; 514/565

(56)   **References Cited**

U.S. PATENT DOCUMENTS

5,523,087 A   *   6/1996 Shlyankevich
6,007,824 A   * 12/1999 Duckett et al.

FOREIGN PATENT DOCUMENTS

AU   WO 9965337   *   1/2000

* cited by examiner

Primary Examiner—Christopher R. Tate
Assistant Examiner—Randall Winston

(57)   **ABSTRACT**

The inhibitors of cyclic guanosine monophosphate (cGMP) phosphodiesterases type 5 (cGMP-PDE5) such as sildenafil citrate (Viagra®) act by increasing the level of cGMP in sexual organs to produce enhanced blood flow and an erectile response of sexual organs. Though sildenafil citrate is a specific inhibitor of cGMP-PDE5, its effects on other body organs produce many side effects including fatalities. Described here is a method of combining cGMP-PDE5 inhibitors with natural sources of nutrients that instantly enhance the levels of endogenous cGMP and thus reduce the therapeutic dose and therefore the side effects of cGMP-PDE5 inhibitors. We have discovered that if sildenafil citrate, as a prototype of cGMP-PDE5, is combined with L-arginine, ginseng, vitamin B6, vitamin B12, and folic acid, all natural and safe ingredients, the dose requirements for sildenafil citrate can be reduced substantially. The specific composition described here assists in the action of sildenafil primarily by increasing the production of cGMP through modulation of nitric oxide pathway (L-arginine→nitric oxide→cGMP) and secondarily by having its own effect on improving blood circulation to sexual organs.

11 Claims, No Drawings

FIGURE 6.25 Issued Patent

7 USPTO: PASAT

INTRODUCTION

One of the major components of the U.S. Patent and Trademark Office's (USPTO) Electronic Filing System (EFS) is the Patent Application Specification Authoring Tool (PASAT). PASAT is used to author electronic versions of specifications documents consisting of content such as text, titles, and pictures in XML (Extensible Markup Language). The structure is the organizational form that determines which content objects are permitted at any point in a document, as well as how these objects are displayed in various viewers (such as Internet Explorer).

Whereas you may choose to convert documents to XML format directly, this practice is discouraged in favor of the use of the free PASAT software available through the USPTO. Recently, the USPTO has allowed five companies to create their own systems of online patent filing as long as they meet the requirements of submission.

PASAT enables you to create patent specifications in the XML format required by the USPTO with little or no XML knowledge. You will be using the familiar Microsoft® Word with a slightly modified interface to create a specification, and then PASAT exports it as an XML file.

As you edit the specification, PASAT handles the XML-required structure of the document behind the scenes, based on the USPTO Document Type Definition (DTD) and Stylesheet (XSL file). The specification is saved as an .s4w file for future editing and can be validated against the DTD. If satisfactory, the specification can be exported in an XML format ready for submission to the USPTO using ePAVE.

PASAT is a plug-in for Microsoft Word 97 or later versions and it is assumed that you are familiar with the various functions of this word processing program. It is further assumed that you are familiar with the traditional paper-based patent application specification authoring process; however, the Appendix provides a detailed glossary of terms for reference purposes.

GETTING STARTED

After you have installed the program on your machine, the PASAT shortcut appears on your desktop. When you use this shortcut, Word will launch, and you will find the following new options on the File menu:

- New Specification prompts you to define the skeleton for the new specification, then displays it as a Word document.
- Load Specification loads a specification saved as an .s4w file and displays it as a Word document.

- Save Specification saves the current specification as an .s4w file. The option is unavailable ("grayed") until you have a created a new specification; it is discussed later in the chapter.
- Import XML Specification imports an XML file and displays it as a Word document.
- Export XML Specification exports the current specification as an XML file. The option is unavailable ("grayed") until you have created a new specification; it is discussed later in the chapter.

By choosing the New Specification, Load Specification, or Import XML Specification option, you initiate the PASAT workflow, which is described in the subsequent sections.

If you select the New or Open option from the File menu, or click the New or Open toolbar button, the application returns control to Word and your regular Word menus and settings will be in effect.

CREATING NEW SPECIFICATIONS

1. From the File menu, select the New Specification option. The Create New Specification dialog box appears (Figure 7.1).
2. This dialog box includes all sections allowed in a specification by the DTD. The required sections are shown in bold. By default, all required sections are selected.

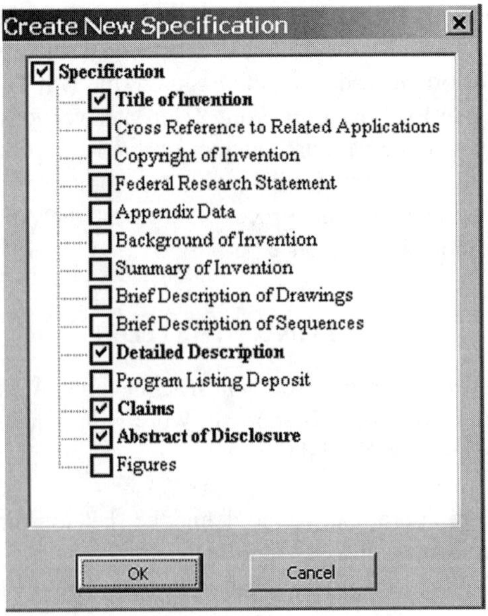

FIGURE 7.1

3. To include a section in the specification select the check box adjacent to its name.
4. When done, click the OK button.
5. The new specification appears in the Word window in the Tags Off mode (looks similar to a regular Word document), ready for editing. The document layout includes the titles of the sections you have selected. Shown below is the screen with tags turned on to demonstrate how PASAT works in the background to insert .xml coding (Figure 7.2).

SPECIFICATION

<specification><spec.title-block> <spec.title> </spec.title>

<spec.version>[Electronic Version 1.2.8] </spec.version>
</spec.title-block> <specification-block>

<title-of-invention>[Insert title of invention]</title-of-invention>

<detailed-description>
<heading>Detailed Description </heading>

</detailed-description><claims>
<heading>Claims </heading>

</claims>
<abstract-of-disclosure>
<heading>Abstract of Disclosure </heading>

</abstract-of-disclosure></specification-block></specification>

FIGURE 7.2

IMPORTING SPECIFICATIONS

1. Select the Import XML Specification option from the File menu, and the Import XML Instance dialog box appears.
2. In the dialog box, locate the XML file you want to import and click the Open button.

If the selected XML instance is valid and conforms to the DTD, it appears in the Word window in the Tags Off mode, ready for editing. If the instance is invalid, the import aborts and a Validation Report message appears. Click the OK button to close the message.

LOADING SPECIFICATIONS

To load a specification that has been saved as an .s4w file:

1. Select the Load Specification option from the File menu, and the Load Specification dialog box appears (this is a standard Windows File Open dialog box).
2. In the dialog box, locate the specification (.s4w file) you want to load and click the Open button.

The selected specification appears in the Word window in the Tags Off mode, ready for editing.

INTERFACE FEATURES

Once you have loaded, imported, or created a new specification, the PASAT features come into play. Some of them are visible in the Word window; some are hidden behind the scenes.

MENUS AND MENU OPTIONS

Although the names of menu bar items remain the same as in Word, some of the menu options are renamed, removed, added, or modified:

File Menu: The added options appear as in PASAT.

Edit Menu: All functions show markup. Paste loads clipboard content (excluding markup); Paste Structure loads markup as well.

View Menu

> **View Tags:** Toggles between the Tags Off and Tags On display modes of the specification.
>
> **View Entities:** Shows/hides entity names.
>
> **View S4/Guide:** Shows/hides the Office Assistant.
>
> **Document Map:** Shows/hides the Specification Map (a tree of the specification sections and elements) at the left-hand side of the Word window.

Insert Menu

> **Symbol:** Displays the dialog box that enables you to insert HTML 4.0 named character entities at the cursor location.
>
> **Picture:** Displays the Figure dialog box that enables you to insert graphics at the cursor location.

Tools Menu

> **Renumber:** Renumbers paragraphs, claims, or both starting from the beginning of the specification.
>
> **Add Sections:** Displays the Edit Specification Sections dialog box, allowing new sections to be added to the specification at any time during the editing process.
>
> **Validate Instance:** Validates the structure of the specification against the DTD and highlights the first error to be corrected.
>
> **Spelling:** Initiates the Batch Mode content spell check feature.

Table Menu: These functions are identical to MS Word Table functions.

TOOLBARS

When you rest your mouse pointer on toolbar buttons, you can view information about them in ScreenTips. These pop-up messages show the function of the toolbar button. Following is a description of the toolbar functions available in PASAT:

Indentation: Claim-text elements support five levels of indentation. The buttons on this toolbar enable management of the claim-text indentation. The indentation mark can be clicked up to five levels.

Shortcut Keys

In applications, a key or key combination used to perform a defined function is called a shortcut key. The following shortcut keys are part of the PASAT interface:

Shortcut	Function
Ctrl+l	Pastes claims or paragraphs
Ctrl+b	Applies bold
Ctrl+c	Copies text and objects
Ctrl+f	Initiates Find and Replace function
Ctrl+o	Opens Microsoft Word document
Ctrl+r	Repeats last Insert Symbol operation
Ctrl+s	Saves specification
Ctrl+t	Toggles tag display mode
Ctrl+v	Paste option
Ctrl+Shift+v	Initiates the Paste Structure function
Ctrl+x	Cut
Ctrl+y	Displays the Symbol Manager dialog box
Ctrl+z	Undo option
Ctrl+--	Applies superscript
Ctrl+ =	Applies subscript
Ctrl+Left Arrow	Moves cursor to next word
Ctrl+Right Arrow	Moves cursor to previous word
Ctrl+Up Arrow	Moves cursor to previous paragraph
Ctrl+Down Arrow	Moves cursor to next paragraph
Fl	Initiates Online Help
F7	Initiates Spell Check
Crtl F5	Renumbers all paragraphs and claims in the specification
Crtl F6	Initiates the Validate Document function
Crtl F7	Initiates the Preview in Browser function
Crtl F8	Exports the specification as XML instance
Crtl+End	Moves cursor to the end of the document
Enter	Splits a paragraph or a claim-text element at the cursor position
Ctrl+Enter	Splits claim or paragraph at the insertion point; in a claim, splits the entire claim where a regular Enter key splits the current claim-text element only; in a paragraph, creates a new paragraph
Home	Moves cursor to the beginning of a line

OFFICE ASSISTANT

When working with PASAT, the familiar Office Assistant feature provides you with context-sensitive PASAT help. To see how the Office Assistant can provide ready help, move the cursor to different headings and see the Office Assistant options change. This is indeed one of the most useful features of PASAT: to remind you of the type of insertion or addition you make to each section.

STATUS BAR

The Status Bar in the top right section of the Word window displays the "ancestry line" of the element the cursor is currently in.

DISABLED MICROSOFT WORD FEATURES

The following Word features are disabled in PASAT in order to facilitate the behind-the-scenes XML activities:

- Allow Accented Uppercase
- AutoCorrect
- AutoFormat
- AutoFormat As You Type
- Automatic Word Selection
- AutoText
- Background Save
- Create Backup Copy
- Drag and Drop Printing
- Fast Save
- Indent Set by Tab Key
- Insert Key for Paste
- Smart Cut and Paste
- Track Changes

The AutoRecover feature is not disabled; however, you should be aware of the fact that the recovered documents will not contain any of the XML markup. They will be regular Word documents. It is therefore a good idea to save the file periodically.

EDITING SPECIFICATIONS

CHANGING TAG AND ENTITY DISPLAY

By default, PASAT files are displayed in the Word window in Tags Off mode (with tags hidden), which makes the specification look like a regular Word document. By default, the entities are displayed as the special characters they represent.

When a table is rendered, the tags of the table elements (row, entry, etc.) are hidden even if the document is in Tags On mode. The tags of the table itself (<table> and </table>) are shown.

If for some reason you want to display the entities embedded in your specification as XML codes, you can do that at any time by turning on this feature from the View menu. If the entities were displayed as special characters, PASAT displays them as codes and vice versa.

USING THE SPECIFICATION MAP

The Specification Map, similar to Document Map in Word, is a tree of the specification sections and elements. It allows you to click on a specification directly without the need to scroll down or up.

MANAGING SELECTIONS

Although not visible in the Tags Off mode, the PASAT specification you are working on is not a single flow of text, titles, tables, figures, etc., but a collection of XML elements such as paragraphs, claims, etc. Each element is wrapped in a pair of tags: the start tag and the end tag. The outcome of a selection operation you perform depends on whether the selection crosses the element boundaries or, in other words, whether it includes any tags.

The possible cases are as follows:

- The part of the specification you highlighted is entirely within a single element. In this case, only the highlighted part is selected, as it would be in Word (without any tags).
- The part of the specification you attempt to highlight includes one or both element tags. In this case, the entire element is selected, together with both tags. The part of the specification you attempt to highlight includes the end tag of one element and the start tag of the other element or, in the other words, crosses the element boundary. When a numbered element (a paragraph or a claim) is selected together with its tags, the number of the element appears highlighted. You can select a numbered element, together with its start and end tags, by double-clicking its number. In the Tags Off mode, to select an unnumbered element together with its tags, extend the selection slightly beyond the visual boundary of the element. In the Tags Off mode, to select a formatted section (bold, superscript, or subscript) together with its tags, position the cursor either immediately before the first character or immediately after the last character of the section and press Shift+Left Arrow or Shift+Right Arrow combination on the keyboard.

MANAGING PARAGRAPHS

Adding Paragraphs

To add a new paragraph to the specification, position the cursor at the required location in the corresponding section. Do one of the following:

- Select Paragraph from the Insert menu.
- Select the Insert New Paragraph option from the Office Assistant.

A new (empty) paragraph appears at the specified location, along with a pair of brackets for the paragraph number (e.g., [*]). The brackets are populated by the Renumber Paragraph operation. You can begin keying the paragraph text.

Splitting Paragraphs

To split a single paragraph into two separate paragraphs, position the cursor at the required split position within the paragraph. Press the Enter key.

- The paragraph formed from the start of the original paragraph to the cursor position retains the original element number
- The paragraph formed from the cursor position to the end of the original paragraph becomes a new element and receives a separate number. This new number does not appear until the Renumber Paragraphs operation is performed. PASAT does not renumber paragraphs automatically after the split. Therefore, the original and the new paragraph have the same number until you perform the Renumber Paragraphs operation.

Pressing the Enter key when the cursor is at the very end of a paragraph (between the last character and the end tag) creates a new paragraph. Pressing the Enter key when the cursor is positioned within a program-listing element adds a hard return to the text just as it would in Word. No element split occurs.

Deleting Paragraphs

To delete an entire paragraph, double-click the paragraph number to select the paragraph. Press the Delete key. The selected paragraph is removed from the specification (together with its number), as well as from the Specification Map. You cannot delete all paragraphs in a section. You may insert a correct paragraph and then go back and delete the incorrect paragraph, or you may delete the section in its entirety and reenter the text.

Renumbering Paragraphs

As a result of adding, deleting, and splitting operations, the paragraph numbers may be out of sequence: [0001] may come after [0003], [0012] may come between [0007] and [0004], etc. Use the following path to renumber paragraphs in a sequential manner, starting from the beginning of the specification: Tools/Renumber/Paragraphs.

MANAGING CLAIMS

Claims have hierarchical structure. The main element in the hierarchy is the claim itself. It is represented by a number and can be referenced from other claims or paragraphs. Under the claim, an unlimited number of claim-text elements can be created. These elements have no numbers and cannot be referenced. The claim-text elements support up to five indentation levels, each of which corresponds to the position in the claim hierarchy.

Adding Claims

Position the cursor at the required location in the Claims section. Select the Insert New Claim option from the Office Assistant. A pair of brackets for the claim number appears at the specified location ([c*]). Claim numbers are inserted by the Renumber Claims operation. You can begin keying the text of the claim.

Adding Claim-Text Elements

Position the cursor at the required location within a claim and do one of the following:

- Select the Claim-text option from the Insert menu.
- Select the Insert New Claim-text option from the Office Assistant.

The cursor moves to the next line. You can begin keying the text.

Indenting Claim-Text Elements

In Tags Off mode, claim-text elements appear as text sections separated by line breaks. Each of these sections can be positioned at one of the five available levels of indentation. Position the cursor anywhere within the required element. Click the Increase Indent or Decrease Indent button on the toolbar. With each click of the toolbar button, the indentation of the selected claim-text element increases or decreases, respectively.

Splitting Claim-Text Elements

Position the cursor at the required split location within the claim-text element. Press the Enter key. The claim-text element splits into two elements at the cursor location. They both stay at the indentation level of the original element.

Deleting Claim-Text Elements

Highlight the claim-text element together with its tags (for details, see Managing Selections). Press the Delete key. The selected claim-text element is deleted. You cannot delete all claim-text elements in a section. You may insert a correct claim-text and then go back and delete the incorrect claim-text or you may delete the section in its entirety and reenter the text.

Splitting Claims

Position the cursor at the required split location within the claim. Press Ctrl+Enter. The claim splits into two claims at the cursor location:

- The claim formed from the start of the original claim to the cursor position retains the original element number.
- The claim formed from the cursor position to the end of the original claim becomes a new element and receives a separate number. This new number appears when the Renumber Claims operation is performed.

Deleting Claims

Double-click the claim number to select the claim. Press the Delete key. The selected claim is removed from the specification (together with its number), as well as from the Specification Map. In accordance with the DTD, the last claim in a section cannot be deleted; you can, however, delete its content.

Renumbering Claims

As a result of adding, deleting, and splitting operations, the claim numbers may be out of sequence: [cl] may come after [c3], [c12] may come between [c7] and [c4], etc. Use the following path to renumber claims in a sequential manner, starting from the beginning of the specification: Tools/Renumber/Claims.

MANAGING CLAIM DEPENDENCIES

Creating Claim Dependency References

1. Do one of the following:
   - Position the cursor at a location from which you want to reference a claim dependency.
   - Select a section of text (without tags).
2. Do one of the following:
   - Select the Dependent Claim Reference option from the Insert menu.
   - Select the Insert Dependent Claim Reference option from the Office Assistant.
3. Highlight the required claim on the list and click the OK button.
4. Optionally, type relevant text (such as "Refer to..."). The text you type inside the dependent claim reference element is underlined in blue; when the specification is viewed as an XML instance, the references are rendered as hyperlinks.

Redefining Reference Targets

1. Position the cursor anywhere within the text of the required claim dependency reference (underlined in blue).
2. Select the Edit Dependent Claim Reference option from the Office Assistant, and the Modify Dependent Claim Reference Target dialog box appears.
3. Proceed as described in the Creating Claim Dependency References section.

Behind the scenes, PASAT changes the value of the "target" attribute of the dependent claim reference element.

Deleting Claim Dependency References

1. Select the reference to be deleted (the text underlined in blue together with the corresponding tags).
2. Press the Delete key. The selected reference is deleted (both the element and the text).

Formatting Text

PASAT supports three formatting options: bold, superscript, and subscript. These options work similarly to their Microsoft Word counterparts. You can superimpose format options (e.g., bold a superscript section). You can remove a format only from the entire formatted section, not from its parts. To remove a format, position the cursor anywhere within the formatted section. Do one of the following:

- On the Format toolbar, click the button that appears active.
- Press the corresponding shortcut key(s) on the keyboard.

It might happen that, as a result of the above operation, the format appears to have been removed from only part of the section. This means that you encountered a series of two or more contiguous, similarly formatted sections. In the Tags Off mode, they look like a single formatted section (Text 1 Text 2). Position the cursor within the part that remains formatted and repeat the operation.

Copy, Cut, and Paste

The Copy operation copies a selection to the clipboard and leaves the original information in place. If the copied selection includes tags, this operation copies markup along with the content.

The Cut operation copies a selection to the clipboard and deletes it from its original location. If the selection includes tags, this operation cuts markup along with the content. To copy a selection to the clipboard and delete it from its original location, select the section to be cut. Do one of the following: select the Cut option from the Edit menu, or click the Cut button on the toolbar, or press Ctrl+x on the keyboard.

The Paste operation copies clipboard content to the cursor position in the specification. Content without markup is pasted as plain content. Content that includes markup is pasted as marked-up content. PASAT supports replacement of a selection with the clipboard content only if neither the selection nor the clipboard content include markup. To paste the clipboard content, position the cursor at the location where you want the content to be pasted. Do one of the following:

- Select Paste from the Edit menu.
- Click the Paste button on the Edit toolbar.
- Press Ctrl+v on the keyboard.

After applying any of these Paste methods, the clipboard content appears at the cursor location in the specification.

If the clipboard contains characters (symbols) not supported by PASAT, they are replaced in the specification by the Unknown Symbol tags. You can delete the signs and replace them with the PASAT-supported symbols. For the replacement procedure, see Replacing Unknown Symbols.

Paste Paragraphs

The Paste Paragraphs operation pastes text sections as paragraphs. This operation is enabled if paragraphs are allowed at the current cursor position. When pasting text copied from a nonstructured document (e.g., from a regular Word file), all text formatting (bold, italics, etc.) is lost. To paste the clipboard content as multiple paragraphs:

1. Copy a section of text to the clipboard.
2. Position the cursor at the location where you want the clipboard content to be pasted.
3. Select the Paste Paragraphs option from the Edit menu. The text from the clipboard is now pasted at the specified location.

Paste Claims

The Paste Claims operation pastes text sections as multiple claims. The text is split based on hard returns. This operation is enabled only in the Claims section. When pasting text copied from a nonstructured document (e.g., from a regular Word file), italics formatting is converted to bold. To paste the clipboard content as multiple claims:

1. Copy a section of text to the clipboard.
2. Position the cursor at the location where you want the clipboard content to be pasted.

3. Select the Paste Claim(s) option from the Edit menu. The text from the clipboard is now pasted at the specified location as multiple claims. The text is split into claims at hard returns.
4. Use the following path to renumber the new claims: Edit/Renumber/Claims.

REMOVING DOUBLE EMPHASIS TAGS

Text that is formatted as both bold and italics will result in double <emphasis> tags when pasted into PASAT. This double tagging scenario causes a validation error and the Validation Report window appears (Figure 7.3). To correct the error:

1. Click the OK button to close the Validation Report window.
2. Click the Tag button to view tags.
   Example: <emphasis><emphasis>**Bold   and   Italic   text**</emphasis></emphasis>
3. Select and cut the text within the tags.
   Result: <emphasis><emphasis></emphasis></emphasis>
4. Paste the text between the <emphasis> tags.
   Result: <emphasis>**Bold and Italic text**<emphasis></emphasis></emphasis>
5. Select and delete the <emphasis></emphasis> tags following the moved text.
   Result: <emphasis>**Bold and Italic text**</emphasis>

Validation Report	[X]
Element 'emphasis' not allowed in the current position. Possible missing tag before or illegal element.	
OK	

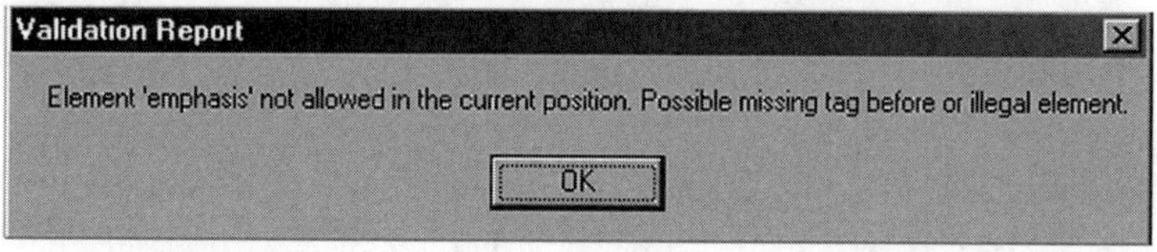

FIGURE 7.3

NONBREAKING SPACES AND HYPHENS

Nonbreaking spaces and nonbreaking hyphens do not translate in PASAT. When these characters are used in Word source documents and pasted into PASAT, the text string after the nonbreaking character is lost.

For example, the degree-like symbol between "winter" and "night" in Figure 7.4 represents a nonbreaking space, and the long dash between "half" and "past" represents a nonbreaking hyphen. In word processing programs, the nonbreaking characters will cause the words around them to be treated as a single word. When this sentence is pasted into PASAT, the text strings of "night" and "past" are lost and the result is "One winter, at half nine." To correct the problem in a Word document, you must replace all nonbreaking spaces with normal spaces, and all nonbreaking hyphens with normal hyphens.

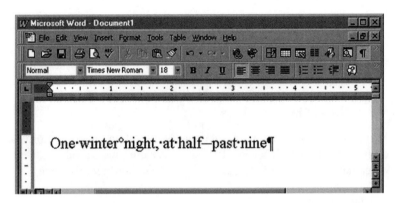

FIGURE 7.4

FIGURE 7.5

To replace nonbreaking spaces with normal spaces in Word:

1. Press Ctrl+H. The Find and Replace dialog box appears.
2. In the Find what field, enter a Shift 6 (^) and a lowercase s.
3. In the Replace with field, enter a space (Figure 7.5).
4. Click the Replace All button.

To replace nonbreaking hyphens with normal hyphens in Word:

1. Press Ctrl+H. The Find and Replace dialog box appears.
2. In the Find what field, enter a Shift 6 (^) and a ~ (you will find this character to the left of the number 1 key).
3. In the Replace with field, enter a hyphen (Figure 7.6).
4. Click the Replace All button.

Tip: You can use the Special button at the bottom of the Find and Replace dialog box to insert the codes for the special characters instead of entering them manually.

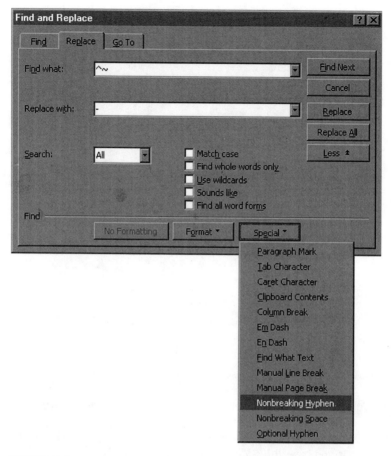

FIGURE 7.6

Smart Quotes, Apostrophes, Fractions, and Double Hyphens

Smart quotes are "curly" quotation marks (different than unidirectional "straight" quotes). Smart quotes and apostrophes do not translate in PASAT. To work with smart quotes in Word, use the following path:

1. Tools menu
2. AutoCorrect submenu
3. AutoFormat As You Type tab
4. Replace as you type group box
5. "Straight quotes" with "smart quotes" checkbox (Figure 7.7; note that the option is not selected in the figure)

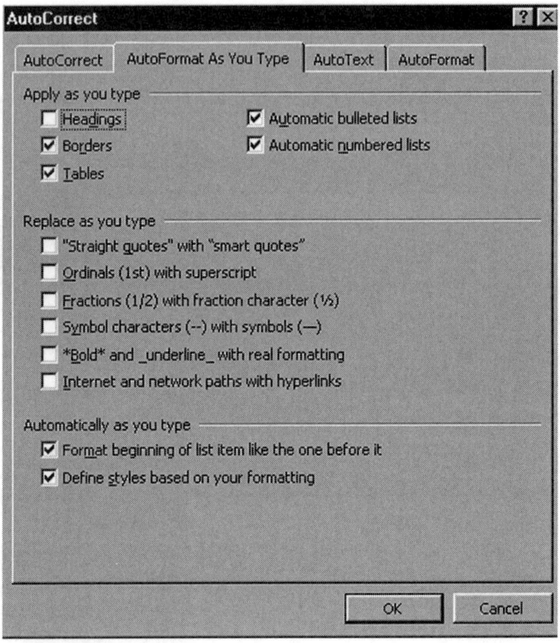

FIGURE 7.7

This AutoCorrect feature causes the following translation issues:

- Smart quotes get lost therefore if you have *"Title of Book"* it will translate to: *Title of a Book*
- With smart quotes on, apostrophes translates to straight quotes, for example: If you have *Bill's bike* it translates to: *Bill's bike*
- With the option that double hyphens (--) becomes an em dash (—), the dash will not translate at all.
- With the option to convert fractions, the space after the converted fraction may be lost: The phrase "*1/2 of the*" becomes "*1/2of the*"

The behavior is a little different between Word 97 and Word 2000 (in Word 2000 the smart quotes translate).

To correct the problem in a Word document, you must disable these features by making sure the AutoCorrect options are not selected (no check in the checkbox). Then replace the smart quotes with normal quotes and the em dashes with normal hyphens:

1. Press Ctrl+H. The Find and Replace dialog box appears.
2. In the Find what field, enter ".
3. In the Replace with field, enter ".
4. Click the Replace All button.
5. In the Find what field, enter Shift 6 (^) and +.

6. In the Replace with field, enter – (hyphen).
7. Click the Replace All button.

Tip: You can use the Special button at the bottom of the Find and Replace dialog box to insert the codes for the special characters instead of entering them manually.

REVERSING OPERATIONS

The Undo operation in PASAT can reverse the following operations (up to six):

- Insertion of text
- Deletion of content
- Cutting and pasting (except for Paste Paragraphs and Paste Claims)
- Formatting text
- Splitting paragraphs

To reverse the last operation on the Undo list, do one of the following:

- Select the Undo option from the Edit menu.
- Press Ctrl+z.

MANAGING COMPLEX WORK UNITS

PASAT recognizes the following Complex Work Units (CWU):

- **Table-CWU:** A Microsoft Word table or a scanned table in a TIFF file
- **Math-CWU:** A math formula in a TIFF file, inserted inline
- **Chemistry-CWU:** A chemical formula in a TIFF file, inserted inline

To insert a Math- or Chemistry-CWU, do the following:

1. Position the cursor in the required location.
2. Select the appropriate option from the Insert menu or select the corresponding option from the Office Assistant. The File Open dialog box appears with a TIFF default extension.
3. Select the required file.
4. Click the OK button. The selected graphic now appears at the specified location.

To insert a Table-CWU, do the following:

1. Position the cursor in the required location.
2. Do one of the following:
   Select the Table-CWU option from the Insert menu.
   Select the corresponding option from the Office Assistant.
   Select the Insert Table option from the Table menu.
3. The Insert Table dialog box appears. Do one of the following:

To insert a Word table, type the required number of rows and columns in the corresponding fields and click the OK button. Behind the scenes, PASAT inserts the required XML table elements at the specified position.

To insert a scanned table in a TIFF file, click the Browse button, select the file, and click the OK button. The table now appears at the specified location.

To delete a CWU:

1. Double-click the required CWU element in the specification.
2. Press the Delete key. The selected CWU is deleted.

Converting Equations, Formulae, Symbols, and Tables to TIFF Images

To convert mathematical equations, chemical formulae, symbols, or tables that were created in Word to TIFF files to be pasted into PASAT, do the following:

1. Open the Word file and copy the equation, formula, symbol, or table (Figure 7.8).
2. Go to the Start Menu and open the Microsoft Windows Paint utility using the following path: Programs/Accessories/Paint.
3. Select Attributes from the Image menu.
4. Size the image using the Width and Height fields. Choose the appropriate unit of measure.
5. Set the Colors to Black and White (Figure 7.9).
6. Click OK. Your drawing area will be reduced to a small white square in the upper left corner of the workspace.
7. Click the small white square.
8. Paste the equation, formula, symbol, or table you created in Word to the white square (by selecting Paste from the Edit menu, or by right clicking your mouse and selecting Paste from the popup menu, or by pressing Ctrl+V). If the area on the square is too small to accommodate the object, a dialog box will ask you if you would like to resize it. Click the Yes button; Paint will resize the image to accommodate your CWU.
9. From the File menu, select Save As and name your newly created CWU.
10. From the File menu, select New or Exit.

The complex work unit you have created has been saved as a bitmap. To convert the bitmap to a TIFF image, do the following:

1. Go to the Start Menu and open the Microsoft Windows Imaging utility using the following path: Programs/Accessories/Imaging. The reader should consult equivalent actions in Windows XP.
2. From the File menu, select Open.
3. In the File of Type list, select bitmap.

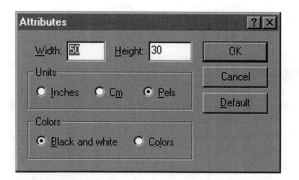

FIGURE 7.8

FIGURE 7.9

4. Open your newly created CWU bitmap (Figure 7.10).
5. From the File menu, select Save As.
6. Select TIFF file from the Save as type list.
7. Type in the CWU name with the TIFF extension, e.g., equation1TIFF.
8. From the Page menu, select Convert or Properties (this will depend on the version of Imaging that you have).
9. Change the Color to Black and White, if necessary.
10. From the Resolution tab, select 300×300 dpi from the drop list and select the OK button.
11. On the Compression tab, select CCITT Group 4 (2d) Fax and click on the OK button.
12. From the File menu, select Save.

This image of your CWU can be entered in the PASAT authoring tool using the Office Assistant's list of Insert Complex Work Unit options.

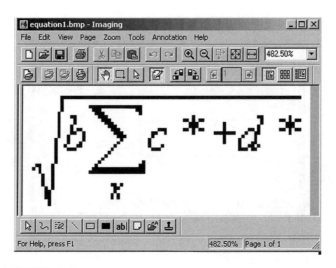

FIGURE 7.10

To create a custom character TIFF image:

1. Open the Windows Paint utility.
   a. From the Image menu, select Attributes.
   b. Size the image at 0.30×0.30 inches.
   c. Select the Black and White options from the Colors group box.
   d. Click the OK button.
   e. Select the text tool from the toolbox (the button with an A on it).
   f. Click the cursor on the workspace of the image.
   g. From the View menu, select Text Toolbar.
2. Select the Font that has the Symbol that you want to use. For example, Math Ext includes many mathematical symbols, Symbol includes the Greek alphabet, and Lucida Sans Unicode include many of the unicode character sets.

   Choose a font size to match your document text; 12 point is recommended.

   Click the cursor again on your screen. In the gray box, type or paste the character that you want. Modify the character as desired using the other functions available from the Paint utility (Figure 7.11).

   If needed, crop the image by using the image attributes.

   From the File menu, select Save As and name your newly created custom character.

   From the File menu, select New or Exit.

The custom character you have created has been saved as a bitmap. To convert the bitmap to a TIFF image, follow the instructions given earlier. This tiny image of your custom symbol can be entered in the PASAT authoring tool from the Custom Character tab of the Symbols tool.

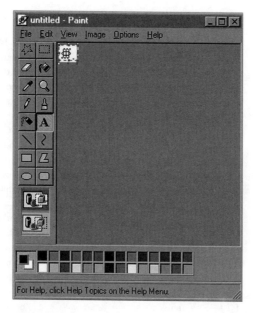

FIGURE 7.11

CHANGING THE BROWSER DISPLAY FONT

If you have a problem viewing the following supported special characters in Internet Explorer, you will need to change the default font.

Although many fonts comply with the Unicode specification, a font may not include a glyph (picture) to display a particular character in this table. This does not mean that content is lost.

1. From the Tools menu in Internet Explorer, select Internet Options.
2. On the General tab, click the Fonts button.
3. In the Language script list box, select Latin based.
4. Select Lucida Sans Unicode for the Web page font.
5. Select Lucida Console for the Plain text font.
6. Click OK to close the Fonts dialog box.
7. Click OK to close Internet Options.

Entity Name	Character	Entity Name	Character	Entity Name	Character
apos	'	pound	£	iexcl	¡
cent	¢	brvbar	¦	curren	¤
yen	¥	copy	©	sect	§
uml	¨	not	¬	ordf	ª
laquo	«	macr	¯	deg	°
reg	®	sup2	²	sup3	³
plusmn	±	micro	µ	para	¶
acute	´	cedil	¸	sup1	¹

(continued)

Entity Name	Character	Entity Name	Character	Entity Name	Character
midddot	·	raquo	»	frac14	¼
ordm	º	frac34	¾	iquest	¿
frac12	½	Aacute	Á	Acirc	Â
Agrave	À	Auml	Ä	Aring	Å
Atilde	Ã	Ccedil	Ç	Egrave	È
AElig	Æ	Ecirc	Ê	Euml	Ë
Eacute	É	Iacute	Í	Icirc	Î
Igrave	Ì	ETH	Ð	Ntilde	Ñ
Iuml	Ï	Oacute	Ó	Ocirc	Ô
Ograve	Ò	Ouml	Ö	times	×
Otilde	Õ	Ugrave	Ù	Uacute	Ú
Oslash	Ø	Uuml	Ü	Yacute	Ý
Ucirc	Û	szlig	ß	agrave	à
THORN	Þ	acirc	â	atilde	ã
aacute	á	aring	å	aelig	æ
auml	ä	egrave	è	eacute	é
ccedil	ç	euml	ë	igrave	ì
ecirc	ê	icirc	î	iuml	ï
iacute	í	ntilde	ñ	ograve	ò
eth	ð	ocirc	ô	otilde	õ
oacute	ó	divide	÷	oslash	ø
ouml	ö	uacute	ú	ucirc	û
ugrave	ù	yacute	ý	thorn	þ
uuml	ü	fnof	ƒ	Alpha	Α
yuml	ÿ	Gamma	Γ	Delta	Δ
Beta	Β	Zeta	Ζ	Eta	Η
Epsilon	Ε	Iota	Ι	Kappa	Κ
Theta	Θ	Mu	Μ	Nu	Ν
Lambda	Λ	Omicron	Ο	Pi	Π
Xi	Ξ	Sigma	Σ	Tau	Τ
Rho	Ρ	Phi	Φ	Chi	Χ
Upsilon	Υ	Omega	Ω	alpha	α
Psi	Ψ	gamma	γ	delta	δ
beta	β	zeta	ζ	eta	η
epsilon	ε	iota	ι	kappa	κ
theta	θ	mu	μ	nu	ν
lambda	λ	omicron	ο	pi	π
xi	ξ	sigmaf	ς	sigma	σ
rho	ρ	upsilon	υ	phi	φ
tau	τ	psi	ψ	omega	ω
chi	χ	upsih	ϒ	piv	ϖ

(continued)

Entity Name	Character	Entity Name	Character	Entity Name	Character
thetasym	€	hellip	…	prime	′
bull	•	oline	‾	frasl	/
Prime	″	image	ℑ	real	ℜ
weierp	℘	alefsym	ℵ	larr	←
trade	™	rarr	→	darr	↓
uarr	↑	crarr	↵	lArr	⇐
harr	↔	bdquo	„	permil	‰
uArr	⇑	empty	∅	dArr	⇓
prod	∏	notin	∉	part	∂
lowast	∗	sum	∑	minus	−
infin	∞	radic	√	ne	≠
int	∫	cap	∩	ge	≥
cong	≅	asymp	≈	sdot	·
equiv	≡	le	≤	lfloor	⌊
otimes	⊗	rceil	⌉	spades	™
lceil	⌈	loz	◊	diams	◆
rfloor	⌋	hearts	♥	Scaron	Š
clubs	♣	oelig	œ	circ	^
OElig	Œ	Yuml	Ÿ	ndash	–
scaron	š	lsquo	'	rsquo	'
tilde	˜	ldquo	"	rdquo	"
mdash	—	dagger	†	Dagger	‡
sbquo	'	lsaquo	‹	rsaquo	›

Managing Tables

You perform most of the table management operations the same way you would perform them in Word. Behind the scenes, PASAT inserts or deletes the appropriate XML elements so that the validity of the table structure is always preserved.

Managing Figures

The only allowed format for the figures is TIFF (not compressed). Once inserted, figures cannot be resized. The MS Word Graphic toolbox is disabled. All figure management operations are performed in the Figures dialog box. To display the dialog box, do one of the following:

- Select the Insert Figures option from the Office Assistant.
- Select the Picture option from the Insert menu. The Figures dialog box appears (Figure 7.12).

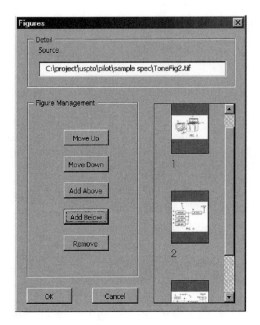

FIGURE 7.12

The dialog box layout is as follows:

- The right-hand pane displays the figures that are already in the specification (if any), in the order in which they appear in the Figures section.
- The Source field (across the top) shows the path and name of the source file for the figure selected in the right-hand section.
- The left-hand pane offers a series of buttons (Move Up, Move Down, Add Above, Add Below, Remove) that perform the corresponding operation on the figure selected in the right-hand section.
- The OK and Cancel buttons at the bottom are used to accept/reject the changes you have made to the Figures section and to close the dialog box

Adding Figures

1. If there are figures displayed in the right-hand pane of the Figures dialog box, highlight the figure adjacent to where you want to insert the new figure.
2. Click the Add Below or Add Above button. The Image File dialog box appears with a default TIFF extension.
3. Select the required file and click the OK button. The selected graphic appears at the specified location in the right-hand pane of the Figures dialog box. The Figures dialog box closes. The new figure is inserted at the specified location in the Figures section of the specification.

Reordering Figures

1. Highlight the figure to be moved in the right-hand pane of the Figures dialog box.
2. Click the Move Up or Move Down button. Each click moves the highlighted figure one position up or down on the list, respectively.
3. When satisfied with the new order, click the OK button. The Figures dialog box closes. The figures in the Figures section appear in the new order.

Removing Figures

1. Highlight the figure to be removed in the right-hand pane of the Figures dialog box.
2. Click the Remove button. The figure is removed from the right-hand pane.
3. Click the OK button. The Figure dialog box closes. The selected figure is removed from the Figures section of the specification.

MANAGING SPECIAL CHARACTERS

PASAT supports special characters defined by ISO 8859-1 (HTML 4.0 named character entities). It also enables the use of custom characters, which should be drawn or scanned and saved as TIFF files.

The special character management activities include:

- Insert
- Search and replace unknown symbols
- Delete

Inserting Custom Characters

1. Position the cursor at the insertion point.
2. Select the Symbol option from the Insert menu. The Symbol dialog box appears.
3. Click the Custom Character tab. The Custom Character page appears.
4. Click the Add button. The Browse for Graphic dialog box appears. This is a standard Windows File Open dialog box.
5. Select the TIFF file you want to use as a custom character and click the Open button. The image contained in the selected file appears on the central panel of the Custom Character page.
6. Highlight the image. The path and name of the corresponding file appear in the Source field.
7. Click the Insert button. The selected image is inserted at the cursor location as a custom character.

Replacing Unknown Symbols

As a result of pasting sections copied from non-PASAT documents, your specification may contain unknown symbols, marked in the text by the Unknown Symbol tag. To replace the unknown symbols with the appropriate special characters:

1. Display the Insert Symbol dialog box.
2. Click the Next Unknown button. The first Unknown Symbol sign in the specification is highlighted.
3. Select the special character or specify the custom character to replace the unknown symbol. For procedure, see Inserting Custom Characters.
4. Repeat Steps 2 and 3 for each unknown symbol.

Deleting Special Characters

1. Highlight the required character in the specification.
2. Press the Delete key. The selected special character is deleted from the specification.

ENTERING BIOLOGICAL DEPOSIT DATA

The Biological Deposit Data is an optional element of the Detailed Description section.

1. Position the cursor anywhere in the Detailed Description title.
2. Select the Insert Biological Deposit Data option from the Office Assistant. The Biological Deposit Data title appears in the specification.
3. Select the Insert Biological Deposit option from the Office Assistant. The Enter Biological Deposit Data dialog box appears. Enter Biological Deposit Data.
4. Fill out the dialog box fields.
5. Click the OK button. The dialog box closes. The data you have entered appears in the specification under the Biological Deposit Data title in a predefined layout.

SPELL CHECK

As in Microsoft Word, you can spell check your specification in real-time and batch modes. In both modes, PASAT uses all custom dictionaries selected in the Word Options dialog box.

Spell Check in Real-Time

As in Word documents, the misspelled words in the specification are underlined in red.

1. Right-click anywhere in the underlined word.
2. Select the correct spelling option from the popup list. The misspelled word is replaced with the word you chose from the list.

Spell Check in Batch Mode

Select the Check Spelling option from the Tools menu. The Content Spelling dialog box appears. The layout and functionality of this dialog box are very similar to those of the Word Spelling and Grammar dialog box. The PASAT spell-checker deals only with the spelling of individual words. It does not check grammatical structures.

The AutoCorrect, Options and Undo buttons are disabled.

FINDING AND REPLACING CONTENT

As in Word, PASAT enables you to search for words and phrases and automatically replace them with other words and phrases. The specialty of PASAT is that its Search and Replace capabilities pertain only to the content of the displayed instance, not to the markup it may include.

VALIDATING AND PREVIEWING SPECIFICATIONS

Before you export a specification to an .xml file, it is strongly recommended that you validate its structure and correct all errors revealed by the validation process. You may want also to preview the specification in the Internet browser window, to get a clear idea of how it is going to look as a rendered XML instance.

VALIDATE SPECIFICATION

1. Select the Validate Structure option from the Tools menu. PASAT starts the validation process from the beginning of the document. When it encounters a structural error, an error message appears (Figure 7.13). The section that caused the error is highlighted in the specification.
2. Click the OK button.
3. Correct the highlighted error.
4. Repeat Steps 1 through 3 until the "Instance is Valid" message appears. Your specification is now XML-valid and is ready to be exported as an XML instance.

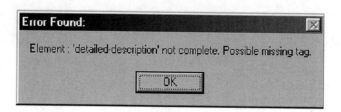

FIGURE 7.13

PREVIEWING SPECIFICATIONS

1. Select the Preview in Browser option from the File menu. Your Internet browser is launched. The specification appears in the browser window as an XML instance.
2. Check the appearance of your specification.
3. To return to the specification in PASAT, close the browser window.

SAVING AND EXPORTING SPECIFICATIONS

The Export XML Specification operation saves specifications in the XML format for submission to the USPTO. The Save Specification operation saves specifications in the PASAT format (.s4w and .s4t). Note that it does not generate the .xml file required by the USPTO. There are two main reasons for storing a specification as a .s4w and .s4t couple as long as you are working on it:

1. An XML-invalid .s4w file can be loaded for further editing in PASAT; an invalid XML instance cannot be imported.
2. Loading an .s4w file is a much faster process than importing an .xml file.

SAVING SPECIFICATIONS

1. Do one of the following:
   Select the Save Specification option from the File menu.
   Click the Save Specification button on the toolbar.
2. If this is the first time you are saving the specification, the Save Specification dialog box appears. This is a standard Windows Save File dialog box.
3. In the dialog box, specify the path and the file name for the .s4w file.
4. Click the Save button.

Specifications are not validated in Save. Each consecutive Save Specification operation updates both the .s4w and .s4t files. Always keep .s4w files and the corresponding .s4t files in the same directory. Do not open .s4w and .s4t files in any editor other than PASAT (this will corrupt the specification).

EXPORTING SPECIFICATIONS

1. Do one of the following:
   Select the Export XML Specification option from the File menu.
   Click the Export XML Specification button on the toolbar. The Export Specification dialog box appears. This is a standard Windows Save File dialog box.
2. In the dialog box, specify the path and the file name for the .xml file to which you want to export the specification.
3. Click the Save button.

If the specification is valid (conforms to the DTD), it is saved at the specified location with the specified name as an XML instance, ready for submission to the USPTO. If the specification is invalid, the appropriate warning appears.

8 USPTO TSA

INTRODUCTION

In addition to the PASAT system for Microsoft® Word, a program to work with Corel® WordPerfect also is available to author electronic versions of the specification, called Template for Specification Authoring. You will need to install the Visual Basic for Applications (VBA) component as part of the WordPerfect Office 2000 setup when using the USPTO-provided WordPerfect XML Template. To see if Visual Basic for Applications has already been installed as part of the WordPerfect Office 2000 setup, open WordPerfect and select the Tools menu. If Visual Basic is unavailable ("grayed"), you will need to run the WordPerfect setup again. Follow the setup procedure given in your WordPerfect software to install Visual Basic. If Visual Basic is available, go to the Macro Setup section to continue installation.

Macro Setup

1. Launch WordPerfect.
2. From the main menu, select Tools, then Visual Basic Editor.
3. In the Project Explorer window, highlight Global Macros. If the Project Explorer window does not appear by default, select View, then Project Explorer from the menu.
4. From the File menu, select Import File.
5. Navigate to the USPTO\WordPerfect Authoring Tool\Version 1.2.5 directory and select TiffInfo.bas to import this file.
6. You should now see this file listed under Global Macros in the Project Explorer window.
7. From the File menu, select References.
8. In the references dialog box, use the navigation arrows to find Microsoft XML,* check the box, then click OK.
9. Be sure Global Macros appears in the References window.
10. In the Visual Basic Editor, click Save.
11. Close the Visual Basic Editor.
12. Copy the file "tiffdll.dll" from the CAProgram Files\USPTO\WordPerfect Authoring Tool\Version 1.2.5 directory to C:\Winnt\System 32 (for Windows NT operating systems) or C:\Windows\System (for Windows 95 and 98 operating systems).

---

* There are many versions of the Microsoft XML DLL 2.0; select whichever version is installed on your machine (this file is installed as part of Internet Explorer 5.0 and above). If there is no Microsoft XML listed, use the Browse button to navigate to the C:\Winnt\System32 directory (on Windows NT workstations) or C:\Windows\System (for Windows 95 and 98 operating systems) and search for msxml.dll.

Setup is now complete. You may optionally copy the shortcut from the C:\Program Files\USPTO\WordPerfect Authoring Tool\Version 1.2.5 directory to the desktop.

TEMPLATE SETUP PROCEDURES

After installing WordPerfect and any provided USPTO files, you must complete the following steps to ensure that all EFS customizations are available as you proceed through the authoring process.

1. Open WordPerfect 9.0.
2. From the Tools menu, select Settings. The Settings window opens.
3. Double-click the Files icon, the File Settings Window opens. If you have installed a previous version of the template, you must set the following options with the new path and file for the settings to become active.
4. Click the Template tab (Files Settings Window: Template Tab)
5. Set the Default template folder to C:\Program Files\USPTO\WordPerfect Authoring Tool\Version 1.2.5\Template\EFS.
6. Set the default template to C:\Program Files\Corel\WordPerfect Office Templates\wp9US.wpt.
7. Leave the Additional template folder as C:\Program Files\Corel\WordPerfect Office 2000\Template\Custom WP Templates.
8. Clear the Update default template option.
9. Select the Update Favorites with changes option.
10. Click the Apply button.
11. Click on the Merge/Macro tab at the top of the window (Files Settings Window: Merge/Macro Tab).
12. Set the Supplemental macro folder to C:\Program Files\USPTO\WordPerfectAuthoring Tool\Version 1.2.5\Macros.
13. Click the Apply button.
14. Click the Document tab.
15. Set the Default save file format by clicking the down arrow and selecting WordPerfect 6/7/8/9 from the drop list.
16. At the bottom of the window, select the On Save, keep document's original file format option.
17. Click the Apply button.
18. Click XML.
19. At the bottom of the window, clear the Use XML/SGML as default option.
20. Click the _Apply button.
21. Click the OK button. The Settings window will appear.
22. Click the _Close button.
23. From the _File menu, select New from Project (select EFS from the Create New tab).
24. On the Create New tab, click the Options button and select Refresh Projects from the list.
25. Click OK to proceed.

26. Click on EFS in the drop-down menu. If EFS does not appear in the list, repeat Step 5, then repeat Steps 22–26.
27. Select Specification 1_2_5 from the window and click on the Create button. (Select Specification l_1.) If the macro warning appears, click the NO button.
28. The Specification document opens.
29. Wait for an Initialization window to appear (Macro Warning). Click OK.
30. Turn off the Attribute Prompt:
    a. Select Insert from the menu.
    b. Select Elements.
    c. Select Options and make sure "Never Prompt for Attributes" is selected (ensure that Never Prompt for Attributes is selected).
    d. Make sure the Auto-Insert option is selected (ensure that Auto-Insert is selected).
    e. Close the Elements box.
31. Select the default Image Style:
    a. From the Format menu, select Graphics Styles. The Graphic Styles window appears (Format Graphic Styles).
    b. Verify that Image is highlighted.

OVERVIEW OF WORDPERFECT XML TEMPLATE

The primary difference between using WordPerfect with XML to author a specification and using a common word processing program is that the specification structured document is designed using Extensible Markup Language (XML). XML uses markup codes, called tags, to categorize parts of a document. The USPTO uses these codes to electronically process the information you submit. Keep your document open as a visual reference while you read the following chapter.

THE TEMPLATE ENVIRONMENT

- If you have not already done so, launch WordPerfect 9.2. Select _File, and New From Project.
- Select the Create New tab.
- Select EFS as the project and double-click on specification 1_2_ 5. If a macro warning box appears, click the NO button.
- Click OK to initialize the template macros.
- The template environment is composed of three sections: a document window on the right; the XML Tree on the left; and customized toolbars and menus at the top. The Document Window on the right displays the text and XML tags. The template provides headings based on MPEP (*Manual of Patent Examining Procedure*) recommendations as well as placeholder tags and text for guidance. Some tags will be indicated by bracketed labels. For example, a paragraph will be indicated by "[p]."

During the authoring process, numbers will be added to these labels for differentiation.

The XML Tree on the left corresponds to the XML tags in the template. For example, Title of Invention on the left corresponds to Title of Invention on the right. Use the XML Tree to navigate quickly through the document. The blue triangle in the XML Tree indicates the position of the cursor in the Document Window. The yellow triangle indicates an authoring error.

EFS TOOLBARS

The toolbars at the top of the screen provide shortcut icons and an XML drop-down list for common tags while authoring. The USPTO has created a custom toolbar to assist you in inserting elements into the specification.

KEYBOARD SHORTCUTS

In addition to toolbar icons, the WordPerfect XML Template also provides keyboard shortcuts for common actions while authoring. Following is a list of keyboard shortcuts for quick reference.

Insert Application Reference	Alt+Ctrl+a
Insert Artwork	Alt+a
Insert Chemistry CWU	Alt+y
Insert Claim	Alt+c
Insert Claim Text	Alt+Shift+C
Insert Claim Dependency	Alt+Ctrl+d
Go to Cross-reference	F3
Insert Cross-reference to CWU	Ctrl+Shift+C
Show Current Element	F7
Go to Previous Element	F9
Go to Next Element	F10
Split Current Element	Alt+Shift+S
Insert List	Alt+l (ell, not one)
Insert List Item	Alt+Shift+L
Insert Math CWU	Alt+m
Open File	Ctrl+o
Insert Paragraph	Alt+p
Insert Patent Reference	Alt+Ctrl+p
Save	Ctrl+s

Save As	F3
Insert Section	Alt+s
Insert Table CWU	Alt+t
Insert Table	Alt+Ctrl+t
Insert Superscript	Alt+keypad 8
Insert Subscript	Alt+keypad 2
Validate	Alt+v
QuickFind Next	Alt+Ctrl+n
Insert Artwork	Alt+Shift+A
Insert Table CWU	Alt+Shift+T

OVERVIEW OF EFS TAGGING

The Display Codes View

In addition to using the XML Tree to view and navigate through the elements in your document, you can use the Display Codes view. When the Display Codes view is activated, start and end tags appear, representing the beginning and end of each element.

To turn on display codes click the Change XML Codes icon on the toolbar, choose Display Codes from the drop-down menu. This view is useful in determining the location of text with respect to the elements.

There are two ways to insert text into the template:

Method 1: Type directly in the Document Window.
Method 2: Copy and paste from another text file.

To type directly into the template, highlight the placeholder text, or click in the desired location and type the text directly into the template.

Copy and Paste from Text Files*

1. Open the original document in WordPerfect (File, Open).
2. From the Window menu, select Tile Top to Bottom.
3. Copy (Ctrl+c) the appropriate text from source document.
4. In the template, click on the desired insertion point. For example, to the right of a [p] label (paragraph tag indicator).
5. Paste (Ctrl+v) the text.

---

* For best results, convert source text from other word processors to CG Times or Times New Roman font before opening in WordPerfect. This provides improved translation when copying and pasting special characters.

Paste and Tag Paragraphs

Paragraphs may be inserted in blocks but must be tagged individually.

1. Copy and paste the desired group of paragraphs.
2. Place the cursor at the end of the first paragraph.
3. Select the Split Element icon or press Alt+Shift+S. The new paragraph will have the same ID number as the previous paragraph. This will be resolved upon renumbering paragraphs (see the Renumber section).
4. Repeat Steps 2 and 3 for each paragraph to be tagged.

Insert Special Characters

1. From the Insert menu, select Text References. The Text References window will open.
2. From the Text Reference list, select the reference code for the character you wish to insert. The character to be displayed in the document will be shown in the Value field at the bottom of the window.
3. Click the Insert button.

Methods of Tagging*

A tag must precede all text in the template. If the appropriate tag is not present, use any of the following methods to insert the tag before entering the text.

Method 1: To use an icon on the toolbar, position the cursor in the template and click the appropriate icon from the toolbar.

Method 2: To use a keyboard shortcut, position the cursor in the template and type the keystrokes, such as Alt+P for a paragraph tag.

Method 3: To use the XML drop-down list, position the cursor at the desired location in the template, click on the drop-down list in the toolbar area, and click on the desired tag. Tags listed with a "?" are optional; tags listed with a "|" are required. "TEXT (PCDATA)" indicates that text may be entered.

Method 4: Right-click at the desired location in the template, select Valid Elements (right-click and Insert Element), and click on the desired tag. You may also use the right-click option in the XML Tree.

Method 5: If a required element is missing, a yellow triangle will be displayed in the XML Tree. Click on the yellow triangle to display and select from a list of valid elements for insertion.

Method 6: To use the Elements dialog box:
   a. Position the cursor at the desired location in the template.
   b. Select Insert from the menu.
   c. Select Elements.
   d. Double-click on the desired element from the list.

---

* For simplicity, the instructions in the Authoring Guide specify a mix of single methods for tag insertion. However, each tag may be inserted using any of the several methods, depending on user preference.

After using any of these methods to insert the tag, type or paste the text into the new tag (see the Inserting Text in the Overview of EFS Tagging section).

Resolving Tagging Errors

A yellow triangle in the XML Tree indicates a required tag is missing or an authoring error has occurred. Hold the cursor over the yellow triangle to display a brief description of the error.

It is strongly recommended that you fix each error immediately.

Display Codes (see the Display Codes View section) is a helpful tool in correcting and preventing errors in tag and text placement.

Correcting a Text Insertion Error

Method 1: Click Edit and select Undo.
Method 2: Use Display Codes to highlight and remove the erroneous text.

Correcting a Missing Tag Error

A yellow triangle displayed upon adding a new element tag or section may indicate a required child element is missing. To add the required element:

1. Click the yellow triangle.
2. A list of valid child elements will appear.
3. Select one of the child elements.

Correcting an Attribute Error

If the error indicated by the yellow triangle is of the form "REQUIRED attribute … not in…," the element has a missing attribute value. This error should be corrected by:

Method 1: Click Edit and select Undo.
Method 2: Use Display Codes to highlight and remove the element including the tags. Reenter the element using the methods described in this chapter.

Using Undo to Correct an Error

Undo is a Windows® command present in WordPerfect that provides valuable error-correcting capabilities when authoring a specification. Undo permits you to cancel previous actions prior to saving your structured document. Once you perform a Save function, the Undo function becomes inactive until you resume working on your structured document.

There are two ways to use the Undo function:

Method 1: Keyboard shortcut command Ctrl+z.
Method 2: From the Edit menu, select Undo.

Using Redo to Correct an Error

You can use the Redo command to restore any element, data, or attribute value that you may have mistakenly deleted while using the Undo function. The Redo function does not allow you to repeat the insertion of an element. Once you save your document, the Redo command button becomes inactive until you use the Undo command. There are two ways to use the Redo function:

Method 1: Keyboard shortcut command Ctrl+Shift+R.
Method 2: From the Edit menu, select Redo.

AUTHORING A SPECIFICATION

CREATE A NEW SPECIFICATION

1. Click File and select New from Project. The PerfectExpert window opens.
2. Click on the Create New tab. Click on the down arrow and select EFS.
3. Select Specificationl 2 5 from the window and click on the Create button. The macro warning may appear. Click the NO button.
4. The Specification document opens.
5. The Initialization message box appears.* Click the OK button. This initiates the USPTO's WordPerfect customizations.
6. The default specification template appears, including only the MPEP required section headings.
7. If you have not already done so, turn off the Attribute Prompt:
   a. From the Insert menu, select Elements.
   b. Select Options and make sure "Never prompt for attributes" is selected.
   c. Make sure that the Auto-Insert option is selected.
   d. Close the Elements box.
8. Save the new Specification file in WordPerfect 6/7/8/9 format (Save File window).
   a. From the File menu, select Save As.
   b. Select the Folder where you wish to save the document.
   c. Type in the File Name.
   d. Select WordPerfect 6/7/8/9 as the File Type.
   e. Click the Save button.

Be sure to save the file intermittently during the process of authoring your document. This ensures that only a limited amount of information is lost in the unlikely case of a computer or software malfunction. To activate the Auto-Save feature:

---

* If the message box in the Initializing figure does not appear, the template installation is corrupt. Repeat the setup. If the problem persists, contact your system administrator to reinstall the WordPerfect XML Template.

1. From the Tools menu, select Settings.
2. Click the Files button.
3. Click the Documents tab.
4. Select the Timed document backup option and enter number of minutes between auto-saves.
5. Select the Save original document as backup option.
6. Click OK.
7. Click Close.
8. Click inside the Document Window to activate the XML Tree.

SELECT SPECIFICATION SECTIONS

1. Click the Template Setup icon (first icon on the left) on the toolbar.
2. In the Template Setup window, select the sections for inclusion. The MPEP required sections are checked by default and cannot be removed.
3. Click OK to insert the selected sections in the template.

While authoring, section headings may be added or removed as needed.

ADD MPEP RECOMMENDED SECTION

1. From the Template menu, click Add and select the desired section. The section with its default heading will be inserted into the specification template.
2. The text of the heading may be modified as needed. For example, "Summary of the Invention" could be changed to "Brief Summary."
3. In most cases the initial tag, such as a <paragraph>, will be provided. Insert the appropriate tags and text, as needed.

REMOVE MPEP RECOMMENDED SECTION

1. From the Template menu, click Remove.
2. Select the desired section. The section with its contents will be deleted from the specification template.

CREATE A NEW SECTION

Additional sections may be required for the specification, such as "Examples" or "Field of the Invention." To create a new section:

1. In the Document Window, click at the desired insertion point.
2. Click the Insert Section icon on the toolbar or press Alt+s.
3. Highlight the "Heading" placeholder, and type or paste the desired section heading text.
4. The first <paragraph> tag has been provided. Click to the right of the [p] label, and type or paste the paragraph text.

TITLE OF INVENTION (REQUIRED)

1. In the Document Window, highlight the default text "Title of Invention."
2. Type or paste the invention's title.

CROSS-REFERENCE TO RELATED APPLICATIONS (OPTIONAL)

Continuity Data

1. Turn on Display Codes.
2. In the Document Window, position the cursor between the <continuity statement> start and end tags.
3. Type or paste the continuity data.

Referenced Applications and Patents

1. Turn on Display Codes.
2. Position your source reference text at the very top of the window.
3. In the Document Window, position the cursor just before the <cross-reference-to-related-applications> end tag.
4. From the XML drop-down list, select Referenced Applications.
5. Insert any text necessary for the Referenced Applications. You may only insert the Referenced Applications tag once.
6. To tag a reference to a patent, select <patent-reference> from the XML drop-down list.
7. To tag a reference to an application, select <application-reference> from the XML drop-down list. Enter the Application Number and Filing Date in the Application Reference window (Application Reference Window).
8. To add additional patent or application references, repeat Steps 6–7 as needed.

Copyright Statement (Optional)

1. If the Copyright Statement was not included during Template Setup, add the section from the Template, Add menu.
2. In the XML Tree, click on <copyright-statement>.
3. The cursor will automatically move to the correct insertion point in the Document Window.
4. In the Document Window, type or paste your copyright statement.
5. If copyright statement includes a copyright date, tag the date:
   a. Highlight the date text.
   b. From the XML drop-down list, select copyright.

Federal Research Statement (Optional)

1. In the XML Tree, click on the <paragraph-federal-research-statement> tag. The cursor will move to the correct insertion point in the Document Window.
2. Insert the statement in the specification.
3. Within the statement, select any grant numbers, contract numbers. or U.S. agency references and tag them with the <grant-number>, <contact-number>, and <US-Agency> elements using the XML drop-down list, respectively.

Compact Disc Appendix (Optional)

The Compact Disc Appendix is used to reference a computer program listing on a CD-ROM or CD-R. The Compact Disc Appendix should be tagged to include the Object ID (identification name/reference for the compact disc); the Object Description (format of the compact disc); and the Object Contents (file listing). To tag the Compact Disc Appendix data:

1. Turn on Display Codes.
2. In the Document Window, position your cursor just to the left of the <appendix-data> end tag.
3. Select <object-reference> from the XML drop-down list, or click the Object Reference icon on the toolbar. The Insert Object Reference window will appear.
4. Type in the identifying Object ID, Object Description, and Object Contents data for the compact disc, and click OK.

To enter additional references:

1. Move the cursor to the right of the <object-reference> end tag.
2. Use the XML drop-down list to insert a new <object-reference> tag.
3. Type in the identifying Object ID, Object Description, and Object Contents data for the compact disc, and click OK.

Background of Invention (Optional)

1. The first <paragraph> tag has been provided.
2. In the Document Window, click to the right of the [p] label (paragraph tag) and insert (copy and paste) the desired block of paragraphs.
3. To individually tag the paragraphs that you have entered:
   a. Place the cursor at the start of a paragraph to be tagged.
   b. Select the Split Element icon or press Alt+Shift+S.
   c. Repeat these two steps for each paragraph to be tagged.
4. Several subelements, such as section, subscript, and superscript, are available for use within the Background of Invention; refer to the Commonly Used Elements section for additional information regarding the use of these elements.

Summary of the Invention (Optional)

Follow the instructions in the Background of Invention section.

Brief Description of the Drawings (Conditional)

If the application includes drawings, this section is required. Follow the instructions in the Background of Invention section.

Brief Description of Sequences (Conditional)

If the application includes a sequence listing, this section is required. Follow the instructions in the Background of Invention section.

Detailed Description of the Invention (Required)

The first <paragraph> element has been provided. Refer to the Background of Invention for information regarding how to use the available subelements.

Deposit of Computer Program Listings (Optional)

1. In the Document Window, click immediately below the Deposit of Computer Program Listings section heading, to position the cursor within the <programlisting> tags.
2. "Text (PCDATA)" will appear in the XML drop-down list.
3. Type or paste the program listing information. The template will automatically insert line numbers in the left margin.

The maximum number of lines allowed for submission is 540 lines at 65 characters per line. This corresponds to the paper practice of submitting computer program listings under 11 pages with the specification. Any listings over 540 lines must be submitted via compact disc.

WHAT IS CLAIMED (REQUIRED)

By law, at least one claim is required in a patent application.

BASIC CLAIM TAGGING

Tagging for the first claim has been provided.

1. Turn on Display Codes.
2. To insert the body of the claim, copy the appropriate text from the source document and paste within the claim-text tag or type directly into the <claimtext> tag.

ADDITIONAL CLAIMS

1. To insert additional claims, place the cursor between the claim start tag and the claims end tag.
2. Click the Insert Claim icon on the toolbar or press Alt+c.
3. A new claim tag, with one claim-text tag, will be automatically inserted in the template.
4. Type or copy and paste the claim text into the claim-text tag.
5. To insert additional claim text sections within the same claim, see Indented Sections.

INDENTED SECTIONS

1. To tag a claim with indented sections, move the cursor to the place within the claim-text where you want to indent the text. Insert a new claim-text tag and paste in text as needed. Or highlight the text of the claim to be indented and insert a new claim-text tag.
2. To create additional indented sections of the same level:
   a. Place the cursor at the end of each phrase within the claim-text tag.
   b. Select the Split Element icon or press Alt+Shift+S.
3. You may insert additional claim-text tags within the existing claim-text tags to create further indented sections within the claim body.
   a. Move the cursor to the desired location and insert the claim-text tag.
   b. Insert a claim-text tag from the XML drop-down list.
   c. Continue to copy, paste, and tag as needed.

DEPENDENT CLAIM REFERENCE

All claims must be entered and numbered properly (see the Renumber section) before inserting a Dependent Claim Reference.

1. Highlight the text of the dependent claim reference.
2. Click the Insert Claim Dependency icon on the toolbar.
3. The Select IDs of Dependent Claims window will appear (see Dependent Claim Reference Window). The displayed Claim IDs represent the unique internal IDs of the claims. These IDs are numbered in the order the claims were entered into the document. The Claim Numbers represent the sequential number of the claims as displayed during final printout.
4. Click on the ID(s) in the Claim ID column to indicate the dependency, then click OK.

DISPLAY CLAIMS

This option counts the claims in the document and displays the number of tagged dependent and independent claims. It is a way to double-check that the proper dependent claim tags have been added.

1. From the Assistant menu, select Display Claims.
2. As each Claim Information box appears, click the OK button until all claims are addressed.
3. A message box appears for each claim, noting its independent status or dependencies
4. Click the OK button to close each Dependencies message box that appears.
5. The last message box totals all dependent and independent claims and lists the claim numbers for each type. *Warning:* The number of independent and dependent claims will be correct only if each dependent claim has been properly tagged.
6. Click the OK button to close the final Claim Information box.

ABSTRACT OF THE DISCLOSURE (REQUIRED)

As this section of the specification should only consist of one paragraph, the <paragraph> element has already been inserted.

1. Click to the right of the [p] label and insert the Abstract text by copying and pasting from a source document or by typing directly into the template.
2. Several subelements are available for use within the Abstract; refer to the Commonly Used Elements section for additional information regarding the use of these elements.

FIGURES (OPTIONAL)

Preparation for Attaching Figures

Figures must be scanned as TIFF images before being attached to the specification. It may also be necessary to crop smaller figures for optimum presentation.

Attaching Figures

1. If you have not already done so, turn on Display Codes.
2. Using the XML Tree, scroll to the Figures section.
3. Click on the yellow triangle next to Figure and select Artwork.
4. Browse to select the desired figure (*TIFF). A thumbnail of your image will appear.
5. Please note that the yellow triangle beside the artwork tag in the XML Tree will be resolved at the end of the authoring process (see the Formatting Images section) when attaching each image/artwork.

Formatting Images

1. Select Insert from the main menu and select File References.
2. In the File Reference section, select the first file.

3. At the bottom of the dialog box, verify the path and file name.
4. Click the Edit button.
5. Verify the File Path.

To replace an attached figure file with a different image file:

1. If you have not already done so, turn on Display Codes.
2. Using the XML Tree, scroll to the Figures section.
3. In the XML Tree, highlight the figure and tags to be deleted. Look in the Document Window to ensure that the highlighting includes the correct Figure start and end tags, and associated image.
4. Press the Delete key.
5. From the main menu, select Insert.
6. Select File References.
7. Click on the Artwork file you deleted. For example, if you deleted Figure2 click on Artwork2. At the bottom of the dialog box, verify the path and image file to be deleted.
8. Click the Delete button.
9. Click the Yes button.
10. Click the Close button.
11. Place the cursor at the correct location in the Document Window and press Alt+F to insert the new Figure tag.
12. Click on the new yellow triangle, and select Artwork.
13. Browse and select the desired image file. A thumbnail of the image will appear to the right.
14. Your image will now display in the template.
15. From the main menu, select Insert.
16. Select File References.
17. Click the User Declared radio button.
18. Click on the Artwork file you replaced. For example, if you replaced Figure2, click on Artwork2.
19. At the bottom of the dialog box, verify the path and image file name.
20. If the path and file name are incorrect:
    a. Click the Edit button.
    b. Change the File Path and file name to refer to the new image file.
    c. Click the OK button.
    d. Click the Close button.

Deleting a Figure

To permanently delete an attached figure file from the template:

1. If you have not already done so, turn on Display Codes.
2. Using the XML Tree, scroll to the Figures section.

3. In the XML Tree, highlight the figure to be deleted. Check in the Document Window to ensure that the highlighting includes the correct Figure start and end tags, and associated image.
4. Press Delete.
5. Perform the following steps only if the figure is not used elsewhere in the document.
6. From the Insert menu, select File References.
7. Click on the Image or Artwork reference corresponding to the figure you deleted. For example, if you deleted the second figure that was added to the specification, click on Artwork2.
8. Verify the File Path is correct. You may need to click the Edit button to view the full file path name.
9. Click the Delete button.
10. Click the Yes button.
11. Click the Close button.

AUTHORING WRAP-UP

After you finish authoring the specification, complete the following steps to ensure a proper submission is created. You may close your source documents at this point.

Save the submission with a unique name. It cannot have the same name as any image files included in the submission.

Renumbering

1. From the Assistant menu, select Numbering.
2. Select Renumber all or select the type of tags to be renumbered, such as Paragraphs. You will be notified if a tag type is not found. Click OK to proceed.
3. Repeat as appropriate for each tag type in your specification.

Validation

After you have authored your specification, run Validation to verify that the USPTO and XML rules have been correctly applied.

1. Click the Validate button on the toolbar.
2. Click the Find Errors radio button.
3. Select all Error Types.
4. Click the Start button.
5. When an error is found, a message box explains the error and moves the cursor to the location of the error in the template.
6. Correct the error, then click on the Next or Close button as appropriate.
7. Repeat the Validation procedure until all errors are resolved.

Correcting Validation Errors

Validation errors usually fall into one of three categories:

1. Incorrect placement of text or tag
   a. Data not allowed at this point
   b. Element not allowed at this point
2. Missing tag
   a. Required element not found
3. Incomplete Authoring Wrap-Up
   a. ID is not unique
   b. Attribute source is not a data entity

Character Mapping Error

This error occurs when a character pasted into WordPerfect cannot be matched to one of WordPerfect's characters. To correct this error, insert a WordPerfect character by selecting Insert, Text References from the menu, then navigate for the character to replace by examining the Value.

Data Not Allowed Error

This error usually occurs when text has been accidentally inserted between elements, such as between two paragraph tags.

1. Turn on Display Codes.
2. Highlight and cut (Ctrl+x) the improperly placed text.
3. Place the cursor within the correct tag.
4. Paste (Ctrl+v) the text.

Element Not Allowed at This Point Error

This error usually occurs when a parent element has been deleted but the child element remains.

1. Turn on Display Codes.
2. Highlight the child element and its text.
3. To insert the parent element, select the appropriate parent element from the XML drop-down list; to remove the child element from the document, press the Delete key.

Required Element Not Found Error

This error usually occurs when a required child element has not been inserted.

1. Click on the corresponding yellow triangle in the XML Tree.
2. Select the appropriate child element for insertion. For example, a figure tag must contain associated artwork. A claim tag must contain a claim-text tag.

ID Is Not Unique Error

This error occurs when the Renumbering step of Authoring Wrap-Up has not been completed. See the Renumbering section for detailed instructions.

Attribute Source Is Not a Data Entity Error

This error occurs when the Formatting Images steps of Authoring Wrap-up have not been completed. See the Authoring Wrap-Up/Numbering section for detailed instructions.

VIEWING THE SUBMISSION

The following guidelines will assist you in viewing your submission, as the USPTO will print it, by displaying the XML specification in the Internet Explorer 5.5 browser. You must view your specification in the browser prior to transmitting it to USPTO.

1. Validate your submission before viewing it.
2. If you have not already done so, save the document as a WordPerfect 9.0 file type (.wpd).
3. Select View XML with Stylesheet from the Assistant menu, or press the save icon on the toolbar. This will save your WordPerfect (.wpd) document as an XML file in the same directory and open it for viewing in Internet Explorer. Note that subsequent viewing can be accomplished by clicking on the XML file through Windows Explorer.
4. You may wish to print a copy, because this will be the same presentation that the USPTO will print for examination.
5. Print the specification. You may wish to use the same margins that the USPTO will use when printing your submission. From the Internet Explorer main menu, select File, then click on Page Setup. In the Margins section (lower right corner), change the settings as needed. Recommended settings: left = 1, right = 0.75, top = 1.25, bottom = 0.75.
6. Click the OK button.

TROUBLESHOOTING: IMAGES DO NOT DISPLAY

If your image files do not display in the brower, install the AlternaTIFF 1.3.5 viewer:

1. For best results, your computer should be connected to the Internet.
2. Close WordPerfect and any other open programs.
3. In Windows Explorer, browse to C:\ProgramFiles\USPTO\WordPerfect-AuthoringTool\Version1.2.5.
4. Double-click on the ALTERNATIFF-1.3.5.exe file.
5. Click the Setup button in the WinZip dialog box.
6. Enter the appropriate information in the AlternaTIFF 1.3.5 registration dialog box.
7. Click the Next button, then click the Send Registration button to upload the information.

8. In the AlternaTIFF 1.3.5 Setup dialog box, select Install into Microsoft Internet Explorer.
9. Click the Install button.
10. Click the OK button when notified that AlternaTIFF 1.3.5 has been installed successfully.
11. Navigate to the XML file through Windows Explorer to view the XML file.

CHANGES AFTER VIEWING

If changes to the document are needed, it is critical that you complete the following steps:

1. Close the browser windows.
2. Make the corrections to the WPD WordPerfect Specification file.
3. Validate.
4. Select View XML with Stylesheet from the Assistant menu, or press the icon on the toolbar. This will save your WordPerfect (.wpd) document as an XML file in the same directory and open it for viewing in Internet Explorer. Note that subsequent viewing can be accomplished by clicking on the XML file through Windows Explorer. Resave the file as WordPerfect 9.0 (.wpd).

COMMONLY USED ELEMENTS

The following sections contain instructions for inserting the most commonly used elements into the specification document.

<Application-Reference>

To enter an <application-reference> element you must activate Display Codes first.

1. Click the Change XML Codes icon and from the XML drop-down menu select Display Codes.
2. Click on the Application Reference icon on the tool bar. The Application Reference window opens.
3. Type the application number in the Application Number field.
4. Type in the Filing Date using the YYYY-MM-DD format.
5. Click the OK button.

<Artwork>

Use the <artwork> element, with a <figure> element, to associate a 300 × 300 dpi TIFF file with your structured document.

1. If you have not already done so, insert the <figure> tag (Alt+F).
2. Insert the <artwork> element (Alt+a).

3. The Insert Image window opens. Browse and double-click on the scanned TIFF image file. *Warning:* Do not move the inserted image by dragging as this causes the document to become invalid.
4. Click the OK button. A thumbnail of the graphic appears.

After you associate an image, a yellow triangle is still visible in the XML Tree. This triangle will be removed when you complete the Formatting Images section.

<Chemistry-CWU>

1. Turn on Display Codes.
2. Double-click on the <chemistry-cwu> element in the XML drop-down list.
3. An ID number appears (a "y" followed by a number) in the Document Window.
4. If the start and end tags are divided by a page break in the Document Window, the start tag must be moved to the next page:
   a. Place the cursor immediately to the left of the start tag.
   b. Press the ENTER key until both tags are on the same page.
5. From the XML drop-down list, double-click on the <image> element.
6. The Insert Image window opens. Browse and double-click on the scanned TIFF image. A thumbnail of the graphic appears.

Warning: Do not move the inserted image by dragging as this causes the document to become invalid.

<Copyright>

The <copyright> element is an optional child element of the <copyright-statement> and <figure> elements.

1. Insert the <copyright> element by double-clicking on it from the XML drop-down list. A [Copyright] label appears.
2. Type or paste the copyright date to the right of the label.

<Custom-Character>

The <custom-character> element is used to attach a TIFF image of custom characters, such as symbols.

1. From the XML drop-down list, double-click on <custom-character> element. The Insert Image window opens.
2. Browse and select on the scanned TIFF image file. A thumbnail of the graphic appears.

Warning: Do not move the inserted image by dragging as this causes the document to become invalid.

<Emphasis>

The <emphasis> element will present the selected text in italics.

1. Select the text you want to be emphasized.
2. Select Emphasis from the XML drop-down list on the toolbar.

Emphasize Common Phrases

This option automatically adds the <emphasis> element to italicize the following common phrases:

a fortiori	a posteriori	a priori
ab initio	ad hoc	cf.
e.g.	et al.	etc.
i.e.	in vitro	in vivo
infra	inter alia	per se
prima facie	q.v.	supra

1. From the Assistant Menu, select Emphasize common phrases.
2. Any of the above phrases found in the document will be automatically tagged for emphasis.
3. Repeat as needed throughout the authoring process.

<Heading>

The <heading> element is an element available for insertion immediately after a major section of the specification, such as <background-of-invention>, or inserted simultaneously along with the <section> element (see the Overview of EFS Tagging section). The <heading> tag increases the point size of your text and gives the text a bold font. Default heading text, such as "Detailed Description of the Invention," may be modified as needed. To insert a <heading> element:

1. Insert the <heading> element from the XML drop-down list.
2. Type or paste the appropriate heading text.

<Lists> and <List-Item>

The <lists> and <list-item> elements create indented text within a <paragraph>. To insert the <lists> element:

1. Turn on Display Codes.
2. Select <lists> from the XML drop-down list or click the list icon. An ID number appears (the letter "l" plus the list number).

To add the first item in the list, select <list-item> from the drop down menu or click the list-item icon. Type or paste the text of the first item within the <list-item> tag. To create additional items in the list:

1. Move the cursor to the right of the <list-item> end tag.
2. Insert the <list-item> element from the XML drop-down list or icon.
3. Repeat as needed.

<Math-CWU>

The <math-cwu> element is added by scanning a formula to a TIFF file and attaching it using the <image> element. The <math-cwu> element may be inserted within <paragraph> elements or between them. To attach a math image:

1. Turn on Display Codes.
2. Insert the <math-cwu> element from the XML drop-down list or click the Math-CWU icon on the toolbar.
3. If the start and end tags are divided by a page break in the Document Window, the start tag must be moved to the next page:
   a. Place the cursor immediately to the left of the start tag.
   b. Press the Enter key until both tags are on the same page.
4. Insert the <image> element from the XML drop-down list. The Insert Image window opens.
5. Browse and select the scanned TIFF image file. A thumbnail of the graphic appears.

Warning: Do not move the inserted image by dragging as it causes the document to become invalid.

Note: After you complete the steps above you will find a yellow triangle is still visible in the XML Tree. This triangle will be removed when you complete the steps for finalizing the specification as discussed in the Formatting Images section.

<Paragraph>

To tag a single paragraph:

1. Press Alt+p or click the Paragraph icon on the toolbar.
2. Click to the right of the [p] label and type or paste the paragraph text.

To tag multiple paragraphs:

1. Insert the first <paragraph> element.
2. Click to the right of the [p] label and type or paste the text.
3. Place the cursor at the beginning of the next paragraph to be tagged.
4. Select the Split Element icon or right-click at the beginning of the paragraph and select Split Element from the menu.

<Patent-Reference>

1. Select the patent number in the Document Window.
2. Select the <patent-reference> element from the XML drop-down list. The [Patent Reference] label appears and the selected data is underlined.

<Section>

Additional sections may be required for the specification, such as "Examples" or "Field of the Invention." To create a new section:

1. In the Document Window, click at the desired insertion point.
2. Click the Insert Section icon on the toolbar or press Alt+s.
3. Highlight the "Heading" placeholder, and type or paste the desired section heading text.
4. The first <paragraph> tag has been provided. Click to the right of the [p] label, and type or paste the paragraph text.

<Subscript>

1. Highlight the subscript text in the Document Window.
2. Insert the <subscript> element from the XML drop-down list or click the Subscript icon on the toolbar. The selected text appears as a subscript.
3. When subscript tags must be added repeatedly, highlight the subscripted character and use the QuickFind Next and QuickFind Previous icons to locate the characters needing tags.

Warning: The <subscript> element cannot be used to create footnotes.

<Superscript>

1. Highlight the superscript text in the Document Window.
2. Insert the <superscript> element from the XML drop-down list or click the Superscript icon on the toolbar. The selected text appears as a superscript.
3. When superscript tags must be added repeatedly highlight the super-scripted character and use the QuickFind Next icons to locate the char-acters needing tags.

<Table>

1. To attach a scanned image of a table, confirm that the image is in 300 dpi, black-and-white, uncompressed or Group 4 compression, TIFF format.
2. Turn on Display Codes.

3. Place the cursor at the desired location in the document.
4. Click the Insert Table CWU icon on the toolbar.
5. If the start and end tags are divided by a page break in the Document Window, the start tag must be moved to the next page:
   a. Place the cursor immediately to the left of the start tag.
   b. Press the Enter key until both tags are on the same page.
6. In the XML Tree, click on the new yellow triangle and select Image.
7. Browse and select the correct table image file. A thumbnail of your image will appear. *Warning:* Do not move the inserted image by dragging as it causes the document to become invalid.
8. Please note that the yellow triangle beside the image tag in the XML Tree will be resolved at the end of the authoring process. No action on your part is required at this time.

TROUBLESHOOTING

This section contains general troubleshooting information and specific solutions to problems that may arise during the authoring process.

APPLICATION CLOSES BEFORE DATA IS SAVED

In the event that your computer or application closes before you can save, you may revert to the last auto-save copy:

1. After reopening WordPerfect, the message box in the Timed Backup Message Box appears.
2. Choose the desired option.

To change your Auto-Save feature so WordPerfect automatically saves files more often:

1. From the Tools menu, select Settings.
2. Click the Files button.
3. Click the Documents tab.
4. Check the Timed document backup option and enter number of minutes between auto-saves.
5. Check the Save original document as back up option. Click OK. Click Close.

WORDPERFECT-SPECIFIC KEYBOARD SHORTCUTS FAIL

The USPTO has created numerous shortcut key combinations that correspond to the actions found on the EFS specification toolbar. These keyboard combinations are the default combinations loaded when you open the specification template. To activate the WordPerfect specific combinations, you must deactivate the specification combinations.

1. Click Tools on the menu.
2. From the XML drop-down menu, select Settings and then click on the Customize button.
3. Click the Keyboard tab.
4. Select WPWin 9 Keyboard from the list.

ONE OR BOTH TOOLBARS ARE MISSING

1. From the View menu, select Toolbars. The Toolbars window will open.
2. Make sure that Property Bar and EFS specification are selected.
3. Click the OK button.

ASSISTANT OR TEMPLATE MENU IS MISSING

1. Right-click in the gray area to the far right of the Help menu option.
2. Check the <Template> option. The Assistant and Template options should now appear at the far right end of the menu.

ONLINE HELP

WordPerfect provides two types of online help: ToolTips and WordPerfect Help.

Tooltips

ToolTips provide a brief description of various fields and icons available while authoring your electronic submissions. The USPTO has created a customized toolbar within WordPerfect to help you quickly accomplish common tasks. ToolTips provide a useful method of investigating the task performed by the icons found on these toolbars. To activate a ToolTip, hold the mouse cursor over an icon (do not click) and a ToolTip appears. ToolTips for the customized toolbar icons also contain the shortcut key combination associated with the toolbar icon. You can also allow your mouse to hover over any yellow triangles that appear in the XML Tree. A ToolTip appears describing the error.

WordPerfect Help

You may access WordPerfect Help by clicking on Help on the menu bar and then clicking on Help Topics (or press F1). This brings up WordPerfect's online help system. There are five tabbed sections that you may use. A description for each _Help Tab follows.

1. **Contents:** Provides help information by nested topics. Click on topics and then click on subtopics until you reach the desired information.
2. **Index:** Provides help by keyword. Type a word in the first field and select topics from those that appear in the second field.

3. **Find:** Similar to the Index tab but provides more comprehensive search capabilities.

4. **Ask the Perfect Expert:** In the first field type your question or search term. Then click on the Search button. Topics appear in the second window, select the topic and click on the Display button. Note: Online Word-Perfect Help has not been customized to reflect any changes the USPTO made to the program interface. Thus some functions or elements described in the online Help may function or appear differently in your customized version of WordPerfect.

5. **Corel Knowledge Base:** Type a search term in the field and then click on the Search button. This searches the Online Corel Database, via the World Wide Web (WWW), for information.

9 USPTO PatentIn

INTRODUCTION

PatentIn is a computer program designed to expedite the preparation of U.S. Patent and Trademark Office (USPTO) patent applications containing nucleic acid and polypeptide sequences. PatentIn complies with all format requirements specified in World Intellectual Property Organization standard (WIPO) ST.25 and the related U.S. final rule, "Requirements for Patent Applications Containing Nucleotide Sequence and/or Amino Acid Disclosures." It runs on Windows® 95/98/NT/2000. Screen displays are in English. Because the sequence listings generated by PatentIn are in compliance with ST.25, this program has worldwide applicability. PatentIn facilitates the creation of sequence listings for inclusion in patent applications sequences. It accepts data about the sequences, validates the data, creates a sequence listing file, and a mechanism for printing out and saving to removable medium for submission. This chapter describes how to use PatentIn. For ease of use, the design follows standard Windows user interface conventions.

PatentIn was designed to be installed on individual computers; it can be downloaded onto your personal computer and, if desired, the project files stored remotely. The program can be downloaded from the USPTO Web page. The Universal Resource Locator (URL) from which the PatentIn 3.1 application can be obtained is: http://www.uspto.gov/web/offices/pac/patin/patentinv3.htm. Follow the instructions to download PatentIn 3.1 and install it on your PC. Upon completing the installation, an icon will be placed on your desktop. Access to the PatentIn 3.1 application program occurs when you double-click on the PatentIn 3.1 icon. Later versions may be available.

A SEQUENCE EDITOR

The primary tool within PatentIn is the sequence editor, which enables you to enter and modify both nucleic acid and protein sequence listings, as well as import sequence listing files created by another editor or word processor (provided they are stored as ASCII text files). When working in PatentIn you may enter data in any order, and also add, remove, or revise sequence listing data at any time. You may also save a partially completed project and finish it at a later time. PatentIn does not require that a project exist or remain on a particular machine or device. Users are free to e-mail files to clients or each other so that they might review and update them.

A SEQUENCE GENERATOR

After you have entered all the data necessary for your patent application, PatentIn enables you to generate your application. The application consists of a computer-readable, ST.25-compliant file containing a sequence listing file.

GETTING STARTED: SEQUENCE SCREEN

When you first access PatentIn by double-clicking on the PatentIn 3.1 icon on your desktop, you have immediate access to the Sequence Screen, which provides you with five drop-down menus, three of which provide access to the real-time system interface. They are Project, Application Steps, and Help. The remaining two drop-down menus, Edit and View, are general Microsoft® Windows-type menus. You may select any one of the three drop-down menus when a project is begun. PatentIn presents an empty project upon startup entitled "Untitled" (Figure 9.1).

PROJECT MENU

The Project menu enables you to create and save a project. Selecting Save displays the Save As Screen where a new project is given a name and is saved. Selecting Open displays the Open Screen where you can select a previously saved project to open. The Exit PatentIn 3.1 selection closes the application. Menu items that require a project to be opened, or an output file to be present, are unavailable ("grayed") until those conditions are met. To create and save a new project, select New from the Project menu; click Save to create the new file. An existing project file (.prj) can be opened by double-clicking the file in the directory.

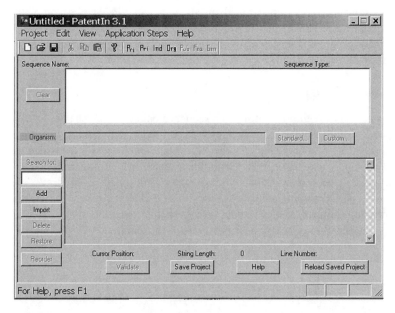

FIGURE 9.1

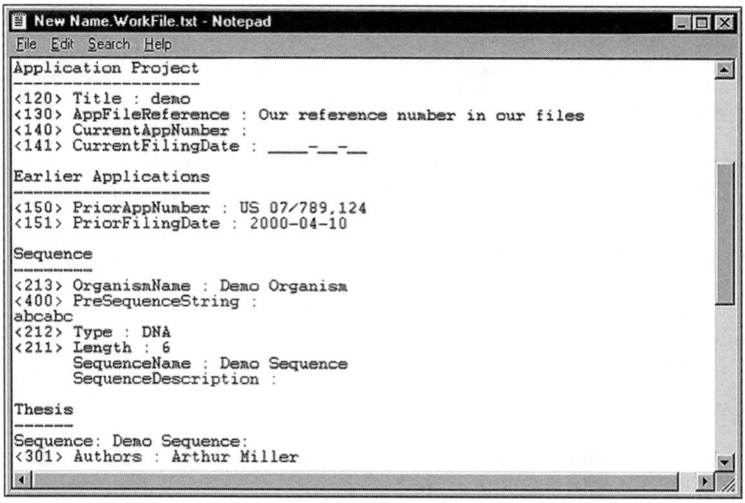

```
┌─────────────────────────────────────────────────────────────────┐
│ 📄 New Name.WorkFile.txt - Notepad                      _ □ ✕    │
├─────────────────────────────────────────────────────────────────┤
│ File  Edit  Search  Help                                          │
├─────────────────────────────────────────────────────────────────┤
│ Application Project                                          ▲     │
│ -------------------                                                │
│ <120> Title : demo                                                │
│ <130> AppFileReference : Our reference number in our files         │
│ <140> CurrentAppNumber :                                           │
│ <141> CurrentFilingDate : ____-__-__                               │
│                                                                   │
│ Earlier Applications                                              │
│ --------------------                                              │
│ <150> PriorAppNumber : US 07/789,124                              │
│ <151> PriorFilingDate : 2000-04-10                               │
│                                                                   │
│ Sequence                                                         │
│ --------                                                         │
│ <213> OrganismName : Demo Organism                               │
│ <400> PreSequenceString :                                         │
│ abcabc                                                           │
│ <212> Type : DNA                                                 │
│ <211> Length : 6                                                 │
│       SequenceName : Demo Sequence                               │
│       SequenceDescription :                                       │
│                                                                   │
│ Thesis                                                           │
│ ------                                                           │
│ Sequence: Demo Sequence:                                          │
│ <301> Authors : Arthur Miller                              ▼     │
│ ◄                                                        ► │     │
└─────────────────────────────────────────────────────────────────┘
```

FIGURE 9.2

Viewing a Work File

You can view the current work in progress by creating a work file. This work file provides a vehicle for you to view the data for the entire project in a single place instead of reviewing each individual screen. Use caution not to confuse the work file with the sequence listing. To see the Work File from the Project Menu, select View/Print Work in Progress. *Note:* This work file was built by selecting Create Work File (Figure 9.2). To view the current patent application: From the Project menu, select View Work in Progress. To print the error report, click on File then Print. To exit the screen, click on File Exit.

Viewing a Sequence Listing

PatentIn provides you with an on-screen view of the Sequence Listing with the View Sequence Listing Windows. To view the sequence listing: From the Project menu, select View Sequence Listing. To print the error report, click on File then Print. To exit the screen, click on File then Exit. *Note:* The sequence must first be generated.

Viewing Error Reports

PatentIn provides you with an on-screen Error Report with the View Error Report Window, if one exists, for the opened project. To view an error report: From the Project menu, select View Error Report. To print the error report, click on File then Print. To exit the screen, click on File then Exit.

Rename Sequence

A new feature of PatentIn is the ability to change the name of a sequence. To open the Rename Sequence screen, click on the Sequence Name. From the Project Menu, select Rename Sequence. Type the new sequence name in the Rename Sequence dialog box. Click on the OK button.

Message Dialog

The Message Dialog Screen is a screen that appears if one of the action buttons (e.g., Add) is pressed and an entry has not been made to the input area of the screen.

Project and Applicant Data

Once the Sequence Listing data file has been created, you can add information to the application.

APPLICATION STEPS MENU

The Application Steps menu selections are available when a project is begun, created, or selected. The project name is visible at the upper left corner of the screen. In this example the project has opened a previously existing file. New Name is shown for the project name (Figure 9.3).

Project Data

The Project Data screen (Figure 9.4) provides you with input fields to establish the identifying information for the new invention. This information is the key that establishes the title of the invention and the filing date. *Note:* The mandatory information fields (Title Of Invention and Application File Reference) are in red.

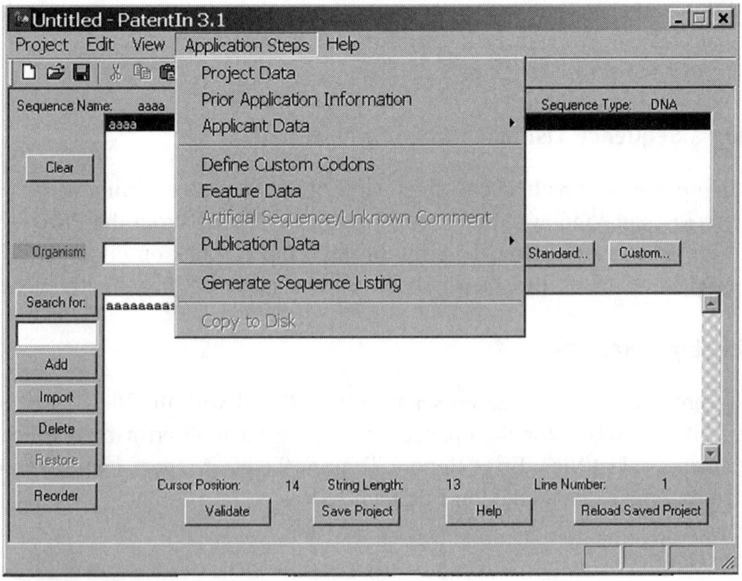

FIGURE 9.3

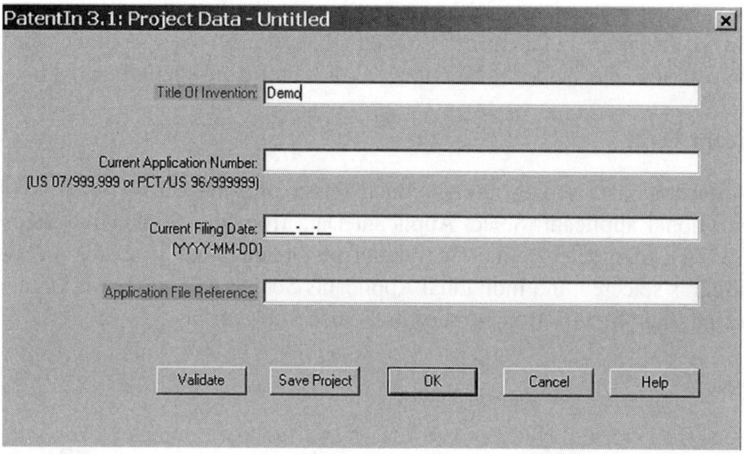

FIGURE 9.4

To enter Project Data, enter the title of the invention. This information is mandatory. Enter the Current Application Number, if one exists. If an application is entered the current filing date becomes mandatory. Enter the Current Filing Date. The date format is numeric: YYYY-MM-DD. Enter the Application File Reference. To validate the information entered, click on Validate. To save the information, click on the Save Project button.

Prior Application Information

Entering information about prior applications is optional because such information is available to the examiner elsewhere in the application file wrapper. Any number of prior applications may be included on the Prior Application Information Screen. They will be displayed in the table in the order entered and may be selected for editing or deleting.

To enter information about a prior application, enter the Prior Application Number. If a prior application number is entered then the prior application date becomes mandatory. Enter the Prior Application Filing Date. The date format is numeric: YYYY-MM-DD.

To clear the information in the Edit Prior Application area, click on Clear.

To insert the information to the list, select the item you want the information to follow, enter the Prior Application Number and the Prior Application Filing Date, and then click on the Insert button.

To replace an entry from the list, select the item, enter the Prior Application Number and the Prior Application Filing Date, then click Replace.

To delete an entry from the list, select the item from the list, and then click on the Delete button.

To validate the information entered, click on Validate. Data entered in the table (Insert) is then validated. Information in the edit area, that has not yet been inserted, is not validated. To validate and close, click on the OK button.

To save the information, click on the Save Project button.

New to PatentIn: In PatentIn 3.1, when OK is clicked the data in the edit field(s) will be inserted into the list when they are different from the selected row.

Applicant Data

The Applicant Data screen allows you to input information for an Individual or Organizational applicant. Select Applicant Data from the Application Steps menu (Figure 9.5), then select either Individual or Organization from the submenu. If Individual is selected, the Individual Applicants Screen will appear. If Organization is selected, the Organization Applicants Screen will appear.

SEQUENCES

The Sequence Screen is where you create and modify sequences. You can create and edit custom codons and custom organism names from this screen. It also provides a search function where a genetic sequence may be entered and searched for in the files for this project. You will access this screen immediately after PatentIn is started. To begin entering a new sequence you must first have a sequence name. To select a sequence for editing, select a sequence name from the list of sequences. The following sequence characteristics are displayed:

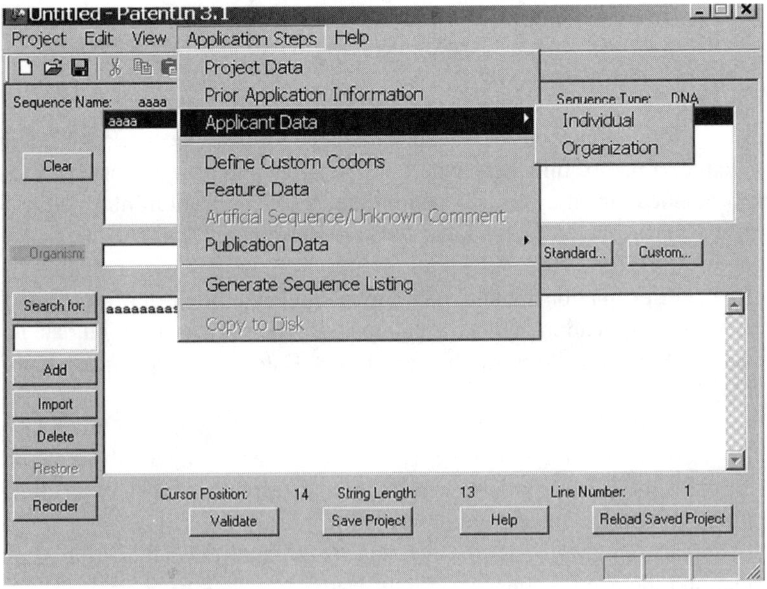

FIGURE 9.5

Cursor Pos: Shows the current cursor position. This field is blank when there is no sequence.

String Length: Shows the length of the sequence string on the line.

Line Number: Indicates the line number of the cursor position relative to the beginning of the string.

Selecting a Standard Organism

This screen enables you to select an organism name from common organisms. Included in its capabilities is an attempt to match on partially input names.

To select an Organism Name, click on the Standard button, begin entering characters for the organism you are looking for. Click on the Apply to all Sequences in the Project checkbox to enable/disable assigning this organism name to all sequences currently in the project. Click on the OK button to enter the selected organism name.

Searching for a Sequence

To search for a specific sequence, enter a particular substring (a feature, for example) in the edit field below the Search for button; click on the Search button. The cursor will move the first instance of that subsequence beginning with its current position. *Note:* Each search is limited/truncated to 60 characters. To clear the entire screen about a specific selected sequence, click on the Clear button.

Adding a Sequence

The Add button on the Sequence Screen provides a means to enter a sequence name and to select a sequence type from a list of radio buttons.

To add a sequence, select the Add button. Enter the sequence name into the dialog box (Figure 9.6). Select the sequence type by clicking on the radio button next to the appropriate sequence type. Click OK.

You can now enter sequence strings in the edit field at the bottom of the screen. If you are using Windows 95, a maximum of 64,000 characters will display in the field. In Windows 98/NT/2000, the upper limit is over 1 million sequence characters. You can work around these limitations by using import files, rather than the Sequence Editor, to create and edit sequences.

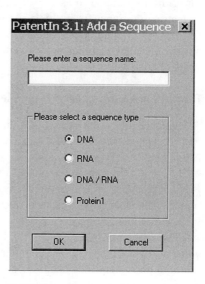

FIGURE 9.6

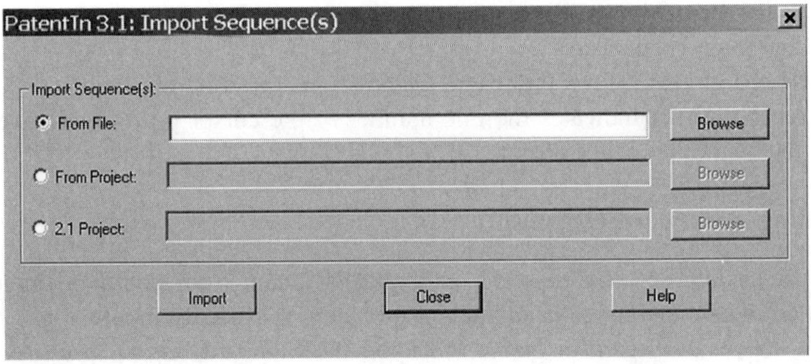

FIGURE 9.7

Importing a Sequence

The Import button on the Sequence Screen provides a means to import sequences from a file, a project, or a 2.1 project by selecting one of three radio buttons (Figure 9.7). *Note:* Importation of a 2.1 Project requires additional software to be installed.

To use a sequence from a text file, click on the Import button on the Sequence Screen, and then click on the From File radio button.

To use a sequence from another project, click on the Import button on the Sequence Screen, and then click on the From Project radio button.

To use a project from a PatentIn 2.1, click on the Import button on the Sequence Screen, and then click on the 2.1 Project radio button. A Browse button is provided for each radio button to assist you in providing the file folder and file name, and formatting the input for multiple file selections. *Note:* For the Protein/3 selection, the data must be imported from a text file that contains only amino acid abbreviated names. The PRT/3 strings are converted to PRT/1 characters for subsequent use in the Sequence Editor.

Format for Multisequence Data Files to Be Imported by PatentIn 3.x

A sequence file is an ASCII text file containing one or more sequences. Each multisequence data file must begin with a header having the format <Sequence-Name;SequenceType;OrganismName>. The header must be the first nonblank text on its line. The sequence type can be DNA, RNA, DNA/RNA, Protein/1, PRT, PRT/1, PRT1, Protein/3, PRT/3, or PRT3. The name of the organism is optional. If it is omitted, the header looks like <SequenceName;SequenceType;>. *Note:* Notice that there are semicolon separators. They are always required.

The sequence data begin on the line following the header. The sequence data are a string of letters appropriate to the sequence type. The sequence data may span multiple lines. Sequence data may not contain spaces. A space signifies the end of the sequence data. The sequence data are terminated by one or more spaces, or by the start of the next header. There may be one or more empty lines between the end of a sequence and the start of the next. A two-sequence file might look like this:

< First Sequence;DNA;Abies alba>

ttttcttattgtttctcctactgcttatcataatgattgtcgtagtggcttc
ctcatcgt

ctcccccaccgcctaccacaacgactgccgcagcggattactaatagtatca
ccaacagc

ataacaaaaagaatgacgaagagggttgctgatggtgtcgccgacggcgtag
cagaagga

gtggcggagggg

< Second Sequence;RNA; >

uuuucuuauuguuucuccuacugcuuaucauaaugauugucguaguggcuuc
cucaucgu

cucccccaccgccuaccacaacgacugccgcagcggauuacuaauaguauca
ccaacagc

auaacaaaaagaaugacgaagagggguugcugauggugucgccgacggcguag
cagaagga

guggcggagggg

Format for Single Sequence Data Files to Be Imported by PatentIn 3.1 (Figure 9.8)

A sequence file is an ASCII text file containing one or more sequences. A single sequence data file does not require a Sequence Header. If the header is missing, you are queried for the sequence type and the file is assumed to be a single sequence data file. *Note:* PatentIn 2.1 ASCII text files used the extension .gbs for its sequence files. While the import feature is running, a screen displays the total number of sequences that have currently been analyzed. A validation errors screen is displayed if validation errors occur.

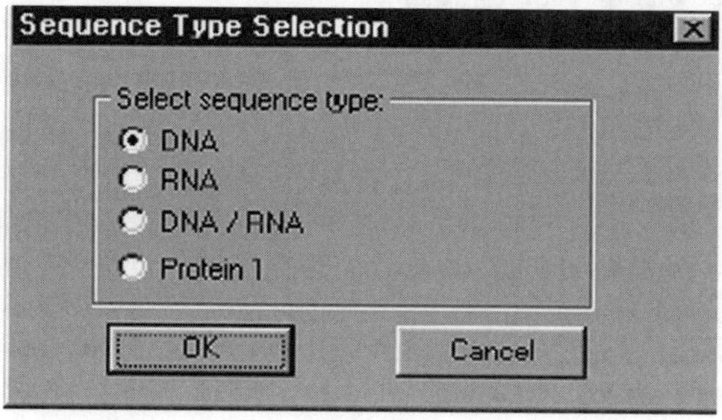

FIGURE 9.8

Importing Sequences from a Project

PatentIn provides a mechanism to import sequences from a PatentIn 3.x project. To use a sequence from a project file, click on the Import button on the Sequence Screen, then click on the From Project radio button. The Browse button is provided to assist you in providing the file folder and file name. When a project has been selected, a list of sequences in the project is displayed. Click on the sequence(s) to be imported. *Note:* By holding the Ctrl key down multiple sequences may be selected; or select the Select All button to select all of the sequences.

Importing a 2.1 Project

To use a sequence from a PatentIn 2.1 project file, click on the Import button on the Sequence Screen, then click on the 2.1 Project radio button. The Browse button is provided to assist you in providing the file folder and file name. Notice that in this case a .dbf file is selected, not a project or text file. After the PatentIn 2.1 project file is identified, the list of project long names is displayed. Click on the project to be imported. Click on the OK button.

Copying a Sequence

PatentIn uses standard Windows-type edit features. When a sequence has been deleted, it can be restored until the current project update is terminated by clicking on the Restore button on the main screen.

Reordering Sequences

The Reorder Sequence Screen (Figure 9.9) provides you with the means to compare the current sequence order and the new sequence order. The Current Sequence Order is displayed on the left of the screen. It displays the sequences in the order that the sequences were entered into the application. The New Sequence Order, displayed on the right, displays the sequences in the order that you specify by selecting a contiguous group of sequences from the left side and selecting a single sequence on the right side that they are to be placed after.

To reorder sequences, select the sequence row(s) from the menu on the left-hand side. Click on the row the sequence will follow. Repeat the steps until the sequences are in the desired order.

Validating Sequences

To validate the sequences, click on the Validate button on the Sequence Screen. A message screen will inform you if there was an error, otherwise Validation OK will appear on the status bar. *Note:* For the Sequence Data, validation is done for the selected sequence name.

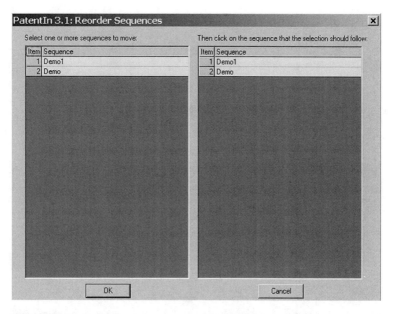

FIGURE 9.9

Saving Sequences

To save a sequence, click on the Save Project button on the Sequence Screen. Your work will be saved in its current state. *Note:* It is important to remember while working with very large or complex projects that saving often can save hours of rework, especially when there is a system failure.

Reloading a Saved Project

The Reload Saved Project button is supplied, at the request of some users, to quickly load the current project from its last saved state.

Adding Custom Codons

The Custom Codons screen (Figure 9.10) provides the means to add Custom Codons to the list of standard codons on your workstation. This screen is accessed from the Application Steps menu by selecting the Define Custom Codons item.

To add a Custom Codon, select the Define Custom Codons item from the Application Steps menu. Select an Amino Acid from the drop-down list. Enter the Custom Codon. Click on the Insert button. *Note:* The format of this screen has changed. It now allows you to see all of the custom codons on a single screen instead of having to select each amino acid individually.

To delete a Custom Codon, click on the Custom Codon in the list. Click on the Delete button.

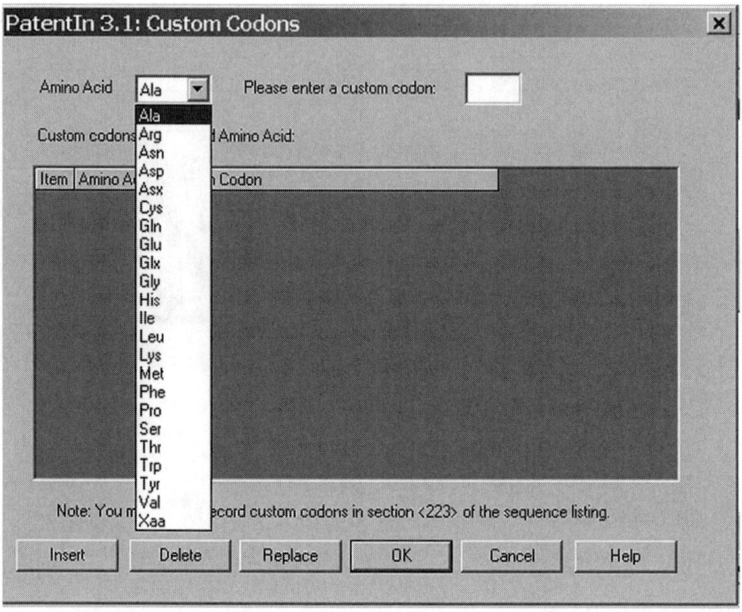

FIGURE 9.10

Adding a Custom Organism

The Custom Organism Input screen provides the means to add a custom organism to the list of custom organisms. It also enables you to select a custom organism to enter on the Sequence Screen. This screen is accessed from the Sequence Screen by selecting the Custom button. You enter the custom organism into the screen, and then can manipulate the list by adding or deleting organisms.

To add a Custom Organism, select the Custom button from the Sequence Screen. Enter the Custom Organism. Click on the Insert button.

To delete a Custom Organism, click on the Custom Organism in the list. Click on the Delete button.

To replace a Custom Organism, click on the Custom Organism in the list. Enter the Custom Organism. Click on the Replace button.

To enter a Custom Organism on the Sequence Screen, Select the Organism so that the name appears in the "Please enter a custom organism name:" box. Click on the OK button.

To apply a Custom Organism to all of the sequences in the project, select the checkbox marked: Apply to all Sequences in the Project. Click on the OK button.

Artificial Sequence or Unknown Organism

An Artificial Sequence or Unknown Organism must have a comment about the organism. After either Artificial Sequence or Unknown is entered into the Organism Name field and you have moved to another field, an automatic popup box will appear. Select the Standard button from the Sequence Screen. Select either Unknown or

Artificial from the list of standard organisms. Tab or move to another cell. The comment box will automatically pop up when a definition of the organism is required. Enter an appropriate comment for the organism. The content of this box should be as descriptive as possible while remaining as terse as possible. This information will be placed in a <223> field when the sequence listing is generated. The <223> section of the sequence listing is updated by using either an Artificial Sequence/Unknown Organism or a misc_feature. The <223> section is the comment or other information, respectively. *Note:* This field can also be accessed by choosing Application Steps/Artificial Sequence/Unknown Comment.

FEATURE DATA

Sequence Features

The Feature screen (Figure 9.11) enables you to create and modify features pertaining to a sequence. You can access this screen by selecting Feature Data, or by selecting the Feature button on the PatentIn toolbar. The features that are displayed apply to the sequence that is currently selected on the Sequence Screen.

To enter information about a Feature, check the Join All CDSs box if the sequence contains more than one CDS and the CDSs are to be joined. *Note:* The Join All CDSs checkbox is available based on whether there is more than one CDS in the Feature List. Click on the Names button to access the list of Nucleotide Names for Feature Name/Key. Enter the "Relevant Residue From" and "To" sequence position numbers. Click in the Other Information box to provide other information.

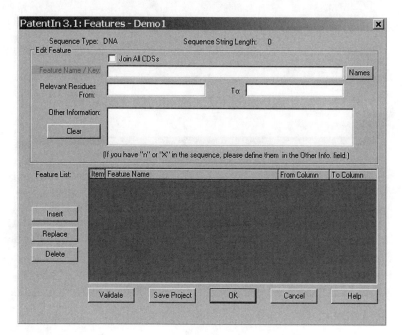

FIGURE 9.11

This is where you would document X in a protein sequence or n in a base sequence. The Feature Name/Key should be misc_feature.

To clear the Edit Feature portion of the screen, click on the Clear button.

To insert an entry from the Feature List, highlight it and click on the Insert button.

To replace an entry from the Feature List, highlight it and click on the Replace button.

To delete an entry from the Feature List, highlight it and click on the Delete button.

To validate the information entered, click on Validate. Data entered in the table (Insert) is then validated. Information in the edit area, that has not yet been inserted, is not validated.

To save the information, click on the Save Project button.

To validate and close, click on the OK button.

To cancel the information, click on the Cancel button.

To access the help information, click on the Help button.

Note: The <223> section of the sequence listing is updated by using either an Artificial Sequence/Unknown Organism or a misc_feature. The <223> section is the comment or other information, respectively. In PatentIn 3.1 there is an automatic expansion of the possible resolutions for "Xaa."

FEATURE KEY SELECTION

The Feature Names/Keys selection screen (Figure 9.12) allows you to select a nucleotide name.

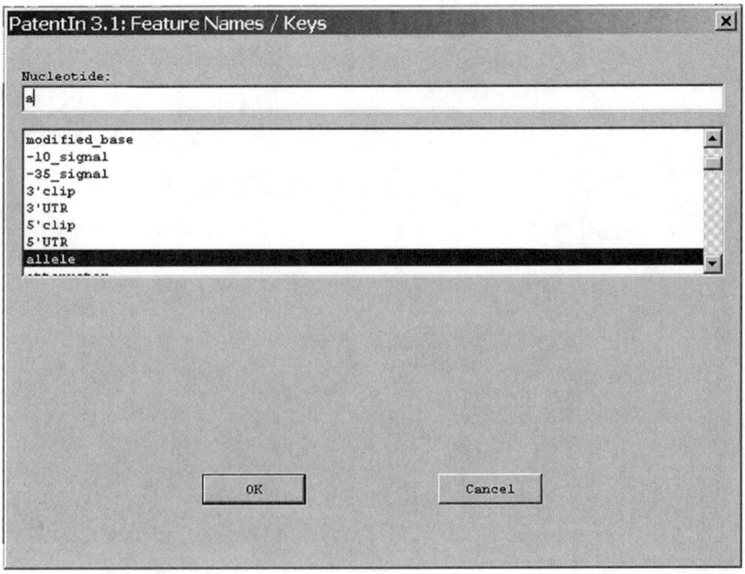

FIGURE 9.12

To select a nucleotide name, select the Names button on the Feature screen, begin typing on the Nucleotide field, or click on the down arrow to open the drop-down list; select a name from the list. Click on OK to accept the selection and return to the Feature screen.

Additional Information Required for Modified_Base

The Feature Names/Keys selection screen (Figure 9.13) automatically reveals an additional window when modified_base is selected.

To add information about the modified_base select the pull down arrow on the box marked "Add the following Modified_base to the Other Information." Select modified_base from the list. Click on OK.

Additional Information on CDS

When a Coding Sequence is specified for a polynucleotide sequence, the DNA sequence will appear in "mixed" format with the DNA split up into codons and the appropriate amino acid beneath each codon. This is exactly what specification of

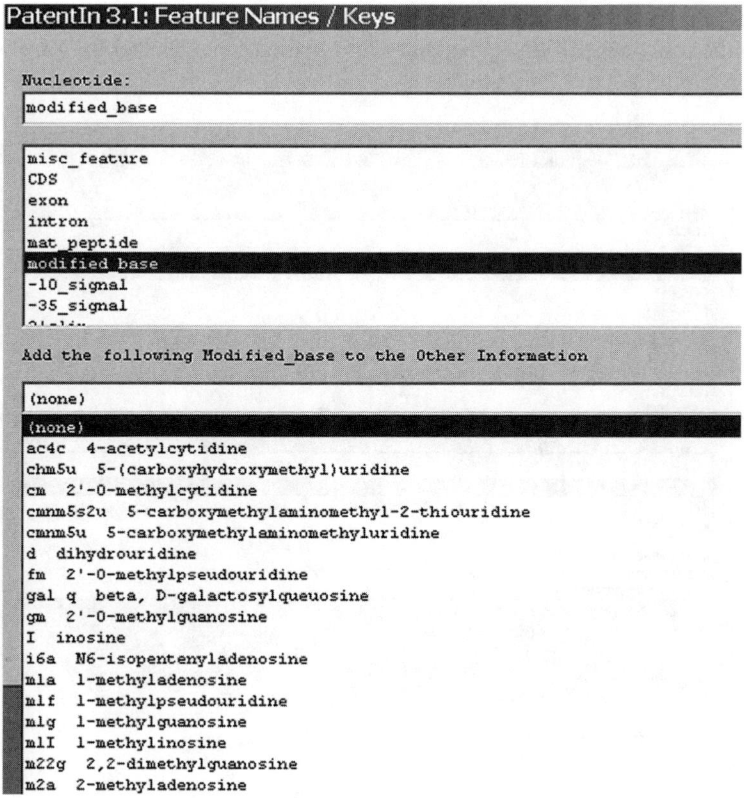

PatentIn 3.1: Feature Names / Keys

Nucleotide:

modified_base

misc_feature
CDS
exon
intron
mat_peptide
modified_base
-10_signal
-35_signal

Add the following Modified_base to the Other Information

(none)

(none)
ac4c   4-acetylcytidine
chm5u   5-(carboxyhydroxymethyl)uridine
cm   2'-O-methylcytidine
cmnm5s2u 5-carboxymethylaminomethyl-2-thiouridine
cmnm5u 5-carboxymethylaminomethyluridine
d   dihydrouridine
fm   2'-O-methylpseudouridine
gal q   beta, D-galactosylqueuosine
gm   2'-O-methylguanosine
I   inosine
i6a   N6-isopentenyladenosine
m1a   1-methyladenosine
m1f   1-methylpseudouridine
m1g   1-methylguanosine
m1I   1-methylinosine
m22g   2,2-dimethylguanosine
m2a   2-methyladenosine

FIGURE 9.13

the "exon" feature will do. Selection of CDS, however, forces PatentIn 3.1 to automatically generate the polypeptide sequence as a "supplemental" sequence.

Further Definition of "n" or "Xaa"

If the variable character "n" appears in a polynucleotide sequence or the variable "Xaa" appears in a polypeptide sequence, ST.25 requires further definition. This is to be provided in the Other Information field using Misc_Feature. PatentIn will copy the definition of "n" into the supplemental polypeptide sequence and translate it to "Xaa."

Selecting an Amino Acid

The Features/Names Key selection screen automatically reveals an additional window when LIPID is selected (Figure 9.14).

To select an Amino Acid name, select the Names button on the Feature screen, begin typing on the Amino Acid field, or click on the down arrow to open the drop-down list; select a name from the list. Click on OK to accept the selection and return to the Feature screen.

To add information about a LIPID, click the down arrow on the box marked "Add the following LIPID to the Other Information field." Select the LIPID information from the list. Click on OK.

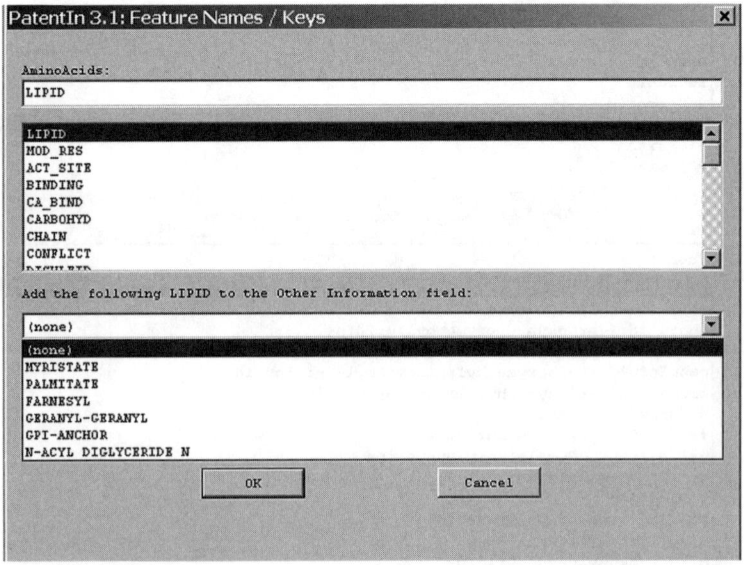

FIGURE 9.14

Additional Information for MOD_RES

The Feature Names/Key selection screen automatically reveals two additional windows when MOD_RES is selected. To select an Amino Acid name, select the Names button on the Feature screen. Begin typing on the Amino Acid field, or click on the down arrow to open the drop-down list; select a name from the list. Click on OK to accept the selection and return to the Feature screen.

To add information about the MOD_RES, select the pull down arrow on the first box in the "Add the following MOD_RES to the Other Information field." Select the appropriate information from the list. Click on OK. Click the down arrow on the second box in the "Add the following MOD_RES to the Other Information field." Select the appropriate information from the list. Click on OK.

PUBLICATION DATA

PUBLICATION DATA SCREEN

The Publication Data screen provides access to four screens for entering publication information: Journal, Database, Patent, and Thesis. You can access this screen by selecting Publication Data from the Application Steps menu (Figure 9.15).

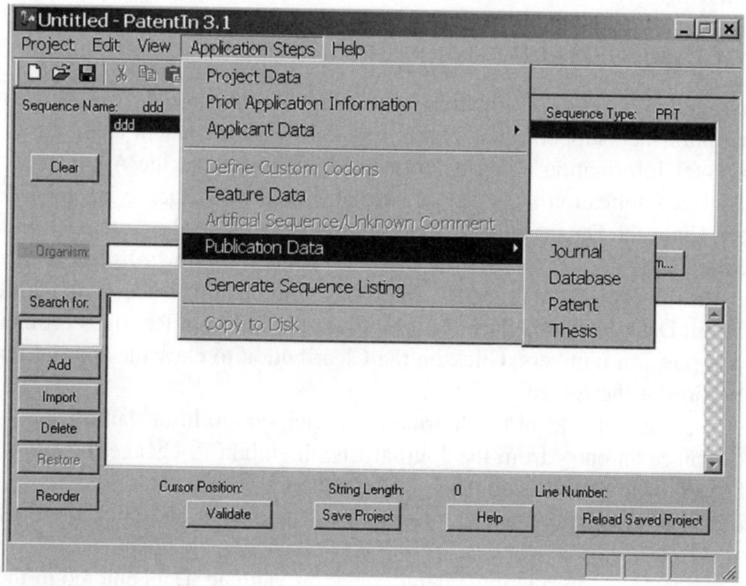

FIGURE 9.15

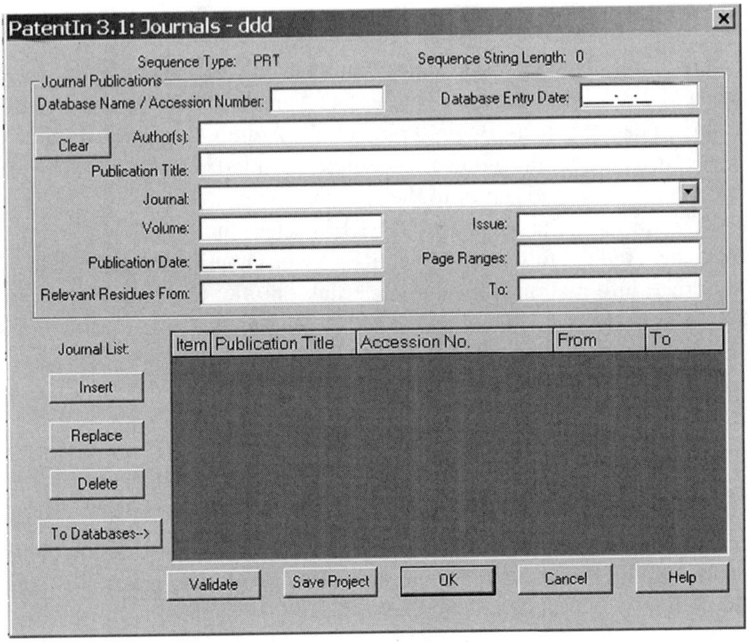

FIGURE 9.16

JOURNAL PUBLICATIONS INFORMATION

The Journal Publications information screen (Figure 9.16) provides you with a means to input published supporting scientific literature with the patent application.

To enter information about a journal publication, from the Application Steps menu, select Publication Data, select Journal. Enter the Database Name/Accession Number. Enter the Database Entry Date. Enter the name of the Author(s). Enter the Publication Title. Select the Journal name from the drop-down list. If the name is not on the list you may enter it. Enter the Volume. Enter the Issue. Enter the Publication Date. Enter the Page Ranges. Enter the Relevant Residues From and To sequence position numbers. Click on the Clear button to clear the Journal Publications portion of the screen.

To insert an entry from the Journal List, click on the Insert button.

To replace an entry from the Journal List, highlight it, change the entry in the top of the screen and click on the Replace button.

To delete an entry from the Journal List, highlight it and click on the Delete button.

To validate the information entered, click on Validate. Data entered in the table (Insert) is then validated. Information in the Journal Publications edit area, that has not yet been inserted, is not validated. To validate and close, click on the OK button. To proceed to the next Publication Data, Database, click on the To Databases → button.

To save the information, click on the Save Project button.

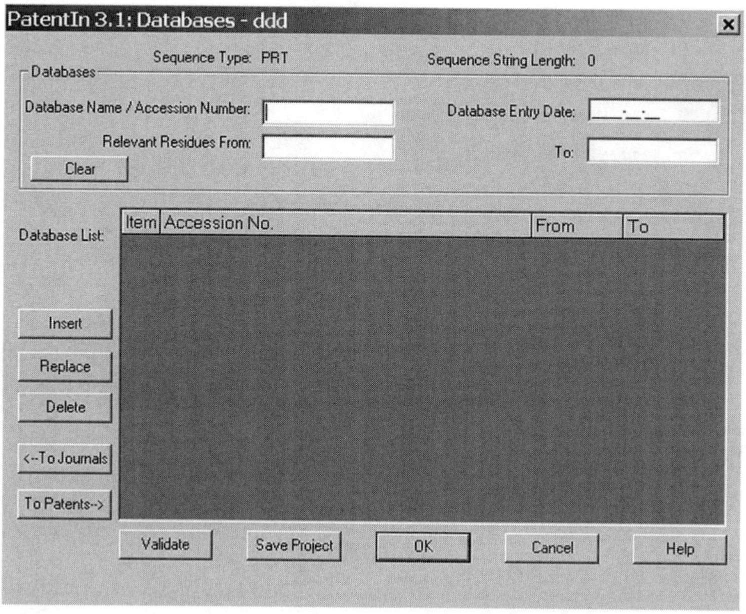

FIGURE 9.17

DATABASES PUBLICATION INFORMATION

The Databases publication information screen (Figure 9.17) provides you with a means to input published supporting scientific database with the patent application. To enter information about a database publication, from the Application Steps select Publication Data, then select Database. Enter the Database Name/Accession Number. Enter the Database Entry Date. Enter the Relevant Residues From and To sequence position numbers. Click on the Clear button to clear the Databases part of the screen.

To insert an entry into the Database List, click on the Insert button.

To replace an entry from the Database List, highlight it, change the entry in the top of the screen and click on the Replace button.

To delete an entry from the Database List, highlight it and click on the Delete button.

To validate the information entered, click on Validate. Data entered in the table (Insert) is then validated. Information in the edit area, that has not yet been inserted, is not validated. To validate and close, click on the OK button.

To go back to the previous Publication Data, Journal, click on the ← To Journals button. To proceed to the next Publication Data, Patent, click on the To Patents → button.

To save the information, click on the Save Project button.

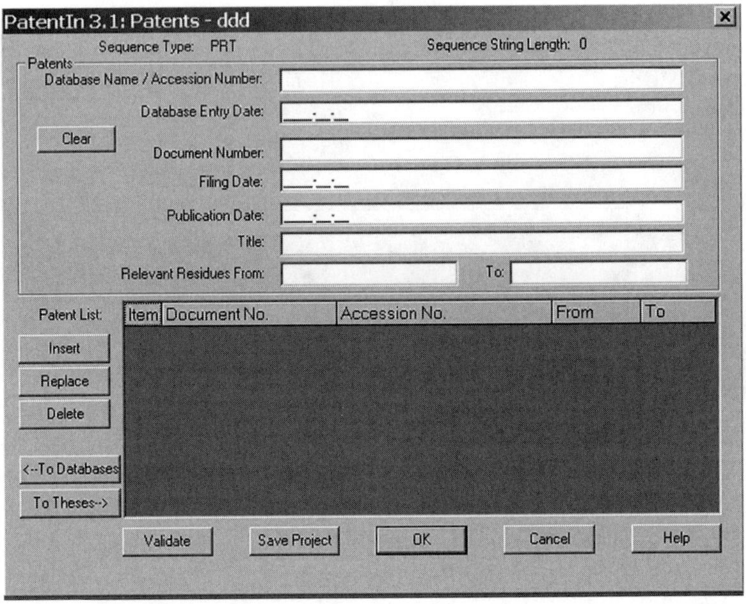

FIGURE 9.18

Patents Publication Information

The Patents publication information screen (Figure 9.18) provides you with a means to input published supporting patent publication information with the patent application.

To enter information about a patent publication, from the Application Steps select Publication Data, then select Patent. Enter the Database Name/Accession Number. Enter the Database Entry Date. Enter the Document Number. Enter the Filing Date. Enter the Publication Date. Enter the Title. Enter the Relevant Residues From and To sequence position numbers. Click on the Clear button to clear the Patents portion of the screen.

To insert an entry into the Patent List, click on the Insert button.

To replace an entry from the Patent List, highlight it, change the entry in the top of the screen and click on the Replace button.

To delete an entry from the Patent List, highlight it and click on the Delete button.

To validate the information entered, click on Validate. Data entered in the table (Insert) is then validated. Information in the edit area, that has not yet been inserted, is not validated. To validate and close, click on the OK button.

To save the information, click on the Save Project button.

To go back to the previous Publication Data, Database, click on the ← To Databases button. To proceed to the next Publication Data, Thesis, click on the To Theses → button.

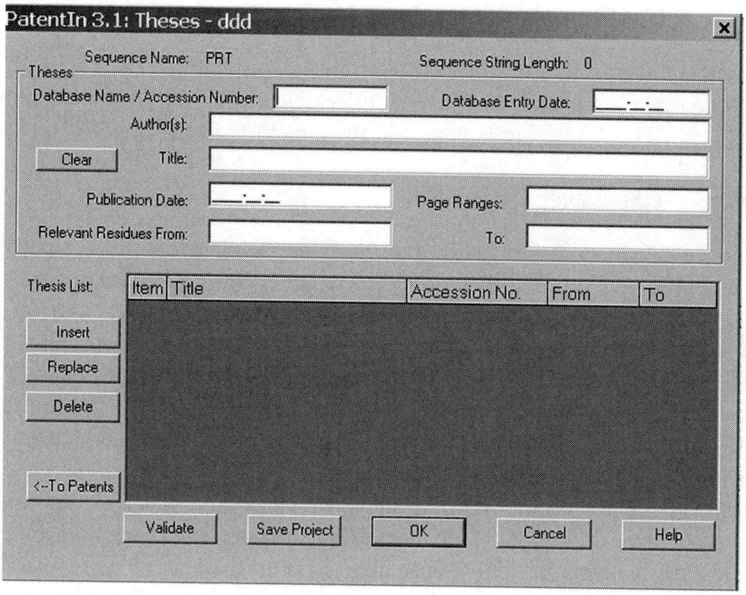

FIGURE 9.19

THESES PUBLICATION INFORMATION

The Theses publication information screen (Figure 9.19) provides you with a means to input published supporting thesis publication information with the patent application.

To enter information about a thesis publication, from the Application Steps select Publication Data, then select Thesis. Enter the Database Name/Accession Number. Enter the Database Entry Date. Enter the names of the Author(s). Enter the Title. Enter the Publication Date. Enter the Page Ranges. Enter the Relevant Residues From and To sequence position numbers. Click on the Clear button to clear the Theses portion of the screen.

To insert an entry into the Thesis List, click on the Insert button.

To replace an entry from the Thesis List, highlight it, change the entry in the top of the screen and click on the Replace button.

To delete an entry from the Thesis List, highlight it and click on the Delete button.

To validate the information entered, click on Validate. Data entered in the table (Insert) is then validated. Information in the edit area, that has not yet been inserted, is not validated.

To save the information, click on the Save Project button. To validate and close, click on the OK button.

To go back to the previous Publication Data, Patent, click on the ← To Patents button.

CREATING A SEQUENCE LISTING PROJECT FILE

The sequence listing file includes all the information required by ST.25. PatentIn 3.x will generate a sequence listing with the extension "ST25.txt" appended to the project name. This ST.25 file is placed in the directory containing the project.

GENERATING A SEQUENCE LISTING FILE

The Sequence Generation screen notifies you that the Generate process is about to occur and gives the option to be notified as errors occur during the process.

To generate a sequence listing, select Generate Sequence Listing from the Application Steps menu or by selecting the Gen button on the PatentIn toolbar. Click in the box next to "Pause after each error message" if you wish to be notified of an error in the sequence data when it occurs. Click in the box next to "View listing or error log when done" if you wish to see the listing or error log immediately after the generation. The listing/log will be automatically displayed when the generation has terminated. Click on the Start the sequence generation. Click on the Continue button to continue validation. Click on the Cancel button to cancel validation. If an error message is displayed and "Pause after each error message" was selected, an error message will appear and validation will pause (Figures 9.20 and 9.21).

VIEWING A SEQUENCE LISTING FILE

To view a Sequence Listing Project File (Figure 9.22), if sequence generation succeeded and "View listing or error log when done" was selected, the sequence

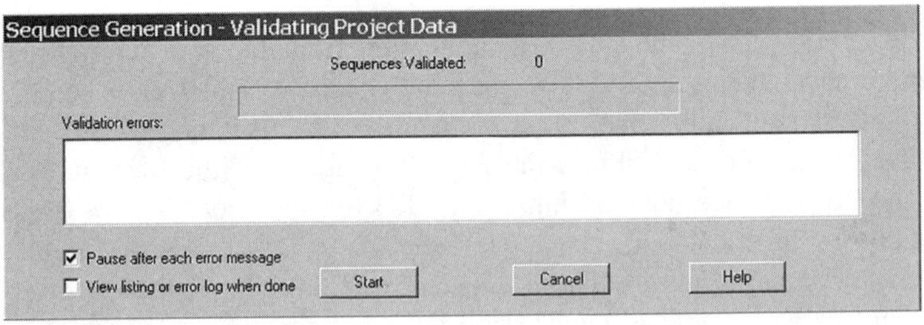

FIGURE 9.20

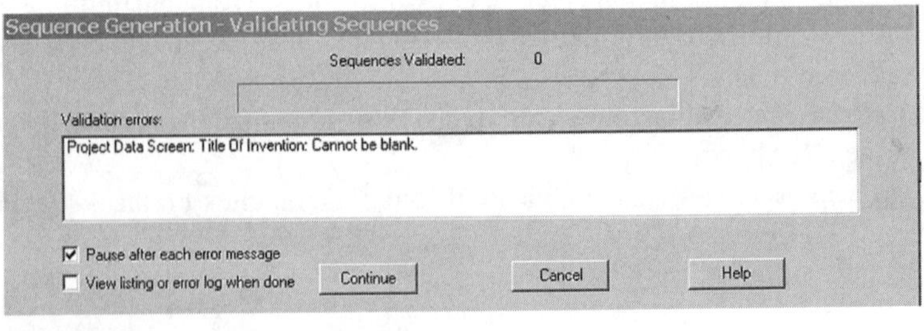

FIGURE 9.21

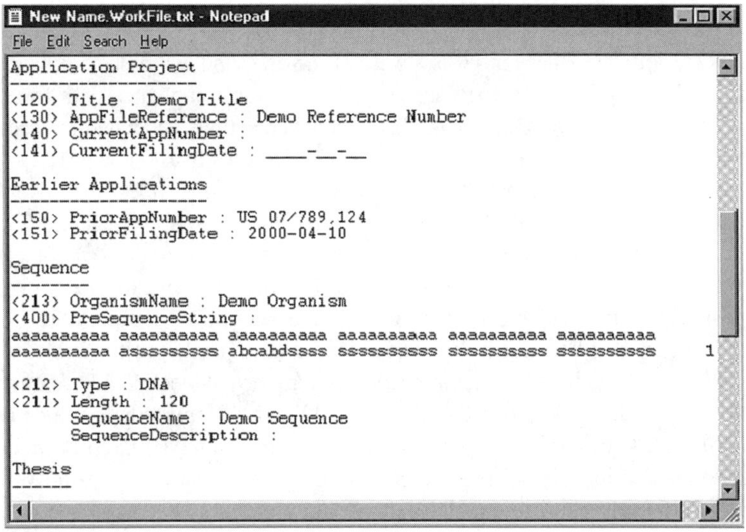

```
New Name.WorkFile.txt - Notepad
File Edit Search Help
Application Project
--------------------
<120> Title : Demo Title
<130> AppFileReference : Demo Reference Number
<140> CurrentAppNumber :
<141> CurrentFilingDate : ____-__-__

Earlier Applications
--------------------
<150> PriorAppNumber : US 07/789,124
<151> PriorFilingDate : 2000-04-10

Sequence
--------
<213> OrganismName : Demo Organism
<400> PreSequenceString :
aaaaaaaaaa aaaaaaaaaa aaaaaaaaaa aaaaaaaaaa aaaaaaaaaa aaaaaaaaaa
aaaaaaaaaa assssssss abcabdssss ssssssssss ssssssssss ssssssssss     1

<212> Type : DNA
<211> Length : 120
      SequenceName : Demo Sequence
      SequenceDescription :

Thesis
------
```

FIGURE 9.22

listing will be shown automatically. If "View listing or error log when done" was not selected, you can view the sequence by selecting View Sequence Listing from the Project menu.

Special note for users with very large sequences and large numbers of sequences: The USPTO has located a viewer that works well for very large text files. A 60-day evaluation version is downloadable at www.fileviewer.com. The viewer is named "V" and the version is 2000 SR-1. It was tested with 60 and 120 MB files and "worked great." It should manage files of almost any size. The USPTO is not recommending this product but is naming it as an example of the type of product available for this use.

Copying the Sequence Listing to Disk

Copy to Disk provides you with the means to name the drive to where the file is to be copied, the file name for the copied file, and the type of copied file. To copy a sequence listing, select Copy to Disk from the Application Steps menu. Enter the drive name in the Save in field. Enter the File name in the File name field. Select the type .txt or .zip in the Save in: field. Click on Save to submit the application. If .txt is selected, PatentIn checks to see if there is enough free disk space to receive the listing file. If so, the file will be copied to the selected location. If not, PatentIn will suggest .zip. *Note:* .zip works only with floppy disk(s) and will format the disk before writing anything to the disk. In general, if a hard drive is selected, you will be prompted to select a removable medium as the target for this copy. The save to a CD expects the CD to function like any other drive, i.e., you can perform Explorer-type commands as if the CD were a disk drive (example: F drive). If your CD does not have such a driver, the file can still be located on your hard drive where it was generated. It is the project name with ".ST25.txt" appended to it.

CHECKER FOR BIOTECHNOLOGY SEQUENCE LISTING

The USPTO software Checker 4.0 is a state-of the-art Windows-based software application for checking biotechnology sequence listings for compliance with format and content rules. Checker Version 4.0 validates sequence listings generated in accordance with the U.S. sequence rules, 37 CFR 1.821–1.825, effective October 1, 1990 (old rules), or the revised version of the US sequence rules (new rules) effective July 1, 1998, as well as World Intellectual Property Organization (WIPO) Standard ST.25.

Checker Version 4.0 replaces the previous version (Checker 3.18) and the earlier DOS-based version of Checker. Checker allows public users to check sequence listings in computer readable form (CRF) before submitting them to the USPTO. Use of Checker prior to filing the sequence listing is expected to result in fewer erred sequence listings, thus saving time and money. Checker 4.0 features full compatibility with the Microsoft Windows 2000 and XP operating systems as well as all Office 2000/XP products. Also, a new setup file named ChkSetup.exe ensures fast, easy installation of the application. A macro for use in Microsoft Word that activates line numbering, to enable viewing line numbers in a sequence listing, is included with the Checker distribution files and is automatically copied to the Checker installation folder. The name of the file is CrfMacros.doc. To access it, open Word, select the open file icon, navigate to the Checker installation folder, and select the macro. Checker does not verify contents of comment fields, only that a required comment is present. Such comments include definitions of any "n"s or "Xaa"s that appear in the sequence listing and comments regarding selection of Artificial or Unknown for the organism. Thus, careful attention needs to be paid to the content of these fields.

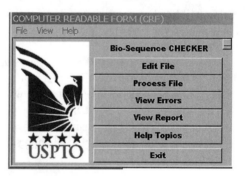

FIGURE 9.23

Checker 4.0 can be downloaded from http://www.uspto.gov/web/offices/pac/checker (Figure 9.23).

Checker Main Menu Window

When you open the Checker application, the Checker Main Menu window (Figure 9.23) appears after clicking Continue from the Welcome screen. The Checker Main Menu includes the following six buttons:

1. Edit File
2. Process File
3. View Errors
4. View Report
5. Help Topics
6. Exit

Checker Edit File Button

To edit a file before running Process File, clicking on Edit opens a Wordpad document window. Select File and then Open from the Main Menu. Click on the file to be edited and click Open. The file is opened in Wordpad or in your default editor.

To edit a file after running Process File, click Edit File on the Checker Main Menu. The WordPad document window displays the input file that was last processed. Edit the file and save.

Checker Process File Button

To process a file, click Process File on the Checker Main Menu. The Open dialog box displays. Click on the file to be processed. Click Open. The Progress Bar dialog box displays. The Progress Bar dialog box closes when validation is complete. If there are errors in the file, the There Are Errors in Your File dialog box displays. If there are no errors in the file, the There Are No Errors in Your File dialog box displays. Click OK. The Checker Main Menu displays.

To view the file errors (if there are errors in your file), click View Errors on the Checker Main Menu.

Checker View Errors Button

To view errors, click View Errors on the Checker Main Menu. The Errors Report is opened in Wordpad or your default editor.

Checker View Report Button

To view the Verification Summary Report (VSR), click View Report on the Checker Main Menu. The VSR is opened in Wordpad or your default editor.

Checker Help Button

To access the Checker online help menu, click Help on the Checker Main Menu. The Checker Online Help menu displays.

Checker Exit Button

To exit Checker, click Exit to exit the Main Menu and return to the main Checker application page. From here, you can use the Checker menu bar.

Checker Properties Dialog Box

To view the Properties Dialog Box, click File or select Alt+F on the keyboard to view the File menu. Click Administration and then Properties to view the Properties dialog box. The Properties dialog box allows you to change the input and output directory paths as well as select an alternate ASCII file editor. To change file editor, you must specify the path and executable file name of a suitable editor to replace WordPad.

About the Checker Dialog Box

To view the About Checker Dialog Box, click Help or select Alt+H on the keyboard to view the Help Menu. Click About Checker to view the About dialog box. The About Checker dialog displays the version number and release date of the installed Checker application, as well as copyright information. The USPTO will periodically update Checker and the current version and release date will be displayed on the Internet site at www.uspto.gov/patents/software.htm.

List of Acronyms

The following acronyms are used in the Checker system.

Acronym	Definition
ABSS	Automated Biotechnology Sequence Search
C.F.R.	Code of Federal Regulations
CRF	Computer Readable Form
MB	Megabytes
PC	Personal Computer
URL	Uniform Resource Locator
USPTO	United States Patent and Trademark Office
VSR	Verification Summary Report

Error Messages

All possible error messages in the Checker software are included in the following list. The legend for the error messages is C = Corrected text string(s); E = error as defined in 32 CFR 1.821–1.825 rules; S = system errors; W = warning as defined in 32 C.F.R. 1.821 – 1.825 rules.

System Errors
100 S: Failure opening input file
101 S: Failure reading input file
102 S: Failure writing output file
103 S: Failure allocating memory

General Messages
110 C: Removed nonprintable characters
111 C: String data converted to upper case
112 C: String data converted to lower case
113 C: Missing blank line
114 E: Unexpected end of input file

General Header Messages
200 E: Mandatory header field missing
201 E: Mandatory field data missing
202 E: Value must be an integer
203 E: Calc# of seq differs from actual; <:input (A), counted (B)>
204 E: Calc# of bases differs from actual; <:input (A), counted (B)>

205 E: Calc length of seq differs from actual; <:input (A), counted (B)>

210 E: Invalid number of sequences

212 E: Invalid or duplicate sequence ID number

214 E: Seq.# missing; <:Seq.ID (A)>

216 E: Seq.#s missing; <:Seq.ID (A) thru (B)>

218 E: Input file vs calc seq length differ; <:input (A), calc (B)>

Alpha Header Messages

220 C: Keyword misspelled

222 E: Mandatory keyword missing

230 E: Invalid or missing general information

240 E: Invalid or missing sequence header field

241 E: Invalid alpha header field

242 E: Mandatory header field value missing

243 E: Alpha header field expected

244 E: Invalid beginning of sequence listing

245.E: Invalid value of alpha general header field

246 E: Invalid value of alpha sequence header field

247 C: Inserted optional header field

248 E: Inserted missing mandatory header field

249 C: Inserted mandatory field

Numeric Header Messages

250 E: Invalid numeric identifier

252 E: Calc# of seq differs from actual; <:input (A), counted (B)>

253 E: Calc# of bases differs from actual; <:input (A), counted (B)>

254 E: Number of bases conflicts running total; <:input (A), counted (B)>

256 E: Numeric Identifier expected

257 W: Sequence data name/key feature missing

258 E: Mandatory feature missing

259 E: Field exceeds allowed number of lines

270 C: Current application number differs

271 C: Current filing date differs

280 E: Numeric identifier already exists

281 E: Numeric fields not ordered

282 E: Numeric field identifier missing

283 E: Missing blank line separator; <before this field identifier>

284 E: Blank line not allowed; <before this field identifier>

285 E: Invalid journal date: wrong YYY-MM-DD, MMM-YYYY or season-YYYY

286 E: Invalid database entry date: wrong YYYY-MM-DD or MMMM-YYYY

287 E: Invalid date; <wrong YYY-MM-DD or MMMM-YYYY>

288 E: Application number is repeated; <prior application number:>

289 E: Numeric identifier mission or out-of-order; <prior application number>

Sequence Data Messages

300 W: Intentionally skipped sequence: sequence ID ()

301 E: No sequence data was shown
302 E: Unknown or misplaced identifier
310 E: Wrong or missing sequence type
320 E: Wrong nucleic acid designator
321 E: "t" not allowed in the RNA sequence
322 E: Invalid residue in sequence
330 E: Wrong amino acid designator
332 E: Invalid/missing amino acid numbering
333 E: Wrong sequence grouping; <spacing>
334 E: Invalid amino acid in coding region
336 E: Invalid amino acid number in coding region
340 E: "n" or "Xaa" used: feature required
341 W: "n" or "Xaa" used
342 E: Invalid stop code on error
344 W: Removed stop code on error
351 E: Sequence data name/key feature out-of-range
360 E: Sequence data overflow
361 E: Invalid split codon

10 USPTO ePAVE

OVERVIEW

Chapters 5 and 6 have provided an overview and various filing scenarios that require use of ePAVE (electronic Packaging and Validation Engine) software. You are advised to read those chapters thoroughly before consulting this chapter, which provides greater detail on how to use ePAVE. It is also advisable that you have ePAVE running while reading this chapter, if possible, to quickly examine the referenced screens and commands; as a result, this chapter does not include detailed graphics presentation of screens.

To file a submission with the USPTO via the Internet, you must be identified as one of the following authorized patent application filers:

- Applicant
- Assignee
- Attorney or Agent
- Assignee undivided part as set forth in 37 CFR 1.33(b)

If you want to use EFS software to submit pre-grant publication filings, please refer to pre-grant publication regulations 37 CFR, 1.211–1.221, for a full description of the process. If you want to file biotechnology sequence listings, you must have a pending paper utility patent application that requires a nucleotide and/or amino acid sequence submission in computer readable form (CRF) (37 CFR 1.824). You must have already created the sequence listing using either the USPTO PatentIn sequence authoring application or another acceptable sequence authoring tool.

In addition to providing electronic forms, ePAVE allows the applicant or practitioner to attach a tagged, structured specification document that includes links to applicable figure image files. Other patent application documents, such as the declaration, are attached as scanned single-page TIFF image files. ePAVE enables patent applicants and appointed practitioners to conduct real-time electronic filing of select new utility patent applications. EFS also enables filing over the Internet of four types of subsequent filings: selected pre-grant publication submissions, information disclosure statements for pending applications, assignment documents for previously filed applications and patents, and submission of CRF amino acid and/or nucleotide sequence listing required during prosecution of a pending biotechnology patent application. The applicant first authors the specification document using a word processing based authoring tool which has the capability to produce an Extensible Markup Language (XML) tagged electronic document. Then the applicant uses ePAVE submission software to attach and send the application specification with any figures to USPTO along with other patent application information.

The submission software accepts ASCII sequence listing files created by a sequence listing authoring tool, PatentIn (as well as accommodating ASCII sequence listing files created by other standard methods or editors). Refer to 37 CFR 1.824 (see Chapter 9). The sequence listing shall be submitted in ASCII text. No other formats are allowed. Using USPTO-developed ePAVE submission software applicants may author XML documents such as fee transmittals or Application Data Sheets, attach electronic documents and image files in specified formats, and validate the completeness of the submission based on patent business rules. The ePAVE program automatically bundles, compresses, encrypts, and digitally signs the submission package once the applicant or appointed practitioner enters an electronic signature and digital certificate authentication information. An acknowledgment receipt is displayed in real-time at the filer's desktop after the submission package is received and validated at the USPTO without error.

INTRODUCTION

The installation and uninstallation procedures of ePAVE follow the general procedures for other Windows®-based software. EFS software components are client applications, and ePAVE can be used with network Internet connections and with networked machines. The most important consideration in effective use of EFS in a network environment is file management. The application files created with the authoring tools (PASAT or TSA) or with ePAVE must reside in network storage that is mapped to all machines working with the application. All EFS files (PASAT and ePAVE) for a given application should be in a dedicated folder. This allows common access to the files from any PC on the network and allows EFS to locate and attach/bundle all the files constituting the application when assembling the submission. Because EFS software associates an application's files with each other based on their path name, their location should not be changed once the files have been stored.

You may receive an error message concerning the calendar functions that are a part of the software. If you receive this error message, or any similar error, your SSCALA32.OCX file is in the wrong location in your directory. To solve this problem, you must correct the location of the file and then uninstall and reinstall ePAVE.

The USPTO will periodically release new versions of the ePAVE software, and you will then need to update your copy. In order to ensure that you are running the most current version of ePAVE, the application automatically gives you the option to check your version each time you launch it. Click Yes to check with the USPTO server for the most recent version. If you want to disable ePAVE's automatic version checking on startup, you may clear it from the File menu. Select the Version Checking Reminder at Startup option to toggle it on and off. The check mark indicates that version checking at startup is active, and is not shown once you disable this feature.

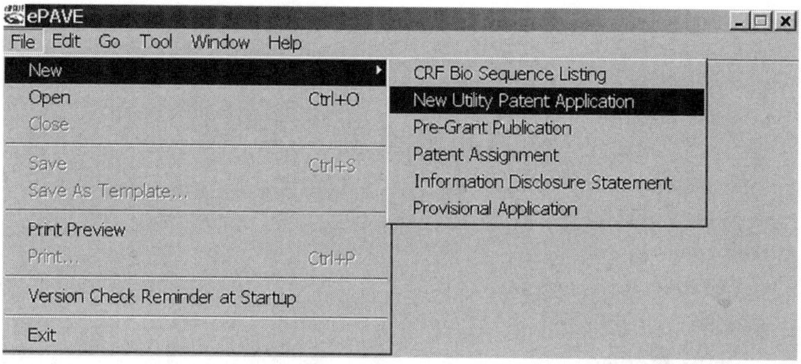

FIGURE 10.1

USER INTERFACE

The ePAVE interface includes the following components: menus, a toolbar, and screens. The menus allow you to perform various functions, including opening and closing documents, saving and printing documents, validating your submission, and sending it to the USPTO. The toolbar provides buttons that allow you to perform various ePAVE tasks without using the menus. The screens contain the data fields where you enter your submission information that is sent to the USPTO.

MENUS

The ePAVE interface has six main menus (File, Edit, Go, Tool, Window, Help; Figure 10.1), each with various submenus:

- File
  - New
    - CRF Biosequence Listing
    - New Utility Patent Application
    - Pre-Grant Publication
    - Patent Assignment
    - Information Disclosure Statement
    - Provisional Application
  - Open [Ctrl+O]
  - Close
  - Save [Ctrl+S]
  - Save As Template
  - Print Preview
  - Print [Ctrl+P]
  - Version Check Reminder at Startup
  - Exit

- Edit
  - Cut [Ctrl+X]
  - Copy [Ctrl+C]
  - Paste [Ctrl+V]
- Go
  - Validate Submission
  - Send to USPTO
- Tool
  - Default User Directory
- Window
  - Show Forms
- Help
  - User's Guide
  - About ePAVE…

TOOLBAR

The toolbar contains the icons that you use to perform various ePAVE tasks. Following is a list of the toolbar icons and their names, as well as a description of the function of each icon:

Biosequence Listing prompts you to save any information you have already entered on the ePAVE screens. Select Yes or No. ePAVE then prompts you to create a new submission folder and begin the process of creating a new CRF biosequence listing submission.

New Utility Patent Application prompts you to save any information you have already entered on the ePAVE screens. Select Yes or No. ePAVE then prompts you to create a new submission folder and begin the process of creating a new utility patent application submission.

Pre-Grant Publication prompts you to save any information you have already entered on the ePAVE screens. Select Yes or No. ePAVE then prompts you to create a new submission folder and begin the process of creating a new pre-grant publication submission.

Patent Assignment prompts you to save any information you have already entered on the ePAVE screens. Select Yes or No. ePAVE then prompts you to create a new submission folder and begin the process of creating a new patent assignment submission.

Information Disclosure Statement prompts you to save any information you have already entered on the ePAVE screens. Select Yes or No. ePAVE then prompts you to create a new submission folder and begin the process of creating a new information disclosure statement for a pending application.

Provisional Application prompts you to save any information you have already entered on the ePAVE screens. Select Yes or No. ePAVE then prompts you to create a new submission folder and begin the process of creating a new provisional patent application submission.

Open an existing EFS submission file that you previously saved. Locate the existing submission folder in the directory path.

Save the EFS submission information you have authored thus far.

Print the information on the active screen.

Cut to remove text from the selected text field.

Copy the selected text.

Paste text to the selected text field.

Validate Syntax and Business Rule to initiate the validation check of all text fields. This identifies errors in data entry or missing information that is required for EFS submission.

Send to USPTO to go to the Submit tab to initiate sending your submission to the USPTO.

SCREENS

Each of the ePAVE screens is represented by a tab below the toolbar. You can access the different screens by clicking on the tab that corresponds to the screen that you want to access. Once you access a screen, you can move through the data fields by using the Tab key on your keyboard or by clicking in each field with the mouse. You can also move backwards through the fields by simultaneously pressing the Shift and Tab keys on your keyboard. The choice of screens that you use is dependent on the type of submission you are filing. The ePAVE data entry screens must collect a minimum amount of information to ensure that your electronic patent application filing is complete and valid for examination and subsequent publication. All mandatory fields or sections in ePAVE are identified by bold type, while optional fields or sections are shown in regular type.

The main screen (Figure 10.2) is organized into a series of tabs (General, Filer, Forms, Attachments, Validation, Comments, Submit) that you must complete regardless of the type of submission you are filing. The information you enter in the fields on each tab is automatically tagged as XML output. The Certificate of Transmittal screen appears as a primary screen only when you select either a CRF Biosequence Listing or Pre-Grant Publication submission, because patent business rules do not allow the use of a Certificate of Transmittal for a new utility or provisional patent application submission. From the Forms tab screen you will select the form or forms that you want to include in this electronic patent application submission. Based on your selection, ePAVE adds any additional screens that are required for your submission.

GENERAL TAB

General Tab fields

Prerequisites: For a Biosequence Listing subsequent to filing of an application, select the type of submission being made from the drop-down list. Choose either Subsequent Filing Before Issue Date or Subsequent Filing After Issue Date. This is required for Biosequence submissions.

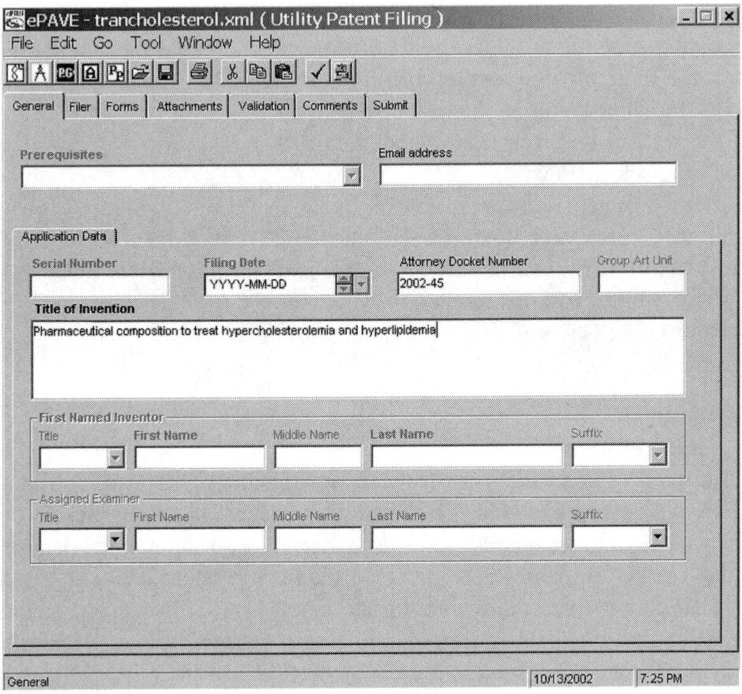

FIGURE 10.2

This field is disabled and grayed out for new filings and Pre-Grant Publication submissions.

E-mail Address: Enter a primary Internet e-mail address that the USPTO can use to send e-mail related to this particular filing only. This address does not supersede the official e-mail address on file as the electronic correspondence address. (Optional)

Serial Number: For Biosequence Listings and Pre-Grant Publication submissions, enter the application serial number that was assigned to this patent application by the USPTO. This is required for Biosequence Listings and Pre-Grant Publication submissions. For new application filings this field is disabled and grayed out.

Filing Date: For Biosequence Listings and Pre-Grant Publication submissions, enter the official (actual) filing date that was granted to this application by the USPTO. This is required for Biosequence and Pre-Grant Publication submissions. For utility patent filings, this field is disabled and grayed out.

Attorney Docket Number: Enter the reference number of your choice as a means of identifying your application. This number is not assigned by the USPTO. (Optional)

Group Art Unit: For Biosequence Listing filings, enter the art unit number where the application is assigned for examination, if known. (Optional)

Title of the Invention: Enter the full title of the patent application for which this filing is being submitted. Include all spaces and punctuation. (Required)

First Named Inventor: For Biosequence submissions enter the first named inventor information in this field. This is required for Biosequence submissions. For new filings and Pre-Grant Publication submissions these fields are grayed out and will be populated when the Application Data Sheet is filled out.

Title: Enter a courtesy title such as Mr., Mrs., Ms., Dr., etc. (Optional)

First Name: Enter the first or given name. (Required)

Middle Name: Enter the middle name. (Optional)

Last Name: Enter the family or surname. (Required)

Suffix: Enter a generational title such as Jr., Sr., III, etc. (Optional)

Assigned Examiner: For Biosequence Listings enter information identifying the Examiner to whom this application is assigned, if known. This entire section is optional; however, if an Examiner is being identified, certain elements in this section are required.

Title: Enter a courtesy title such as Mr., Mrs., Ms., Dr., etc. (Optional)

First Name: Enter the first or given name. (Required if any information is entered in this section)

Middle Name: Enter the middle name. (Optional)

Last Name: Enter the family or surname. (Required if any information is entered in this section)

Suffix: Enter a generational title such as Jr., Sr., III, etc. (Optional)

FILER TAB

The fields on this screen vary depending on the type of filer that you specify. The filer information that you enter on this screen becomes part of the transmittal form that ePAVE automatically produces as an XML form document. In accordance with 37 CFR 1.33(b), the filer or filers can be attorneys or agents, applicants, or assignees. Assignees are people or organizations who sign the transmittal on behalf of another party. If you are filing as an organization, you must also provide the Organization name and the Title at Organization of the person signing the application. The following combinations of filers are acceptable: one or more attorney(s) or agent(s), one assignee only, one or more applicant(s) and assignee(s) of undivided part.

Type of Filer fields

Applicant: Identifies the filer as an inventor or an applicant acting for an inventor under 37 CFR 1.42, 1.43, or 1.47.

Assignee: Identifies the filer as the owner to whom the rights and interest of the invention has been assigned by the applicants. The owner may be a person or an organization. If the assignee is an organization, a person

authorized to sign on behalf of that organization must be identified by
name and title.

Attorney or Agent: Identifies the filer as a practitioner or party under 37
CFR 1.34 who is authorized to prosecute the invention on behalf of the
applicant(s) and/or assignee(s).

Assignee Undivided Part: Identifies the filer as the owner to whom an undivided part interest of the invention has been assigned by applicant(s).
The owner may be a person or an organization. It the assignee is an organization, a person must be identified by name and title that is authorized to sign on behalf of that organization.

Registration Number: Enter the individual registration number of the
practitioner(s) filing this submission on behalf of the applicant(s)
and/or assignee(s). (Optional)

Assignee radio fields

Person: Select this choice if the assignee filing this transmittal is a person.

Organization: Select this choice if the assignee filing this transmittal is a
business entity or nonprofit institution.

Organization Name: Enter the name of the organization if the assignee or
assignee of undivided part interest filing this submission is an organization. The organization may be a business entity or a nonprofit institution. (Required for organizations)

Title at Organization: Enter the official title of the person who is signing
on behalf of the identified organization if the assignee or assignee of undivided part interest filing this submission is an organization. (Optional
for organizations)

Other fields

New: Click this button to clear all of the fields on the Filer screen and begin creating a new filer.

Delete: Click this button to delete a filer you select from a list of filers.

Applicant: Click this button to identify the filer as an inventor or an applicant acting for an inventor under 37 CFR 1.42, 1.43, or 1.47.

Assignee: Click this button to identify the filer as the owner to whom the
rights and interest of the invention have been assigned by the applicants. The owner may be a person or an organization. If the assignee is
an organization, a person authorized to sign on behalf of that organization must be identified by name and title.

Attorney or Agent: Click this button to identify the filer as a practitioner
or party under 37 CFR 1.34 who is authorized to prosecute the invention on behalf of the applicant(s) and/or assignee(s).

Assignee Undivided Part: Click this button to identify the filer as the
owner to whom an undivided part interest of the invention has been assigned by applicant(s). The owner may be a person or an organization.
If the assignee is an organization, a person authorized to sign on behalf
of that organization must be identified by name and title.

CREATING A NEW FILER

Use the following procedure to create a new Filer:

1. Click the Filer tab to go to the Filer screen. ePAVE opens the Filer screen.
2. Select the type of filer by clicking the appropriate radio button in the Type of Filer section. ePAVE disables any fields that are not required for the type of filer that you have selected.
3. Complete the remaining fields in the Filer Information section. *Note:* If the new filer is an Assignee or Assignee Undivided Part, you must also select either Person or Organization from the appropriate radio buttons to indicate whether this assignee is an actual person or a business or nonprofit entity.
4. Click the Add button. The filer is added to the list of filers shown on the left side of the screen.
5. Repeat Step 2 through Step 4 for any additional filers.

CHANGING FILER DATA

ePAVE allows you to change the filer information for filers that you have already added. Use the following procedure to change filer information:

1. Go to the Type/Name field, and click the name of the filer that you want to edit. The current information for the selected filer appears in the Filer Information fields.
2. Enter any changes in the appropriate fields.
3. Click the Update button to update the filer information with your changes.

DELETING A FILER

ePAVE allows you to remove filers from the list of filers. Use the following procedure to remove a filer:

1. Click the name of the filer that you want to delete in the filers list, shown in the Type/Name field on the left side of the screen.
2. Click the Delete button. The filer is removed from the list of filers, and all of the information about this filer is deleted.

FORMS TAB

The Forms tab has two sections: (1) Form Description and Usage and (2) Simple Form List. The Form Description and Usage section displays text that describes the selected form and its intended use. The Simple Form List section shows all forms that are available for electronic filing in the Available Forms list, and shows forms in the EFS submission folder that you have selected to send to the USPTO during your electronic filing transaction in the Selected Forms list. When a form title appears in bold letters, it indicates that the form is required for the type of patent application submission electronic filing you are creating. If, for example, you are filing a CRF Biosequence Listing, the Biosequence Transmittal form is required and is therefore shown in bold letters in both the Available Forms and Selected Forms lists. When you click on the name of a form in either the Available Forms or Selected Forms list, a description of the form and its usage appear in the Form Description and Usage text display box.

The forms listed in the Available Forms text box are (1) Application data, which will assist you in authoring XML documents such as the application data form as defined in 37 CFR 1.76 (Application Data Sheet); (2) a Fee Transmittal; (3) a Patent Assignment Recordation document for a patent provisional application; and (4) the Biosequence Transmittal for a CRF Biosequence Listing filing. *Note:* The Application Data sheet is the equivalent of a provisional application. When a form is highlighted in the Selected Forms field, you may click the Open button. ePAVE will then assist you in preparing an XML form for inclusion in your submission by opening another set of screens where you can enter the information appropriate to the submission you are electronically filing.

Available Forms and Selected Forms

Application Data: A form to enter bibliographic data and create an Application Data Sheet per 37 CFR 1.76. The date entered will be published on the front page of patent application publications. This is required for new utility filings and Pre-Grant Publication submissions. It is not a permissible form for submission with Biosequence Listing submissions.

Biosequence Transmittal: A form to create a transmittal form to accompany Biosequence submissions for previously filed patent applications or issued patents.

Fee Transmittal: A form to enter and calculate fee and payment data and create a fee transmittal for new utility applications and certain Pre-Grant Publication submissions. No fee is required for subsequently filed Biosequence submissions so this form is not appropriate for submissions of this type. In addition, no fee is required for original publications in amended or redacted form so this form should not be included with those submission types.

Information Disclosure Statement: Placeholder text.

Patent Assignment Recordation Form: A form to enter data to submit assignment recordation data and create an assignment recordation cover sheet along with a new patent application filing. This form is not appropriate for Pre-Grant Publication or subsequent Biosequence submissions.

Form Description and Usage: This box contains information about a highlighted form and when it should be included.

ADDING A FORM

Use one of the following procedures to add a form to the Selected Forms list:

Click on the name of the form that you want to add in the Available Forms list. Click the Add button. The form is added to the Selected Forms list.
OR
Double-click the name of the form that you want to add in the Available Forms list. The form is added to the Selected Forms list.

REMOVING A FORM

Use the following procedure to remove a form from the Selected Forms list:

1. Click on the name of the form in the Selected Forms list that you want to remove.
2. Click the Remove button. The form is removed from the Selected Forms list.

You can remove any form listed in the Selected Forms box from the submission, but if you remove a recommended/required form you may cause validation errors. If you have already saved the form, which automatically attaches it to the electronic submission package, you must also remove the form from the electronic package after you remove it from the Selected Forms list. To completely remove the form from the submission, select the Attachments tab, select the form again, and then click the Remove button.

COMPLETING AN APPLICATION DATA FORM

If you want to open an Application Data Form, highlight the name of the form in the Selected Forms field and click the Open button. The window that opens shows the following screens: Application Details, Inventors, and Representative. After you enter the information requested on each Application Data screen, close the form by clicking the X in the upper right hand corner of the screen or by selecting the X icon on the toolbar. When closing the screen you will be prompted by a dialog box to save the form. After the program successfully saves the document you will be automatically returned to the Forms screen. The completed Application Data and Fee Transmittal XML forms will automatically be attached to the submission. If an Assignment Recordation Form has been authored, it too will be automatically attached to the submission. These forms are listed on the Attachments screen with the associated directory path for each XML form.

Application Details Tab

1. Select the type of submission you want to make from the drop-down list in the Application Type field. The selected filing should be either utility or plant.
2. Enter the Attorney Docket Number.
3. Enter your customer number in the Customer Number for Correspondence field. You must have a correspondence customer number to make an

electronic submission. You identify a Customer Number when you request a digital certificate.

Fields

Title of Invention: This field is populated by the information entered in the General Tab.

Attorney Docket Number: This field is populated by information entered in the General Tab.

Application Type: Select the type of submission you want to make from the drop-down list. The selected filing should be either utility or plant. (Required)

Utility: Utility application filing.

Plant: Plant application filing.

Application Filing Date: This field is populated by information entered in the General Tab for Biosequence submissions and Pre-Grant Publication submissions.

Customer Number for Correspondence: Enter your USPTO-assigned Customer Number in this field. This information is required. The correspondence address associated with your Customer Number will become the address that the USPTO uses to communicate with you. You must have a correspondence customer number to make an electronic submission. You identify a Customer Number when you request a digital certificate.

Application Confirmation Number: For Pre-Grant Publication submissions, enter your USPTO-assigned confirmation number in this field. This is required for Pre-Grant Publication submissions. This field is disabled for new utility filings. You can obtain the confirmation number for a pending application from the PAIR (Patent Application Information Retrieval) system.

Inventors Tab

In some circumstances an authorized individual may file an application for an inventor. These circumstances are covered by 37 CFR 1.42, 1.43, and 1.47. If this is such an instance, enter the necessary information indicated by rule.

To delete an inventor from the Application Data Sheet, highlight the inventor's name and address in the top field, and press the Delete button.

To reorder the list of inventors, use the Up and Down buttons. Select an inventor's name in the list, and click on the appropriate button to move the name to a higher (Up) or lower (Down) position in the list.

Fields

Address1: Enter the first line of the inventor's address. (Optional)

Address2: Enter the second line of the inventor's address, if any. (Optional)

City: Enter the city. (Optional)

State: Enter the state or province. (Optional)

Postal Code: Enter the zip or postal code. (Optional)

Country: Enter the country. (Optional)

eMail Address: Enter the inventor's e-mail address. (Optional)

Telephone: Enter the inventor's telephone number. (Optional)

Fax: Enter the inventor's facsimile number. (Optional)

Inventor's Residence: Select either the US or Non-US radio button.

City: Enter the inventor's city of residence. (Required for new filings and Pre-Grant Publication submissions unless Military Service)

State: Enter the inventor's state of residence. (Required for new filings and Pre-Grant Publication submissions unless Military Service or non-U.S. resident)

Country: Enter the country where the inventor resides. (Required for new filings and Pre-Grant Publication submissions unless Military Service)

Citizenship: Enter the country of citizenship of the inventor. (Required for new filings and Pre-Grant Publication submissions unless Military Service)

Military Service checkbox: If the inventor is on active duty in the U.S. Military this box may be selected in lieu of providing residence information.

Authority for Applicant under 37 CFR 1.42, 1.43, or 1.47: In certain circumstances an inventor is unable to file his or her own patent application and an authorized individual must do so. In these cases, the regulation number that this filing is being made under should be entered here.

Publication Data-1 Tab

Fields

Request for Early Publication: Indicate a desire to have a new application published earlier than 18 months from first priority claim under 35 USC by selecting this checkbox. Not available for Pre-Grant Publications.

Publication Filing Type: Indicate the type of Pre-Grant Publication being submitted. The various types are available from the drop-down list.

Corrected: Pre-Grant Publication to correct errors in a previously published patent application.

Original Publication Amended: A Pre-Grant Publication submission which will constitute the original patent application publication that has been amended during patent prosecution and will be published instead of the application as filed per 37 CFR 1.215(c).

Original Publication Redacted: A Pre-Grant Publication submission which will constitute the original patent application publication in redacted form and will be published instead of the application as filed per 37 CFR 1.217(d).

Republication-Amended: Request for Pre-Grant Republication of the application as amended during prosecution as per 37 CFR 1.215(c) and 37 CFR 1.221.

Republication-Redacted: Request for Pre-Grant Republication of the application as redacted as per 37 CFR 1.217(d) and 37 CFR 1.221.

Voluntary: A request for Pre-Grant Publication of an application pending on November 29, 2000, as per 37 CFR 1.221.

Suggested Figure for Publication: Suggested figure for publication on the front page of the Pre-Grant Publication. (Optional)

Request not to Publish: For new applications, indicate that the USPTO is not to publish this application because applicant does not want the application published and applicant certifies that the invention disclosed in the attached application has not and will not be the subject of an application filed in another country, or under a multilateral agreement, that requires publication at 18 months after filing per 37 CFR 1.213. This option is available for new utility filings only.

Publication Data-2 Tab

Use this tab to indicate the address and assignment information that you want published in your patent application publication.

Published Correspondence Name and Address section fields

Name1: Name of individual or organization which will be published on the published patent application under correspondence address (e.g., Joe Jones). (Optional)

Name2: Name of individual or organization which will be published on the published patent application under correspondence address (e.g., Smith and Jones, LLP). (Optional)

Address1: First line of the correspondence address which will be published on the published patent application. (Optional)

Address2: Second line of the correspondence address which will be published on the published patent application. (Optional)

City: City of the correspondence address which will be published on the published patent application. (Optional)

State: State or province of the correspondence address which will be published on the published patent application. (Optional)

Postal Code: Zip or postal code of the correspondence address which will be published on the published patent application. (Optional)

Country: Country of the correspondence address which will be published on the published patent application. (Optional)

eMail Address: The e-mail address of the correspondence address which will be published on the published patent application. (Optional)

Telephone: The telephone number of the correspondence address which will be published on the published patent application. (Optional)

Fax: The facsimile number of the correspondence address which will be published on the published patent application. (Optional)

Published Assignee Information section fields

Title: Enter a courtesy title such as Mr., Mrs., Ms., Dr., etc., for the assignee for publication. (Optional)

Given: Enter the first or given name of an assignee for publication. (Optional)

Middle: Enter the middle name of an assignee for publication (Optional)

Family: Enter the family or surname of an assignee for publication. (Optional)

Suffix: Enter a generational title such as Jr., Sr., III, etc., for publication. (Optional)

Address1: Enter the first line of the assignee's address for publication. (Optional)

Address2: Enter the second line of the assignee's address, if any for publication. (Optional)

City: Enter the assignee's city for publication. (Optional)

State: Enter the assignee's state or province for publication. (Optional)

Postcode: Enter the assignee's zip or postal code for publication. (Optional)

Country: Enter the assignee's country for publication. (Optional)

eMail Address: Enter the e-mail address of the inventor for publication. (Optional)

Telephone: Enter the assignee's telephone number for publication. (Optional)

Fax: Enter the assignee's facsimile number for publication. (Optional)

Representative Tab

If the representative has a Customer Number and associated address information that is different than the application correspondence address, and wishes to have the representative's address published on the patent application publication, then select this radio button and enter that Customer Number. If multiple attorneys or agents are to be published as being associated with this application, then select the Attorney or Agent radio button and enter data as described above.

1. Select the Representative Customer Number radio button and enter the Customer Number associated with the submission being filed in the field.
OR
If the representative is an attorney or agent, select the Attorney or Agent radio button and enter the attorney or agent name information in the name fields. Insert the attorney or agent registration in the Registration Number field.
2. Click the Add button to add that name and registration to the list of representatives.

To delete an attorney or agent from the list of representatives, highlight the name and click the Delete button.

Continuity Data Tab (Optional)

Fields

Preface Phrase section: Select the radio button associated with the desired phrase.

Relationship section: Select the radio button associated with the desired relationship type.

Application section

Doc Number: Enter the application serial number of the related application.

Kind Code: If the related application was published enter the kind code as described in World Intellectual Property Organization standard ST.16, e.g., A1 for the first publication of an application.

Document Date: Enter the application filing date of the related application.

Country: Enter the country where the related application was filed.

Patent/Status Phrase section

Patent radio button: Select if the related application has matured into a patent.

Doc Number: Enter the patent number.

Kind Code: Enter the patent kind code, e.g., B1 for a patent that was not previously published as a patent application publication or B2 if the patent was previously published as a patent application publication. See MPEP 1851.

Document Date: Enter the patent issue date.

Country: Enter the country where the patent issued.

Status Phrase radio button: Click if the related application has not issued as a patent.

Status Phrase: Enter the status of the related application, e.g., now abandoned, or pending.

Foreign Priority Benefit Tab

Fields

Foreign Application Number: Enter the foreign filing application number.

Country: Enter the foreign country where the application was filed.

Foreign Filing Date: Enter the foreign filing date.

Priority Claimed: Click the appropriate radio button indicating whether priority is claimed or not claimed.

Plant Information Tab

Fields

Latin Name: Enter the Latin name of the plant described in the attached submission.

Variety Denomination: Enter the Variety Denomination of the plant described in the attached submission.

Fee Transmittal Form Tab

Use the following procedure to complete a Fee Transmittal form:

1. Click on Application Data in the Selected Forms list.
2. Click the Open button.
3. Three tabs are now visible: File, Fee Calculation, and Method of Payment.

Filer Status Tab

Select the filer status from the drop-down list. The Filer Status is defined by the classification of the person or entity filing the patent. This is important, as it determines which schedule to use for fee calculation for provisional applications. A small entity is either an independent inventor, a small business, a nonprofit organization, and/or a noninventor. Select either Filing-as-small-entity or Filing-as-large-entity. If Filing-as-small-entity is selected, two more pieces of information are required. At the bottom of the Filer Status drop-down list, select all of the checkboxes that apply to the filer.

Fields

Filer Status checkbox: Using the drop-down list, select large or small entity as appropriate.

Small Entity checkbox: If the filer is a small entity, select the appropriate checkbox to indicate whether the filer is an independent inventor, a small business, a nonprofit organization, or a noninventor. (Optional)

Total Fees Due: Indicates fees due for associated submission.

Fee Calculation Tab

The Fee Calculation tab is where the fees associated with the submission are calculated. If a new application is being filed, select New Utility from the Basic Filing Fee drop-down list. The top-most Fee Amount field is the Basic Filing Fee, a noneditable field where the value is determined by the Fee Type selected on the previous tab.

For a provisional application filing, you may pay either a small entity fee or a large entity fee as applicable.

Next are the Extra Claim Fees. Up to 20 total claims and 3 independent claims can be requested for no additional fee; however, each additional claim or independent claim is charged to the total fee due, based once again on the entity size of the filer. A Multiple Dependent Claims checkbox is provided. An additional fee is charged if this is selected. Do not insert any information in these fields for Pre-Grant Publication submissions.

The Extra Filing Fee section allows additional selections. Select from the drop-down list any additional fees required such as the processing fee for voluntary publication or the publication fee for any Pre-Grant Publication submission. Click on the Add button to indicate that selected fee is due. The Fee code, amount of the fee, and a description will appear in those fields. Repeat for each additional fee that is required. To delete a Fee type, highlight that Fee in the Fee Type field and click Delete.

Fields

Basic Filing Fee: Select submission type from the drop-down list.

Extra Claim Fees section

Total Claims Box: Enter the total number of claims filed in a new application.

Independent Claims Box: Enter the number of independent claims for a new application.

Multiple Dependent Claims: Select this checkbox if multiple dependent claims are being submitted in a new application.

Fee Amount: Displays the fee due for this category.

Additional Fees section

Additional Fees: Select any additional fees that may be required for your submission.

Fee Code: Displays the fee code associated with the additional fee.

Amount: Displays the amount of the additional fee.

Description: Displays the description of the additional fee.

Fee Type: Indicates the additional fees that have been added.

Method of Payment Tab

1. Select the payment method by clicking either the Deposit Account or Credit Card radio button. This provides the information the USPTO needs to collect the applicable fees for the patent submission.
2. If you select Deposit Account as your payment type you may authorize USPTO to charge additional fees (as allowed by CFR sections cited next to each button) not calculated on this sheet at the time of submission by checking the checkboxes provided.
3. Enter Deposit Account Number and Name of the account that is to be charged by the USPTO. These fields are required for Deposit Account transactions.
4. Enter the name of the individual who is authorized to sign for use of deposit account, as well as the electronic signature of the authorized user in the fields provided for that data.
5. If you select Credit Card payment, indicate the card type by clicking on the radio button associated with it.
6. Enter the credit card number, expiration date, the name on the credit card and the billing address in the fields provided. The Deposit Account or Credit Card will be charged the amount that appears in the Total Fees Due field in the upper right-hand corner of the screen. The Fee XML file will be created when the Fee Tab is closed.

Fields

> **Deposit Account radio button:** Select to pay fees via deposit account.
>
> **37 CFR 1.16 & 1.17 checkbox:** This is selected if USPTO is allowed to charge additional fees not calculated using ePAVE.
>
> **37 CFR section 1.18 checkbox:** This is selected if USPTO is allowed to charge additional fees not calculated using ePAVE.
>
> **Deposit Account Number:** The number of the deposit account from which the USPTO is to deduct funds. Should be a six digit number submitted in either ##-#### or ###### format.
>
> **Deposit Account Name:** The name associated with the deposit account.
>
> **Authorized User Name:** Enter the name of the individual who is authorizing the payment of the fees.
>
> **Electronic Signature Mark:** Identifies the signature mark of the authorized user.
>
> **Credit Card radio button:** Select if Credit Card payment is desired. Select the radio button for the desired credit card type.
>
> **Credit Card Number:** Enter the credit card number by which fees are being paid.
>
> **Expiration Date:** Enter the credit card expiration date.
>
> **Name as it Appears on Credit Card:** Enter the name on the credit card.
>
> **Billing Postal Code:** Enter the credit card billing postal or zip code.

ATTACHMENTS TAB

The Attachments tab allows you to attach (1) your authored XML specification document with or without figures; and (2) your separate TIFF image file(s) containing the declaration for the new utility patent application to your submission or the optional small entity statement as a TIFF image file and/or the text files cited in the specification document as appendix data (i.e., computer listings, tables) per rule 37 CFR 1.52(e) and 1.58. Forms authored in ePAVE (such as the Application data form) are automatically attached by the application. After viewing an XML document you may close the viewing screen by clicking the X button in the upper right corner of the displayed screen or select the Exit option from the File menu.

To view the Submission Transmittal Form select the Print Preview option from the File menu. The Submission Transmittal Form acts as the cover letter for your electronic submission. The attached declaration document and small entity statement must be single-page TIFF images. For example, if the declaration document is comprised of three pages, then there would be three TIFF image files attached to the EFS submission, each containing one page of the declaration document. Figures or graphics associated with the specification XML document also are scanned as single TIFF image files. Please refer to EFS Authoring User Manuals for a discussion of figures associated with the specification XML document.

If you are submitting a text file as part of a new utility patent application filing, the sequence listing contained in the CRF text file must be referenced in the patent application specification document to be electronically filed. Also, any appendix data (as attached text files) must also be referenced in the specification document.

The Transmission Documents box on the Attachment tab screen contains information identifying all the documents included in this submission. You will view a list of the electronic files you have attached to the submission package. At the bottom of the Attachment tab screen there is a box that displays details about the selected attached electronic document. The Selected Document's Details shows the file name, size, date/time, and document type.

Fields
Transmission Documents: Contains information identifying all of the documents that are currently included in the submission.

Selected Document's Details: Contains information about the file selected above including its file name, size, date/time, and the document type.

Transmittal XML: Identifies the path and name of the XML transmittal file being created in the background by ePAVE.

Attach button: Allows you to attach other documents such as a specification, a declaration, supporting documentation for assignment recordation requests, and Biosequence Listing files.

Remove button: Allows you to remove attached files from the current submission folder.

View button: Allows you to View and Print any of the attached files.

THE EMBEDDED FOLDER

To facilitate the easy organization and transmission of patent applications, ePAVE keeps items attached in the Attachments tab in an automatically created folder labeled "embedded" in the specified project folder that is created at the time of the first attachment. During the creation of a project in ePAVE, you will need to attach the specification document that was created in the authoring tool and, depending on the situation, may need to attach other TIFF images (such as a small entity claim). When any attachment is made in the Attachments tab of ePAVE, the "embedded" folder is created in the open project folder and the attachment is copied into that folder. For a specification this means that any TIFF images, the specification's .dtd and .xsl files along with the selected .xml document itself, are automatically copied into the embedded folder. For other stand-alone attachments, such as a small entity claim, only the image itself is copied into the embedded folder. The embedded folder does not separate the specification files from other attached files (such as a small entity claim). *Note:* Attachments that are made as part of a form (such as an attachment in the Signature tab of the Patent Assignment Recordation Form) are not stored in the embedded folder. ePAVE maintains the link to the attachment and sends it along with the rest of the files at the time of transmission.

ATTACHING A FILE

Click one time on the Attach button with your computer mouse. A dialog box will open to allow you to view the computer directories where you have stored the file to be attached.

Locate and select the drive and folder where you have stored the authored patent application specification document. Attach the XML file containing the new utility patent application specification document and any associated TIFF image files containing figures by double-clicking on the file name, or by selecting the file and clicking Open. If you are filing a new utility application, a dialog box will next appear asking for the file name of a scanned image of the declaration statement. (This file is not required for filing, but is recommended.) This image file needs to be in TIFF image format. This box can be closed without selecting an image file. *Note:* When removing the specification XML file, the declaration statement TIFF file will be automatically removed as well. If the declaration statement TIFF file needs to be updated, the specification XML file must be deleted and reattached.

REMOVING A FILE

1. Select the file you want to remove. The entire file should be highlighted blue on the screen.
2. Click the Remove button to remove the attachment.

Note: To reattach a document that you have removed from the submission package, you must go back to the Forms tab and reselect the form you removed, and then go to the Attachments tab and reattach the form.

VALIDATION TAB

Errors/Warnings: This window shows the errors or warnings that are present in the current submission. By double-clicking a listed validation error, you can display a detailed explanation of the error, including where it occurred in the ePAVE application, what the problem was, and a suggested fix.

> **Type:** Text describing the portion of the electronic transmittal information is missing or defective.
> **Screen:** Text describing the ePAVE screen tab where the error occurred.
> **Field:** Text describing the specific location within the ePAVE tab where the error occurred.

Message: Error message text describing the error.

> **Launching ePAVE:** Prompt to check if you are using the current version; ignore it by choosing NO. ePAVE will terminate if a DLL is missing; contact the USPTO at 1-703-305-3028 or reinstall; also reinstall if the animation file (*.avi) is missing. Error also appears if the Help file or Internet Explorer is missing.

Saving the Submission: Message to replace existing file or this file could not be created at the requested destination: '%1'(error flag).

Printing the Submission: Default printer not available, printer command currently disabled or print command error: %1.

Creating a Submission: The folder already exists (choose a unique name); either the file does not exist or format is incorrect; invalid project, please create a new submission folder; the project template could not be opened.

Filter Tab: CFR describes who can file: attorney or agent, assignee only, one or more applicants and assignees of undivided part.

Forms Tab: Only the following documents are allowed to be attached.

Fee Transmittal Tab: ePAVE cannot find Fee Document Type Definition (*.dtd) file: '%1'. Please run Version Examiner from the USPTO Web site to fix.

Attachment Tab: The declaration image file(s) should be attached to this package. Use attach buttons, select Declaration from the Files of type drop-down list, then select the proper file; error accessing the user directory; ePAVE detects one or more attached files have been moved or deleted. Check the files and references on the Attachment Tab.

Suggestion/Comments: Text describing a possible solution to the error.

Error File box: Identifies the path and name of the file containing the error log displayed above.

Print Errors Button: Use this button to print a list of the errors received with an error number, the file name where the error was detected, the type of document where the error was detected, the location of the error in the particular document, the error message, and a comment that should assist you in correcting the error.

Validate Button: Use this button to check your submission for errors.

Details Button: Select a particular error from the list of errors described in the Errors/Warnings box and click on this button to view details of the error received with the file name where the error was detected, the type of document where the error was detected, the location of the error in the particular document, the error message, and a comment that should assist you in correcting the error.

COMMENTS TAB

You can include any additional data that you would like to submit. The information will appear on the transmittal forwarded to the USPTO.

SUBMIT TAB

At the top of this tab are two certifications that are required before a submission can be made. The first indicates that the system is being used for official correspondence. The second indicates that the signer has viewed a display of the documents being electronically submitted.

Fields

> **Signature:** Displays information related to the identity of the individual signing the submission. The Name field is populated by information provided at the Filer Tab.

> **Name:** Identifies the name of the filer signing the submission. Highlight the name to activate the sign and date dialog box.

Sign and Date Dialog Box

> **Signature:** The electronic mark that the identified filer intends as signature under 37 CFR 1.33(b). (Required)

> **Date:** Identifies the date that the submission was signed.

> **Package Zipfile:** This box identifies the path and file name of the zipped (compressed) package being submitted to the USPTO. A copy of this file is retained in the folder previously created for this submission.

> **Encrypted File:** This box identifies the path and file name of the encrypted package being submitted to the USPTO. A copy of this file is retained in the folder previously created for this submission.

SAVING SUBMISSIONS IN PROGRESS

You can save your ePAVE submission document at any time. Saving preserves your patent application data so that you can change or print it at a later date. Use one of the following procedures to save your electronic file: click the Save icon on the toolbar (this immediately saves your work) or go to the File menu and select Save. When you close a form screen, a dialog box prompts you to save changes to the submission folder as an XML document with a message similar to the following:

Save changes to C:\Program Files\USPTO\EPAVE*name of submission folder\submission folder name with form extension and XML extension*

When you click YES, a second dialog box will appear confirming that your information is successfully saved in the submission folder. Click OK in this dialog box to return to the Forms screen. If you look in the Selected Form field, you can see the directory where the form was saved next to the name of the form.

OPENING A PREVIOUSLY CREATED SUBMISSION

1. Go to the File menu and select Open.
2. Browse your directories to locate the submission folder that you created earlier.
3. Highlight the folder and click the Open button. The folder will contain an .epp file.
4. Highlight the .epp file and click the Open button.
5. The previously created submission opens and displays the information that you entered. The information in the submission can now be added to or modified.

TEMPLATES

SAVING TEMPLATES

Some data used in ePAVE may reoccur often enough to warrant creating a template. Data such as inventors' names, contact and e-mail addresses, and filer name may be entered into the appropriate fields and then saved in template form. You can reuse this template for new submissions, and it will already contain the information that you saved. A saved template should only be used to create new documents that are the same type of application submission as the template.

CREATING A TEMPLATE

Use the following procedure to create a template:

1. Enter the information that you want to save as a template in the appropriate fields.
2. Go to the File menu, then select Save As Template.
3. Enter a name for the template, and choose the location where you want to save the template.
4. Click the Save button.

USING A TEMPLATE

Use the following procedure to open and use an existing template:

1. Go to the File menu and select New. The New submenu appears.
2. Select the type of application that you want to create. The New Submission dialog box appears.
3. Click the Browse button to locate the template file that you want to use.
4. Double-click the template file. Template files have the extension .ept. The template file name is placed in the Template File field on the New Submission window.
5. Enter a name for your submission folder in the Submission Folder field. Click the OK button. The file opens with the template data already entered in the appropriate fields.

PRINTING

PRINTING DATA ENTRY SCREENS/SUBMISSION

You may print any of the ePAVE interface screens by selecting Print from the File menu, or by clicking the Print icon in the toolbar. To print the Validation screen or the acknowledgment receipt, click the Print button at the bottom of the respective screen.

VIEWING AND PRINTING SUBMISSION

To view and/or print the Submission Transmittal Form, select Print Preview from the ePAVE File menu. This allows you to view the form on the screen. Click the Print button to print the form to your default printer.

PRINTING FORMS

When you are working in the tabs on the ePAVE main screen (General, Filer, Forms, Attachments, Validate, Comments, or Submit), you can print the application transmittal form by selecting Print from the File menu. This applies unless another type of form is open. When the Application Data Sheet, Fee Transmittal, Biosequence Transmittal, Information Disclosure Statement, and Patent Assignment Recordation Forms are open, those forms will print when you select Print from the File menu. After validation, you can print a complete list of validation errors and descriptions by clicking on the Print Errors button. You can print a specific form on the Attachments tab by selecting the form name and clicking the View button. This applies to the Application Data Sheet, Fee Transmittal, Biosequence Transmittal, Information Disclosure Statement, and Patent Assignment Recordation Forms. You can then print the attachment from the viewer.

INFORMATION DISCLOSURE STATEMENT FORM

NEW APPLICATION

Up to 50 U.S. patents and 50 U.S. published patent applications citations may be included on each Information Disclosure Statement (IDS) filed via EFS. Paper copies of U.S. patents and published applications are not required for electronically submitted Information Disclosure Statements as outlined in the EFS Legal Framework. The Examiner will be provided with a mechanism for accessing these documents electronically. Timely filed paper copies of foreign patent documents and nonpatent literature must still be provided for consideration by the Examiner.

Launch ePAVE and open a new IDS submission. Complete the required fields on each of the tabs in the ePAVE main screen (General, Filer, Forms, Attachments, Validation, Comments, and Submit).

Citing a U.S. Patent on the IDS

1. Enter the patentee name in the Patentee field. (Required)
2. Enter the U.S. patent number in the U.S. Patent Citation field. (Required)
3. Enter the Kind Code of the U.S. patent in the Kind Code field. (Optional) A Kind Code is a recommended standard code for the identification of different kinds of published patent documents.
4. Enter the issue date of the U.S. patent in the Issue Date field. (Required)
5. Enter the class and subclass where the patent is classified in the U.S. patent classification in the class and subclass fields. (Optional)

6. Click the Add button to add the U.S. patent to the list of citations.
7. Repeat for each additional U.S. Patent. Up to 50 U.S. patents may be cited on each IDS.

To edit a citation, highlight the patent in the list. The previously entered information will appear in the fields. Edit the information as desired and click the Edit button to reenter the citation in the list.

To delete a citation, highlight the patent in the list and click the Delete button.

Citing a Published U.S. Patent Application on the IDS

1. Enter the name of the published applicant in the Applicant field. (Required)
2. Enter the U.S. published patent application number in the US Pub-Application Number field. (Required)
3. Enter the kind code of the U.S. published patent application in the Kind Code field. (Optional)
4. Enter the publication date of the U.S. published patent application in the Publication Date field. (Required)
5. Enter the class and subclass where the published patent application is classified in the U.S. patent classification system in the class and subclass fields. (Optional)
6. Click the Add button to add the U.S. published patent application to the list of citations.
7. Repeat for each additional U.S. published patent application. Up to 50 U.S. published patent applications may be cited on each IDS.

To edit a citation highlight the published application in the list. The previously entered information will appear in the fields. Edit the information and click the Edit button to reenter the citation in the list.

To delete a citation, highlight the published application in the list and click the Delete button.

Including Remarks in the IDS

Enter any remarks you wish to have considered, such as statements of relevance, in the Paragraph field. This section is not intended for entering a response to an Office action.

Completing the IDS Certification

1. Enter the confirmation number of the application in the Confirmation Number field. (Required)
2. No certification is required if the IDS is being submitted in the time period specified in 37 EFS 1.97(b). Move on to the next tab.

3. If the IDS is being submitted in the time period specified in 37 CFR 1.97(c) and one of the two certifications can be made, that certification should be checked. If the certification cannot be made, the fee outlined in 37 CFR 1.17(p) is due. Include a fee transmittal in this case.

4. If the IDS is being submitted in the time period specified in 37 CFR 1.97(d), one of the two certifications must be made and the fee outlined in 37 CFR 1.17(p) must be paid. Include a fee transmittal in this case.

Certification Statements

37 CFR 1.97 and 1.98 outline the requirements for information disclosure statements.

(a) In order for an applicant for a patent or for a reissue of a patent to have an Information Disclosure Statement in compliance with §1.98 considered by the Office during the pendency of the application, the information disclosure statement must satisfy one of paragraphs (b), (c), or (d) of this section.

(b) An Information Disclosure Statement shall be considered by the Office if filed by the applicant within any one of the following time periods:
   • Within 3 months of the filing date of a national application other than a continued prosecution application under §1.53(d)
   • Within 3 months of the date of entry of the national stage as set forth in §1.491 in an international application
   • Before the mailing of a first Office action on the merits
   • Before the mailing of a first Office action after the filing of a request for continued examination under §1.114

(c) An Information Disclosure Statement shall be considered by the Office if filed after the period specified in paragraph (b) of this section, provided that the Information Disclosure Statement is filed before the mailing date of any of a final action under §1.113, a notice of allowance under §1.311, or an action that otherwise closes prosecution in the application, and it is accompanied by one of the following:
   • The statement specified in paragraph (e) of this section
   • The fee set forth in § 1.17(p)

(d) An Information Disclosure Statement shall be considered by the Office if filed by the applicant after the period specified in paragraph (c) of this section, provided that the Information Disclosure Statement is filed on or before payment of the issue fee and is accompanied by:
   • The statement specified in paragraph (e) of this section
   • The fee set forth in §1.17(p)

(e) A statement under this section must state either:
   • That each item of information contained in the Information Disclosure Statement was first cited in any communication from a foreign patent office in a counterpart foreign application not more than 3 months prior to the filing of the information disclosure statement.

- That no item of information contained in the Information Disclosure Statement was cited in a communication from a foreign patent office in a counterpart foreign application and, to the knowledge of the person signing the certification after making reasonable inquiry, no item of information contained in the Information Disclosure Statement was known to any individual designated in §1.56(c) more than 3 months prior to the filing of the information disclosure statement.

(f) No extensions of time for filing an information disclosure statement are permitted under §1.136. If a *bona fide* attempt is made to comply with §1.98, but part of the required content is inadvertently omitted, additional time may be given to enable full compliance.

(g) An Information Disclosure Statement filed in accordance with section shall not be construed as a representation that a search has been made.

(h) The filing of an Information Disclosure Statement shall not be construed to be an admission that the information cited in the statement is, or is considered to be, material to patentability as defined in §1.56(b).

(i) If an Information Disclosure Statement does not comply with either this section or §1.98, it will be placed in the file but will not be considered by the Office.

PREVIOUSLY FILED APPLICATION

Serial Number (under General Filer) is for Information Disclosure Statement submissions filed as subsequent filings; enter the application (serial) number that was assigned to the corresponding patent application by the USPTO.

Filing Date: For Information Disclosure Statement submissions, enter the official (actual) filing date that was granted to the corresponding application by the USPTO.

Attorney Docket Number: Enter the reference number that you want to use to identify your application. This number is not assigned by the USPTO, and can be any number of your choice.

Group Art Unit: Enter the group art unit where the application is being examined.

ASSIGNMENT RECORDATION FORM

To record an assignment in the USPTO, specific information is required. The data elements required on the Assignment Recordation Cover sheet Form 1595 used in paper and fax filings are required in electronic filings. In order to comply with the Government Paper Elimination Act, the Delivery Method tab provides you with the option of delivery via fax. Delivery via fax is the currently preferred method desired by the Office of Public Records to communicate with the correspondent(s). The default delivery method is fax and requires a fax number to be entered in the appropriate field. This will eliminate possible delays in returning official communications to the correspondent and will provide faster turn-around processing. The Assignment Services Division in the Office of Public Records may not modify your electronic data (with the exception of modifying the Customer Number for correspondence address). Each of the tabs, the associated data elements, and the requirement status of each data element are described below.

The EFS 4.1 release that includes new ePAVE software allows you to submit single or multiple assignment documents for electronic submission. You can file these assignments along with a new utility patent application, a patent provisional application, or as a subsequent filing. Subsequent assignment filings must identify the patent property(s) being assigned. A property tab has been added to the assignment form for subsequent assignment filings. Subsequent assignment filings provide the capability to submit related or unrelated assignment cover sheets. All multiple cover sheets will be treated as individual assignment documents after receipt at the Assignment Services Division. To submit an electronic assignment for recordation, you must complete the assignment cover sheet form required for an electronic assignment recordation.

AUTHORING MULTIPLE COVER SHEETS

You may complete up to 15 assignment cover sheet forms for recordation and submit them in one submission. Each cover sheet will be processed individually after receipt at the Assignment Services Division.

FORM VALIDATING REQUIRED DATA ELEMENTS

It is essential for the recordation of your assignment(s) that all required data elements are provided. To ensure the presence of data for the required data elements of each authored assignment cover sheet form, form validation routines for the assignment cover sheet have been provided. This capability provides you with form validating routines that will automatically occur when you navigate between authored cover sheets. When exiting the Patent Assignment Recordation module, the routines will be applied to all cover sheets once you choose to save the assignment XML file. A message will be displayed only if a cover sheet is lacking any of the required data. Additionally, you may execute the validation routine on demand by selecting or clicking the Verify button on the Delivery Method tab or by selecting the menu item Check Current Cover sheet or Check All Cover sheets from the Verify menu on the menu bar. When the Verify button is used or when selecting Check Current Cover sheet from the Verify menu, only the contents of the current cover sheet are validated. To validate all authored cover sheets select Check All Cover sheets from the Verify menu.

NAVIGATIONAL CONTROLS

The Assignment Recordation Form provides the following navigation buttons:

Previous: Move to the previous cover sheet.
Next: Move to the next cover sheet.

Insert: Insert additional assignment cover sheet forms (there is a limitation of 15 assignment recordation forms per patent assignment electronic filing).

Delete: Delete any authored assignment cover sheet form prior to transmission. The current cover sheet is identified between the Previous and Next buttons. If required data is missing from the current cover sheet, a message is displayed identifying the elements lacking data. Select yes to continue or select no to return to the current cover sheet.

Insert button: Click on the Insert button to create an additional assignment cover sheet or to insert a new form between two already authored forms. A message is displayed requesting that you specify where the insert should occur in relationship to the current form. Select Yes to place the new form before the current form. Select No to place the new form after the current form. Select Cancel to return to the current form.

Delete button: Click the Delete button if you want to remove the current cover sheet from the batch of cover sheets in this filing. When the Delete button is selected, a confirmation message is displayed asking you to confirm the delete request. Select Yes to delete the cover sheet and continue. Select No to cancel the delete and return to the current cover sheet.

Previous button: Click the Previous button to move to the previous assignment recordation form.

Next button: Click the Next button to move to the next Assignment Recordation Form. When you click the Next button from the last cover sheet, a confirmation message is displayed to determine if you are attempting to create an additional assignment cover sheet. Click Yes to create the next cover sheet form. Click No to return to the current cover sheet. If you select Yes to create a new cover sheet form and the current cover sheet has attachments, the Copy Attachments Dialog Box opens to confirm whether you want to copy the attachments from the current cover sheet to the new cover sheet. Click Yes to copy the attachments from the current cover sheet to the new cover sheet. The attached TIFs in the current cover sheet will automatically be referenced/attached to the new cover sheet. If the same file name is attached in multiple cover sheets (consecutive or nonconsecutive), the file will only be attached to the final package once. The identification of the attachments inside the Assignment cover sheet is only a reference; the ePAVE software will not allow duplicate file names to be attached to the electronic package. When the assignment package is received in the USPTO and the XML file (specifically the attachments data element(s)) contains one or more references to the same file name, Assignment internal processing procedures will generate a copy or copies as needed. The internal procedures will attach the required conveyance document (TIFs) to each cover sheet based on the references contained within each cover sheet. Click No to continue without copying the attachments. Select this option if different conveyance documents will be used for the two cover sheets.

ASSIGNMENT FEE INFO

The total fee information is shown at the lower right-hand corner of each screen. The Total Fee window provides a cumulative summary of the total fee due for this assignment filing. As cover sheets are authored and/or properties are added on the Properties tab, the Total Fee is adjusted. The Assignment Fee Info button provides a detailed listing for all cover sheets in this filing. Click on the Assignment Fee Info button to display the assignment fee information calculated for the assignment cover sheets in this package. Once you have viewed this information, click OK to return to the cover sheet form. The fee information includes the following items:

1. Cover sheet number.
2. Number of properties per cover sheet.
3. Fee amount per assignment cover sheet form due for each form.
4. First property number entered on each cover sheet.
5. Total property numbers for all cover sheets.
6. Total fee required for all authored assignment cover sheets. If the fee transmittal XML is authored prior to the authoring of the assignment cover sheet(s), the Patent Assignment Fee window on the Fee Calculation Screen will not reflect any assignment cover sheet fee data or assignment fee payment authorization. To have the assignment fee payment and authorization included in the fee transmittal XML, you must revisit the fee form to update. Any Assignment Recordation Cover sheet received with no payment authorization will be nonrecorded and returned to the submitter.

The Assignment cover sheet form is divided into 6 main tabs: Correspondence Data, Conveying Party Data, Receiving Party Data, Properties, Signature, and Delivery Method.

CORRESPONDENCE DATA TAB

The Correspondence Data tab contains three sections: (1) Submission Type, (2) Nature of Conveyance, and (3) Correspondence Address Data. The Submission Type defaults to New Assignment for all submissions. The Nature of Conveyance data contains a drop-down list of frequently used types of assignment transactions and a free form type for assignment transactions that do not fall into one of the standard types. When you select the free form option, a field labeled Conveyance Text is provided for free form data entry. The Correspondence Address section provides you with the option to enter either a Customer Number (which will be padded with leading zeroes if the number is less than 6 digits) or the standard name and address fields. There are nine fields in the Correspondence Address section of the tab, which allow you to enter either the USPTO-provided Customer Number or the name and address information for the person or persons to whom the USPTO should direct official communication. This address will be used in addressing the correspondent(s) with the resulting communication from this assignment filing. You must enter either a Customer Number for correspondence address or a correspondence name and address.

Submission Type: The default value is New Assignment. You cannot change this field at this time.

Nature of Conveyance: This field contains a drop-down list of basic conveyance types commonly used in the USPTO. If the list does not contain the appropriate pre-formatted text that describes the interest conveyed or the assignment transaction, select Free Form Text at the bottom of the list. Upon selecting Free Form Text, a Conveying Text window appears.

Conveying Text: Enter text that accurately describes the nature of conveyance. This field is limited to 250 characters. This field is required if Free Form Text is selected in the Nature of Conveyance field.

Customer Number: Enter the customer correspondence address number provided by the USPTO. When you enter data in this field, the remaining Name and Address fields are disabled. During the examination processing of the assignment, the Office of Public Records will electronically retrieve the official address associated with the Customer Number. Characters are not allowed in this field. This field is limited to six digits. If the Customer Number is less than six digits, the number will be padded with leading zeroes. If you want to enter the Name and Address data, simply delete the entry in Customer Number. *Note:* Please ensure that the Customer Number for correspondence address is provided; do not use the Customer Number for an attorney registration or the attorney registration number. You must complete either the Customer Number field or the Name and Address fields. Assignment recordation practices allow entry of a State Name or a Country Name but not both. Selection of one will eliminate the capability of selecting the other element. If an entry has been made into one of these fields and it is in error, you must delete the entry in the erred field in order to access the desired field.

CONVEYING PARTY DATA TAB

The Conveying Party tab consists of two primary sections, the Conveying Party Name fields and the Execution Date field. The conveying party may be either an individual or a business or organization. You must provide at least one conveying party name and execution date. Please note the detailed formatting information provided below. Following the specified format allows the data to be placed into the USPTO Assignment database records correctly and maintained accordingly. This is also required to accommodate current search and retrieval functions performed by USPTO employees and support search capabilities used by the public within the Assignment Search Room.

It is important to enter data in the prescribed formats to facilitate search and retrieval functions.

RECEIVING PARTY DATA TAB

The Receiving Party tab consists of the receiving party name and address. You must enter at least one receiving party, and for each receiving party you must complete the name and address fields. The receiving party may be either an individual or a business or organization. Please note the detailed formatting information provided below. Following the specified format allows the data to be placed into the USPTO Assignment database records correctly and maintained accordingly. This is also required to accommodate current search and retrieval functions performed by USPTO employees and to support search capabilities used by the public within the Assignment Search Room. It is important to enter data in the prescribed formats to facilitate search and retrieval functions.

SUBSEQUENT PATENT ASSIGNMENT

Enter the name that you want to use to identify the submission folder for your new submission in the Submission Folder field. You can also specify the location of this folder by browsing in the directory on the left side of the window. ePAVE will automatically save files for this submission in this folder. This folder may include the following XML documents: a transmittal, a fee document, an assignment document, an application data document, an error log containing any validation errors, the acknowledgment receipt received from the USPTO, and both an encrypted file and a .zip file containing the package of the entire submission you will send to the USPTO. *Note:* You cannot begin creating a new submission unless you have created a new folder for that submission and related documents.

1. Click on the Assignment Recordation in the Selected Forms list.
2. Click the Open button. The Assignment screen appears, showing new tabs: Correspondence Data, Conveying Party Data, Receiving Party Data, Properties, Signature, and Delivery Method.
3. Complete the required fields on each of these tabs.
4. Close the form by clicking the X box in the upper right-hand corner of the screen, or by selecting Close from the File menu. A dialog box appears, asking if you want to save the form.
5. Click Yes to save the form. After the program successfully saves the document, you are automatically returned to the Forms tab. ePAVE automatically creates an Assignment Recordation Form document based on your saved data, which is automatically attached to the submission. The file is also shown on the Attachments tab, along with the directory path for the form.

FEE TRANSMITTAL FORM

The Filer Status tab is not applicable for a patent assignment filing. Do not complete any fields on this tab. The Fee Calculation tab is where ePAVE calculates the fees associated with your submission. You are not required to enter any information on this tab when you are submitting a subsequent patent assignment. Please note limited information will be available in the Revenue and Accounting System when multiple cover sheets are authored and the payment method selected is credit card. Please note that the property number used in the RAM system may not accurately reflect the first property from each cover sheet if unrelated cover sheets are authored and submitted as one package. Entries made into the RAM system for multiple (related or unrelated) cover sheets using the Deposit Account payment method will have an individual entry made for each cover sheet and the first property number will be used from each cover sheet.

PROPERTIES TAB

The Properties tab contains the following property number fields:

Application Number: An assignment relating to a national patent application must identify the national patent application by the application number (consisting of the series code and the serial number, e.g., 07123456. Please do not separate the series code and the serial number with a slash (/).

Patent Number: An assignment relating to a patent must identify the patent by the patent number.

Patent Cooperation Treaty (PCT) Number: An assignment relating to an international patent application, which designates the United States of America, must identify the international application by the international application number (e.g., US9001234). Please do not separate the country code and the year of filing (US90) with the five-digit number (01234) with a slash (/). Do not enter the application number once the patent number has been entered. You may only enter one of the three property numbers at a time. When an entry is made into one of the fields, the other two fields will be temporarily disabled. Do not provide an entry for an application number and then enter the associated patent number. Do not provide an entry for an application number and then enter the associated Patent Cooperation Treaty number. Do not provide an entry for a Patent Cooperation Treaty number and then enter the associated application number. Do not provide an entry for a patent number and then enter the associated application number.

Adding a Property

1. Tab to the desired field, or click the mouse in the field to place the cursor there.
2. Enter the appropriate property number.
3. Click the Add button. The number is listed in the properties list.

Changing a Property

1. Select the property from the property list.
2. Click the Update button.

Deleting a Property

1. Select the property from the property list.
2. Click the Delete button. If a property number is entered and you attempt to enter the same property number, a message will be displayed indicating

that duplicate numbers are not permitted. Currently there is no method to determine if a relationship exists between the entered property numbers. Do not enter the application number and the patent number for the same patent property. As each property number is added to the property list, the order of entry is maintained. As property numbers are added or removed from the property list, the value in the Number of Properties window and the Recording Fee window is automatically adjusted to reflect the action performed.

SIGNATURE TAB

The signature tab contains three fields: (1) Name of Person Signing, (2) Date Signed, and (3) Attachments. You cannot enter any data in the Attachments field. Click the Attachments button to attach the conveyance document that supports the data entered in the current cover sheet form. The TIFF files attached must be black-and-white single-page images. Image compression format must be 300 dpi, Group 4 compressed. Microfilm media is the standard archival method used by the Assignment Services Division. Microfilm format requires single-page black-and-white TIFF images.

Adding an Attachment

1. Click the Add button.
2. Locate and select the file(s) that you want to attach as part of this submission.
3. Click the Open button. The files are attached. The entry for the total number of attachments is automatically calculated based on your selection of files, and is displayed in the Attachment field. Please ensure that the list of attachments is in the proper page order for this electronic submission. This will ensure proper page order within the microfilm media. The recorded document will be placed on microfilm in the order the document is received. Upon receipt by the USPTO, the electronic XML assignment document and assignment attachments will enter the Patent and Trademark (automated) Assignment System. During PTO preprocessing, the assignment XML document is rendered using an XSL Stylesheet. This rendered document is then converted into a TIFF image and merged with the assignment attachments in an electronic folder that contains one assignment cover sheet document (may consist of multiple pages) and one assignment document (pages determined based on attachments). This process allows the electronic assignment submission to be entered directly into the automated Patent and Trademark Assignment System. A legal supporting (conveyance/assignment) document is required to be attached to each authored cover sheet.

Removing an Attachment

1. Select the attachment(s) that you want to remove from the current cover sheet.

2. Click the Remove button to remove the TIFF attachment from the current cover sheet, or click the Remove All button to remove all TIFF attachments from the current cover sheet.

Rearranging the Attachments

Use the Up and Down arrow buttons on the Attachments dialog box to rearrange the order of the TIFF attachments (pages of the conveyance document) that are attached to the current cover sheet.

DELIVERY METHOD TAB

The Delivery Method tab contains the delivery method options and the Verify button. The default delivery method is Fax Number, and is automatically checked when the Delivery tab is selected. The Email Address option is intended for future use and is not available at this time.

Verifying Cover Sheets

1. Go to the Verify menu.
2. Select Check Current Cover Sheet to verify the current cover sheet, or select Check All Cover Sheets to verify the contents of all cover sheets. You can access either of these menu items at any time during data entry.
3. If data is missing from the Check Current Cover Sheet task, a message is displayed indicating the elements lacking data. If data is missing from the Check All Cover Sheet task, a message is displayed indicating the data element and the number of the cover sheet that is lacking the element. A display message is only shown when data is missing.

VIEWING THE ASSIGNMENT RECORDATION FORM

To view the electronic assignment submission XML document, a Stylesheet document has been provided and will render (in a single-page display format) the data that you have entered in the electronic assignment form. When you author multiple cover sheets, the display shows the contents of all cover sheets on one screen. To render the assignment XML document (all cover sheets), go to the View menu and select Recordation Cover Sheet or click on the Print Preview icon located on the toolbar under the menu bar. If multiple cover sheets are authored, the Assignment Services Division automated programs will parse through the XML file and create individual XML files for each cover sheet authored, then using XSL render the document and create a TIFF image or images from the rendered document.

VALIDATION TAB

The Validation tab provides an automatic validation of your submission to identify any errors before you send your submission to the USPTO. You can manually validate the submission at any time by clicking on the Validate button or by clicking the check mark icon on the ePAVE tool bar. You can print a list of current errors at any time during the authoring stage of the submission process. ePAVE's validation messages are produced by a computer validation program that reads the XML-tagged data that you are submitting. The error messages that ePAVE provides identify specific errors in your submission.

Validating Submission

1. Verify that your computer is connected to the Internet. You must be connected to the Internet before you can validate your submission.
2. Click the Validate button. ePAVE validates your submission and lists any errors that it identifies during this process in the Errors/Warnings field.
3. Double-click on an error that is listed in the field, or select an error and click the Detail button. The Error Message Detail window appears, providing additional information about the error and instructions for correcting the error.
4. Correct the error as suggested in the Error Message Detail window.
5. Repeat Step 3 for each error.
6. Click the Close button or the X button at the top of the page when you are finished. The Error Message Detail window closes, and you return to the Validate tab.
7. Click the Validate button to revalidate your corrected submission.

Common Validation Errors

If you attempt to use a version of ePAVE that is not the most current version available, you will receive an error message during validation that is similar to the following messages:

The local version is not correct.

The XML files DTD does not match any server's. Please check if you need to update your DTD.

If you receive one of these error messages during validation, please download the latest ePAVE software. You can check your version by going to the Help menu in the ePAVE interface and selecting About ePAVE.

Printing Identified Errors

Click the Print Errors button. The list of errors that ePAVE identified during validation are printed on your default printer.

Validation Override

The ePAVE software will allow you to override certain validation errors. USPTO strongly discourages overriding validation errors, because this may affect the completeness of your submission and may affect the USPTO's ability to properly match the submission with the appropriate application or patent. You can only override certain types of errors. Errors such as a missing serial number, a missing signature, or inappropriate file type extension on an attachment must be corrected prior to uploading. *Note:* The validation override is not applicable to Pre-Grant Publication submissions. To return to the ePAVE data entry screens and correct the outstanding errors, use the mouse to click on the Fix the Errors button. Use the following procedure to override the ePAVE validation errors and submit the package to the USPTO:

1. Use the mouse to select the I Accept box after reading the warning message text to acknowledge that the warning message has been read. Checking this box will enable the Override and Submit button. If you have erroneously checked this box, you can clear it by clicking on the box again with the mouse.
2. Click on the Override and Submit button to continue the submission despite the errors. ePAVE bundles your submission. If successful, you will receive a confirmation message.
3. Click OK. *Note:* If you receive an error message stating that your submission exceeds 10 MB, see Filing Large Submissions.

COMMENTS TAB

The Comments tab contains a text box where you can author any additional comments that you want to include on your XML transmittal. For example, if you are filing a Pre-Grant Publication to correct errors in a previous publication, you should indicate the changes you are submitting for republication. For a subsequent filing, such as the CRF biotechnology sequence listing submission or the new utility patent application submission, you should include any detailed information about the patent application that you are filing that is not already contained in the documents and forms attached to your submission. The following examples show notations for citing corrections made to a publication submission. You must identify the internationally agreed number for identification of data (INID) code, drawing page, paragraph number, or claim number. You can also include the title of the application, although it is also captured on the transmittal form.

Example 1: Correction Information: Correction of US 2001–0029557 A2 Mar. 1, 2001.

Example 2: Correction Information: Correction of US 2001–0019557 A2 Mar. 1, 2001; See Drawing Figures 3 and 4; See (3) Foreign Application Priority Data, See Paragraphs 27, 42, 98, and 103.

Another instance where you would use the Comments tab is when you are filing a Pre-Grant Publication redacted application via EFS to indicate that you have met the concurrent paper requirements of the new rule 1.217(c).

SUBMIT TAB

The Submit tab is where you sign and date your submission with your electronic mark. It provides two mandatory checkboxes to indicate that the filers who have signed this submission have reviewed it and can attest to the accuracy of the legal statements to the right of each box.

Signing Your Submission

If you have reviewed the legal statements and have completed your electronic submission, you are ready to sign your document. Each listed filer must personally make an electronic mark and sign the submission prior to uploading to the USPTO. Use the following procedure to sign the document:

1. Click the Submit tab to go to the Submit page.
2. Read the first legal statement and click the corresponding box to indicate your acceptance, placing a check mark in the box.
3. Read the second legal statement and click the corresponding box to indicate your acceptance, placing a check mark in the box.
4. Select your filer name in the Signature field.
5. Click the Sign & Date button. The Signature dialog box for the filer that you selected opens.
6. Enter the electronic mark you intend as your signature under 37 CFR 1.33(b) in the Signature field.
7. Enter the signing date in the Date field. You can change the date using the Up and Down arrows.
8. Click OK to accept this signature or click Cancel to return to the previous screen.
9. Repeat Step 4 through Step 8 for each filer.

SENDING YOUR FILING TO THE USPTO

Once you have completed all of the screens in ePAVE and have successfully validated them, you are ready to file your submission directly with the USPTO over the Internet. Click on the Send to USPTO button on the Submit tab. If you do not receive any error messages, go to Digital Certificate Login. If you receive an Invalid Submission Warning message, go to Validation Override. If you receive an error message stating that the submission exceeds 10 MB, go to Filing Large Submissions.

DIGITAL CERTIFICATE PROFILE LOG-IN

The last step that ePAVE requires is that you log in with the Entrust profile and password that you designated when you created your digital certificate using the USPTO Direct Security software. The ePAVE application will automatically save the location of the last profile used for a submission. If you have more than one profile on a specific computer or have never filed, you may browse to the location of the specific profile.

ACKNOWLEDGMENT RECEIPT

After the package has been transmitted, the USPTO server dates and time stamps the package, and uses digital signature technology to verify that the contents of the package have not been altered in transit. The USPTO server also returns information to ePAVE that ePAVE then uses to create your acknowledgment receipt — including a unique EFS Transaction ID and the date and time received at USPTO. This receipt is returned to you in real-time. The receipt is automatically saved in the folder you created for this submission, and should be printed and, if applicable, included in your formal amendment filed in paper when submitting a CRF sequence listing copy. The acknowledgment receipt establishes the date of filing for new utility patent application or the date of receipt for subsequent filing. The acknowledgment receipt does not grant an official filing date for the new utility patent application.

FILING LARGE SUBMISSIONS ON COMPACT DISC

If you attempt to file a utility patent application or Pre-Grant Publication submission that exceeds the EFS system limit of 10 MB, ePAVE generates an error message and advises you to submit the large application on a compact disc (CD or CD-R). You cannot send submissions larger than 10 MB electronically. If a large Biotechnology Sequence Listing, a table, or a computer program listing is causing the large application size, you may submit the application according to the requirements of 37 CFR 1.52(e) with the large section on CD and the rest in paper. However, regardless of the cause of the large size of the submission, you can use EFS to file the application on CD. The process requires that your workstation is connected to a compact disc recorder, and can only be used for submissions that fit on a single compact disc.

Before saving the .zip files and sending the CD to the USPTO, verify that your image files are compressed. If the application figure images are not compressed, you can compress the images and submit your application electronically. Use the following procedure to compress your application figure images:

1. Remove the specification XML document from the attachments in ePAVE.
2. Load the specification (.s4w document) in PASAT.
3. Remove the figures section from the specification: Go to Tools/Edit Sections and deselect the Figures section. This removes all figures. Once the section and figures have been removed, go back to Tools/Edit Sections and reselect the Figures section.
4. Open one of the images in Windows Imaging, which is located under the Start menu in Program Files/Accessories/Imaging.
5. Click Page/Convert or Properties, depending on the version of Windows Imaging that you have.

6. Specify the following settings for the image: file type: TIF; color: Black & White; compression: Group 4; resolution: 300 × 300 dpi.
7. Save the image.
8. Repeat Step 4 through Step 6 for each image.

Using PASAT, load the specification and add the newly created TIFF figure images. You will need to view the specification in the browser again, validate the specification, and export to XML. Once all of this has been done, you will be able to reattach the specification XML in ePAVE. If the TIFF image problem is caused by the declaration TIFF image file, follow Steps 3 and 4.

There is a possibility that you will have to reenter your information in ePAVE. Occasionally, if you have reached the point during submission where ePAVE bundles and encrypts the package, you will be unable to edit the information.

Saving Your Submission on CD

Use the following procedure to submit your EFS submission that is larger that 10 MB on CD:

1. Print out the Transmittal Form.
2. Copy your submission folder that contains your entire application from the workstation to compact disc-recordable (CD-R) media.
3. Wrap the CD in a jewel case within a padded protective mailing envelope, and attach a copy of the transmittal form.
4. Enclose a cover letter explaining that the submission contains an application that was too large to be submitted electronically.
5. Hand deliver or mail the CD-R and a copy of the paper transmittal form and cover letter to the USPTO. You can also send them via the U.S. Postal Service under the Express Mail procedures of 37 CFR 1.10.

A certificate of mailing may be used in the same manner as the certificate of transmission described above. USPTO advises that you keep a copy of the CD and transmittal form for your records. In step 2 above, you can also make a backup copy of the CD and send both copies to the USPTO. Label the CDs "Copy 1" and "Copy 2" and include a signed statement that the two copies are identical. Copy 1 will be used for processing, unless it is unreadable. Please compare the files that you write to CD with the files that you have on your computer to verify that the write to CD was successful.

Once the USPTO receives the CD in the mailroom, the date of receipt is recorded and your submission is uploaded to the EFS server, where the files are decrypted and unzipped. Your application files will then be processed as EFS submissions. If the submission was a new application (as opposed to a resubmission of an application under 18-month publication), the USPTO prints an acknowledgment receipt that is modified to indicate that the USPTO mailroom date of receipt or the Express Mail date is the date of receipt, rather than the later date of upload to the EFS server. The acknowledgment receipt is placed in the file with the printed application, and a copy is sent back to you for your records

If the files contain large tables, sequence listings, or computer program listings, the Office has the option of not printing the large files, but rather burning two CD-Rs of such data and treating them under the CD practice of 37 CFR 1.52(e). If the file is an amino acid/nucleotide sequence listing, then one additional copy of such a sequence listing will be created and sent to STIC as the CRF. In any case, one CD is placed in the file, and one is put in the CD repository.

If you are paying by credit card or deposit account, the fee information is processed by the Office of Initial Patent Examination's Electronic Application Review Office in the same manner as an online submission. The files provided on CD are signed and encrypted, so the patent application data is protected during mailing and any storage time at the USPTO. Once the Office of Initial Patent Examination's Electronic Application Review Office receives the CD, the electronic files are uploaded to the EFS secure database and made available for publication. From this point, processing continues as if the application were submitted electronically.

NOTES TO SPECIFIC APPLICATION TYPES

PROVISIONAL

While many of the components of a provisional patent application submission are similar to a new utility application, provisional patent applications are unlike new utility applications in that they are not published. The first cursor on the General tab for a patent provisional application will appear in the Email Address text field because this is the starting point for entering application information on this tab screen. The Prerequisites selections on the General tab screen do not apply to a new utility patent application filing or provisional patent application submission. The following also does not apply: Serial Number, Filing Date, and Assigned Examiner.

NEW UTILITY

You cannot begin creating a new submission unless you have created a new folder for that submission and related documents.

Publication Data-1 Tab

When filing a new utility application, you may request early publication under 37 CFR 1.219 (prior to 18 months from earliest priority under 35 USC) by clicking the Request for Early Publication checkbox. The publication filing type new utility is automatically entered when completing a new utility application electronic submission. If you are electronically filing a new utility patent application or voluntary publication, select a suggested figure for publication on the front page of the patent application publication and enter it in the Suggested Figure for Publication field. Alternatively, if you are filing a new utility application and you have not and do not plan to file it in another country or with an authority that publishes the application at 18 months from filing, you may make such a request by checking the Request Not to Publish box.

Publication Data-2 Tab

This tab screen allows you to enter the Assignee Name and Address you would like to have USPTO publish as part of the patent application publication front page. The assignee name and address entered on this screen is for publication purposes only.

Continuity Data Tab

1. Select the phrase that you want to include in your continuity data from the choices in the Step 1 Preface Phrase portion of the tab.
2. Select the relationship that you wish to establish between the earlier field application and this submission from the Relationship portion of the tab.
3. Insert the application serial number for the related application in the Doc Number field. If the application has been published, insert the kind code of the publication in the Kind Code field. See MPEP Section 1851 for a description of kind codes. A kind code is a recommended standard code for the identification of different kinds of published patent documents. The World Intellectual Property Organization (WIPO) published Standard 16, which provides for groups of letter codes in order to distinguish patent documents published by industrial property offices. The letter codes also facilitate the storage and retrieval of such documents. Published patent documents have kind code notation. Examples of kind code entries that will be updates to WIPO Standard 16 for U.S. Patent Documents after pre-grant application begins:
   * Publication filing type/Kind Code for Utility or Plant Kind of Patent document publication
   * New utility A1 (published document)
   * Note: Not accepting new plant applications via EFS at this time
   * Voluntary (filed before Nov 29, 2000) A1 P1 (for plant application to be published)
   * Original-publication-amended A1 P1
   * Original-publication-redacted A1 P1
   * Republication-amended A2 P4
   * Republication-redacted A2 P4
   * Corrected A9 P9
4. Enter the filing date of the related application in the Document Date field.
5. Enter the country of filing in the country field. If the related application has issued into a patent, click the Patent radio button and enter the patent number, its kind code, the patent date and the country where it was patented in the Step 4 portion of the tab. If the related application did not issue as a patent, click the Status Phrase radio button and insert the status of the application, usually pending or abandoned.
6. Click the Add button to include the data in the list in the parent field.
7. Repeat for any additional related applications.

To delete an application from the continuity data, highlight the entry to be deleted in the parent window and click the Delete button.

Foreign Priority Benefit Tab

1. Enter the application number of an associated foreign-filed application in the Application Number field.
2. Enter the country where the application was filed in the Country field.
3. Enter the foreign filing date in the Filing Date field.
4. Indicate whether or not foreign priority is claimed by selecting the appropriate radio button.
5. To add the application to the list of foreign priority application, click the Add button.
6. To delete a reference to a foreign-filed application, highlight the application in the list and click the Delete key.
7. Return to the Forms Tab screen.

Fee Calculation Tab

The Fee Calculation tab is where the fees associated with the submission are calculated. If a new application is being filed, select new utility from the Basic Filing Fee drop-down list. The top-most Fee Amount field is the Basic Filing Fee, a noneditable field and the value is determined by the Fee Type selected on the previous tab. For a provisional application filing, you may pay either a small entity fee or a large entity fee as applicable.

Next are the Extra Claim Fees. Up to 20 total claims and 3 independent claims can be requested for no additional fee. However, each additional claim or independent claim is charged to the total fee due, based once again on the entity size of the filer. Finally, a Multiple Dependent Claims checkbox is provided. An additional fee is charged if this is selected. Do not insert any information in these fields for pregrant publication submissions.

Below the Extra Filing Fee section is the Additional Fees section. Select any additional fees required such as the processing fee for voluntary publication or the publication fee for any pre-grant publication submission from the drop-down list. Click on the Add button to indicate that selected fee is due. The fee code, amount of the fee, and a description will appear in those fields. Repeat for each additional fee that is required. To delete a fee type, highlight that fee in the Fee Type field and click Delete.

PRE-GRANT PUBLICATION

Pre-grant publication submission filed using EFS will contain publication-ready text of patent application information including the specification document and the appropriate fee information. You will author the front cover of the patent application using the Application Data form provided in ePAVE. You will author the publication-ready specification text with or without figures using one of the EFS authoring tools.

Before you can enter the requested information for a new EFS submission, you must first create a new folder in which you will store all ePAVE created files and submission attachments. In the General Tab, enter the Application Number of the pre-grant publication submission that you are creating. In the Filing Date field, enter the filing date associated with the pre-grant publication submission.

11 USPTO Direct

The USPTO Direct program allows secure access to your patent applications in progress. This is an extremely useful tool as it gathers all the elements of following up on the progress of a patent application, including maintenance of fees. You can download the program from the USPTO Web site at http://www.uspto.gov/ebc/efs/downloads/ptodirect.htm.

There are restrictions on who can use this program and the countries to which the program can be exported. It is illegal to export or download this software to Afghanistan, Cuba, India, Iran, Iraq, Libya, Montenegro, North Korea, Pakistan, Serbia, Sudan, or Syria. This software shall be used only to perform business with the USPTO, as described in the PKI Subscriber Agreement (http://www.uspto.gov/ebc/documents/subscribersagreement.pdf).

USPTO Direct includes cryptographic software, which is subject to U.S. export license requirements. The USPTO has obtained an export license, which permits distribution of the USPTO Direct software by download from its Web site. Before downloading the software, you must complete and return the Subscriber Agreement and Certificate Services Request Form, which are available through links on the Web page. You will receive a single-use password permitting download, as well as the information that you need to complete the USPTO Direct enrollment process that installs the downloaded software. Although this download is licensed by the Department of Commerce Bureau of Export Affairs, the software itself is still subject to U.S. Export Administration Regulations and may not be exported outside the U.S. and Canada without an export license. If you are contemplating downloading the USPTO Direct software from a location outside the U.S. or Canada, you should be aware that many nations impose import restrictions on downloading and/or use of cryptographic software. You should understand and comply with the local requirements regarding the import and use of cryptographic products before any such download. You are responsible for procuring all required local permissions for any subsequent export, import, or use of the software or related information.

After downloading and installing the program, click on the "two key" symbol of USPTO Direct, and the main screen appears (Figure 11.1).

Enter your password for the default user name displayed. The password is case sensitive; if you insert a wrong password, it might cripple your key and require you to obtain a key validation from the USPTO. After entering the correct password, USPTO Direct opens a new browser window and a message appears (Figure 11.2).

You are now connected to the Patent Electronic Business Center (Figure 11.3) and ready to browse through your application records in a secure platform. Notice additional information regarding changes to hours of operation, holidays, and a link to check for any system alerts.

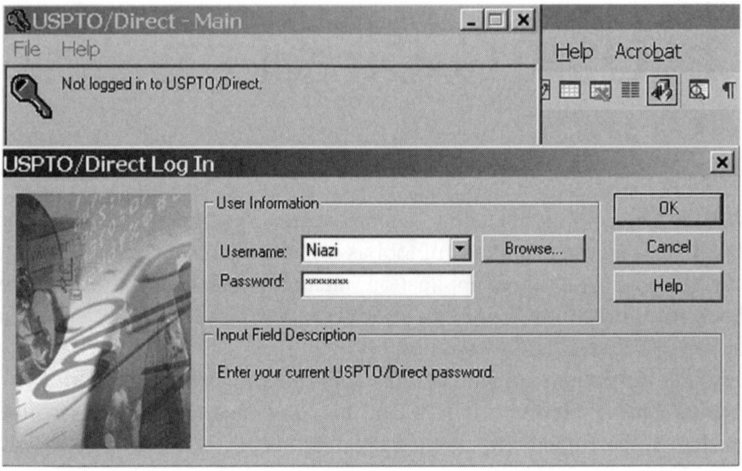

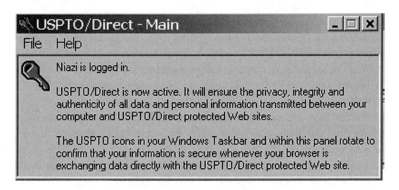

FIGURE 11.1

FIGURE 11.2

Clicking on New Users takes you to information about the PAIR (Patent Application Information Retrieval System) and the EFS (Electronic Filing System) information. You are most likely to begin with the PAIR system. The PAIR screen appears with the default customer number already inserted (Figure 11.4).

From the PAIR screen, you can insert an appropriate Application Number, Patent Number, Publication Number, or Attorney Docket Number to do the search. Note that application numbers are made available as a public record because these applications are still pending. A newer feature of USPTO Direct is access to your Customer Number record to check if the USPTO has the right address and to get procedures on how to correct it. This is an important step because the USPTO generates address labels automatically using the given Customer Number if the Filer is identified with this number. This may supercede in some instances the information given in the Application Data Sheet (Figure 11.5).

The fastest way to get to all of your current records is by Customer Number Search, which will display all applications filed using your Customer Number

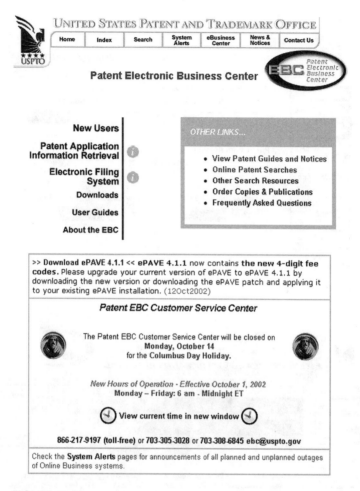

FIGURE 11.3

(Figure 11.6). You can sort the data by any one of the column categories, such as Filing Date or Status Date. To learn more about the status of your application, click on any application number to see the entire prosecution history.

Notice that only three buttons are available for pending applications: Foreign Priority, Continuity Data, and Publication Review (Figure 11.7); if this is an issued application as shown below, there will be additional tabs pertinent to an issued patent (Figure 11.8).

The first button is PTA (Patent Term Adjustment) History. The PTA provisions of the American Inventors Protection Act (AIPA) became effective May 29, 2000, and apply to utility and plant applications filed on or after May 29, 2000. The patent term extension (PTE) provisions of Public Law 103-465 (URAA) apply to utility and plant applications filed before May 29, 2000, but on or after June 8, 1995. Patent term adjustment or extension under 35 USC 154(b) does not apply to design applications or to any application filed before June 8, 1995 (Figure 11.9).

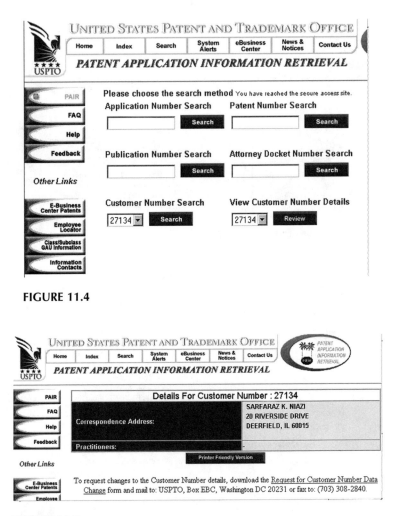

FIGURE 11.4

FIGURE 11.5

The Continuity Data of record can be retrieved (Figure 11.10).

Clicking on Maintenance Fee to Pay brings the pending schedule and logs on to the Finance page (Figure 11.11), from where you can retrieve additional information on payment of fee.

The View Maint. Payment Windows button displays the date payments were made (Figure 11.12).

Clicking on the View Maint. Statement button will produce an error if there are no statements in the past year (Figure 11.13).

Whether you are a *pro se* single application author or represent a large patent attorney group, you will soon learn the power of USPTO Direct to keep your records straight and provide continuous monitoring of your filings and responses. As a result, you will be the first one to know when the patent issues.

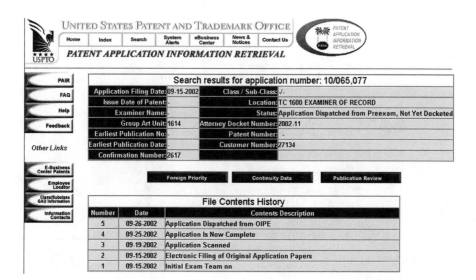

FIGURE 11.6

FIGURE 11.7

Search results for application number: 09/681,362	
Application Filing Date: 03-26-2001	Class / Sub-Class: 424/728.000
Issue Date of Patent: 01-15-2002	Location: FILE REPOSITORY (FRANCONIA)
Examiner Name: WINSTON, RANDALL O	Status: Patented Case
Group Art Unit: 1651	Attorney Docket Number: 20020
Earliest Publication No: -	Patent Number: 6,338,862
Earliest Publication Date: -	Customer Number: 27134
Confirmation Number: 5294	

PTA History   Continuity Data   Web Patent Database

Retrieve Maint.Fees to Pay View Maint. Payment Windows Payment Window: 4 View Maint. Statement

Maintenance Fees Available: Mon-Fri 5:30 AM to Midnight, Sat-Sun-Hol. 7:30 AM to 8:00 PM E.T.

File Contents History		
Number	Date	Contents Description
27	01-15-2002	Recordation of Patent Grant Mailed
26	10-02-2001	Workflow - File Sent to Contractor
25	12-28-2001	Weekly Patent Issue Receipt
23	12-13-2001	Receipt into Pubs
22	12-11-2001	Application Is Considered Ready for Issue
21	10-09-2001	Mailroom Date of Issue Fee Payment
20	12-11-2001	Receipt into Pubs
19	11-19-2001	Receipt into Pubs
18	09-28-2001	Receipt into Pubs
17	09-28-2001	Receipt into Pubs
16	09-28-2001	Mail Notice of Allowance
15	09-28-2001	Notice of Allowance Data Verification Completed
14	09-28-2001	Notice of Allowability
13	07-30-2001	Case Docketed to Examiner in GAU
12	08-10-2001	Date Forwarded to Examiner
11	08-07-2001	Supplemental Response
10	08-10-2001	Date Forwarded to Examiner
9	08-07-2001	Response after Non-Final Action
8	07-31-2001	Mail Non-Final Rejection
7	07-30-2001	Non-Final Rejection
6	06-18-2001	Case Docketed to Examiner in GAU
5	05-22-2001	Case Docketed to Examiner in GAU
4	05-17-2001	Application Dispatched from OIPE
3	05-15-2001	Correspondence Address Change
2	04-04-2001	Application Scanned
1	03-26-2001	Initial Exam Team nn

FIGURE 11.8

Patent Term Adjustment (PTA) for application number: 09/681,362		
		Days
Application Filing Date: 03-26-2001	USPTO Delay (PTO):	0
Issue Date of Patent: 01-15-2002	Three Years:	-
Pre-Issue Petitions (days): +0	Applicant Delay (APPL):	0
Post-Issue Petitions (days): +0	Total PTA:	0
USPTO Adjustment (days): +0	Explanation of Calculations	

File Contents History	Continuity Data	Web Patent Database

FIGURE 11.9

Search results for application number: 09/681,362		
Application Filing Date: 03-26-2001	Class / Sub-Class:	424/728.000
Issue Date of Patent: 01-15-2002	Location:	FILE REPOSITORY (FRANCONIA)
Examiner Name: WINSTON, RANDALL O	Status:	Patented Case
Group Art Unit: 1651	Attorney Docket Number:	20020
Earliest Publication No: -	Patent Number:	6,338,862
Earliest Publication Date: -	Customer Number:	27134
Confirmation Number: 5294		

PTA History	File Contents History	Web Patent Database

Retrieve Maint.Fees to Pay	View Maint. Payment Windows	Payment Window: 4 ▾	View Maint. Statement

Maintenance Fees Available: Mon-Fri 5:30 AM to Midnight, Sat-Sun-Hol. 7:30 AM to 8:00 PM E.T.

Parent Continuity Data			
Description	Parent Number	Parent Filing Date	Parent Status
No Parent Continuity Data Found.			

Child Continuity Data
PCT/US02/02189 filed on 01-23-2002 which has status of Pending claims the benefit of 09/681,362

FIGURE 11.10

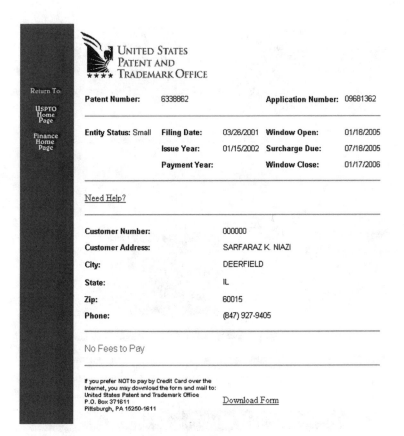

FIGURE 11.11

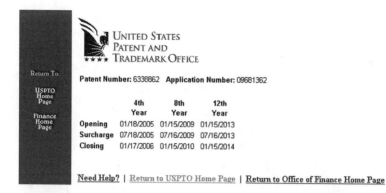

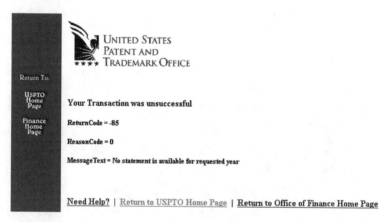

FIGURE 11.12

FIGURE 11.13

12 WIPO PCT-EASY

BACKGROUND

The PCT system is an attractive alternate to multiple national filings until validity or patentability is established. As a result, PCT filings increased by more than 14% between 2000 and 2001 with more than 100,000 PCT applications filed in 2001. Annual PCT filings originating from the U.S. represent about 40% of all PCT filings worldwide. The number of PCT Contracting States is currently 115. Expansion of PCT filing opportunities continues in other ways as well (e.g., designations for Eurasian patents, extension of European patents to certain States).

From January 1, 1998, through January 1, 2002, PCT fees have decreased by more than 30%. The PCT system is now more cost efficient than ever. Also on January 1, 2002, the maximum number of designation fees required to be paid (even if all 115 PCT countries are designated) was reduced from six to five.

The PCT system offers multiple advantages to the discerning applicant and practitioner compared with the traditional route for filing patent applications abroad. For example, since April 1, 2002, it delays the national phase (and the costs associated with it) until the end of 30 months from the priority date in most Contracting States.

Although 115 PCT Contracting States can be designated at the low cost of designating only five, for which of those countries patent protection should be further pursued can be decided late in the proceeding. The decision can be based on a full awareness of the state of the art, which is cited in the international search report, and on the reasonable likelihood of obtaining a patent in view of the opinion contained in the optional international preliminary examination report. The technical advantages of an invention and its economic prospects can thereby be determined more accurately due to the experience and increased knowledge acquired during the additional time provided under the PCT.

A U.S. applicant can file an international application in English and obtain an international search from the U.S. Patent and Trademark Office (USPTO) or the European Patent Office (EPO) with worldwide effect in 115 countries. An international preliminary examination under Chapter II of the PCT gives the U.S. applicant the benefit of an examination by the USPTO or the EPO. The U.S. applicant may receive a written opinion to which response may be made. Thereafter, a preliminary examination report prior to 28 months from the priority date is provided. This report states for each claim examined the novelty, inventive step, and industrial applicability it may or may not have.

Proceeding in this manner, the U.S. practitioner can fully control the progress of the application from the filing, through the search and optional preliminary examining stages. This can facilitate the patenting process before the elected national or regional offices.

The U.S. patent practitioner's control of international patent practice is accompanied by substantial cost savings, through delayed costs of translations, National Office and agent fees, as well as through having the international phase work done centrally by the U.S. practitioner rather than in the offices of foreign patent attorneys and agents.

The terms *Article, Rule, Chapter,* and *Section* refer to the provisions of the PCT, the PCT Regulations, and the PCT Administrative Instructions, respectively. *Paris Convention* refers to the Paris Convention for the Protection of Industrial Property. It is further assumed here that you are familiar with the rules and regulations governing PCT filing and are aware of the legal and technical limitations of the paper filing of PCT. For an update on PCT filing and to understand how PCT operates, you are advised to visit http://www.euspto.com.

ONLINE FILING OVERVIEW

PCT-EASY (Electronic Application System) is software designed to facilitate the preparation of PCT international patent applications and other related documents in electronic form and, ultimately, the transfer of the same by electronic means. You can download the current version of PCT-EASY at http://pcteasy.wipo.int/en. This version of the PCT-EASY software, however, will be limited to:

- A Request Form module providing for the input and validation of Request Form data and the writing, editing, and attachment of the abstract in electronic form.
- Printout of a PCT computer-generated Request Form, replacing the existing PCT/RO/101 form for the purposes of PCT-EASY filing.
- Possibility of copying the PCT-EASY Request Form data file and attached abstract to diskette for submission with the complete paper filing.
- Online updating feature which facilitates the downloading and installation of PCT-EASY updates (Internet access required).
- Printout of a PCT power of attorney from the Names page of the Request Form module.

If you did not register before installing the software, print and submit the registration form using the following the steps after you have installed PCT-EASY:

1. Open the PCT-EASY File Manager.
2. On the menu bar, select Tools, Options, PCT-EASY, PCT Registration.
3. Check that your contact details are correct and click the Register button and then the Print button.
4. Return the completed form by fax, mail, or e-mail registration information to the PCT-EASY Help Desk.

Starting **PCT-EASY**

Double-click the EASY icon on your screen to open the program. You will see the Easy File Manager on your screen.

Creating a New Request Form

To create a Request Form, double-click the PCT-EASY directory inside the EASY File Manager to open it, and then double-click New PCT Forms. Double-click Normal to open a blank Request Form. Follow the instructions.

Fill in the PCT-EASY form by using the notebook pages and use the validation function to verify the input data.

Templates

PCT-EASY can generate templates from saved PCT-EASY Request data. Templates can contain as much or as little data as you are likely to reuse.

To create a template:

1. Locate a previously created PCT-EASY Request to copy from the EASY File Manager.
2. Using the mouse, drag the document to the New PCT Forms folder. A message will request the reference under which the template is to be stored into the database. Give the new template a unique file name and select OK to continue.

You can also create templates by creating a new PCT-EASY Request, adding the data to be included with the template, and then selecting the Save as Template command from the File menu.

To use a template, simply select the desired template file instead of the Normal template when creating a new PCT-EASY application.

Right Mouse Button

Use of the right mouse button within the File Manager and on the Notebook pages allows access to menus including cut, copy, paste, and delete functions as well as PCT-EASY specific functions.

Request Form Notebook Pages

The PCT-EASY Request Form notebook contains nine pages as follows:

1. Request: To indicate the Receiving Office, the International Searching Authority, the language used, the title of invention and earlier search.
2. States: To indicate the designation of States
3. Names: To indicate details concerning applicants, inventors, agents, common representative, etc.

4. Priority: To indicate priority claim details
5. Biology: To indicate the details of biological material
6. Contents: To indicate the number of pages and attached documents
7. Fees: To calculate the prescribed fees
8. Payment: To choose mode of payment
9. Annotate: To indicate/view supplemental information (e.g., validation log, signatories)

VALIDATION FUNCTION

It is recommended that you complete the notebook pages in the sequence in which they appear. Use the validation function to check and confirm that data entered on these screens are consistent and meet the PCT requirements. Validation lights function as traffic lights relating to what has been indicated on the PCT-EASY notebook page:

- Missing indications mandatory for according of international filing date
- Incomplete or erroneous indications also mandatory for according of international filing date or other obvious error
- Missing indications, the omission of which could prompt further communication from the Receiving Office
- Incomplete or erroneous indications, which could prompt further communication from the Receiving Office
- No indication required, nevertheless applicant should evaluate the need to make such indications
- A reminder questioning the need for indications or verification
- The indications appear to be in order

ADDRESS BOOK

You can create your own PCT-EASY Address Book containing a list of legal and natural persons. Once you have created your own Address Book, you can import names from it to the Names page by dragging and dropping or by using the Address Book button on the Names page to open the Address Book Exchange box.

PREVIEWING AND PRINTING A DRAFT OR DUPLICATE REQUEST FORM

A Request Form suitable for submission is printed as part of the Preparation for Submission Process. However, it is possible to preview the Request Form data formatted for print output, and to print draft and duplicate forms using the following functions:

1. Preview function: You can preview Request Form data by clicking the Preview button or by selecting the Preview command from the File menu.
2. Print function: Click the Print button or select the Print command from the File menu to print a draft of a selected form or a duplicate of a form previously printed for submission. *Note:* Draft forms, identified with the header Draft (not for submission), are intended for applicant use only and

should not be submitted. Duplicate forms are identified with the header Duplicate of Original, and may be submitted in the absence of the original printed forms.

Saving Forms before Submission

If you want to save your Request Form before preparing it for submission, select the Save command from the File menu. You can open this form for further editing and to prepare it for submission from the Saved PCT Forms folder in the EASY File Manager by double-clicking the row containing the form details.

Preparing Requests for Submission

Once you have completed your Request Form, you can prepare to submit your document. The Submission button becomes available when your form data no longer contains validation errors (shown in red). However, you should determine the suitability of form data before submitting. Click this button and the submission process will be launched for your form. During this process, you will:

- Indicate who will sign the printout of the PCT-EASY Request Form.
- Print a PCT-EASY Request Form suitable for submission.
- When prompted, create and copy a PCT-EASY zip file of the Request Form and the abstract to diskette for transmittal to the Receiving Office.

Fee Reduction

As indicated in the Schedule of Fees as in force from January 1, 1999, the total amount of the international fee is reduced by 200 Swiss francs (or the equivalent in the currency in which that fee is paid to the Receiving Office) if the international application is, in accordance with and to the extent provided for in the Administrative Instructions, filed on paper together with a copy thereof in electronic form.

Filing a PCT Application Using PCT-EASY

International patent applications prepared using the PCT-EASY software must contain at least the following items:

1. A printout of the completed Request Form with the indication For Submission in the header of each page. This printout replaces the printed Request Form.
2. The application documents (description, claims, abstract, and drawings, if any) in paper form.
3. Any other documents, as appropriate.

The diskette(s) containing the completed Request Form and the abstract should be submitted together with the application papers, labeled PCT-EASY, with the applicant's or agent's file reference and the first applicant's name. If the application concerns nucleotide and amino acid sequences, the relevant listings must be presented on paper as part of the description and on a separate, clearly labeled machine-readable data carrier containing the listings in the prescribed form. Applications may be filed by post, via facsimile in some cases, or in person. If in doubt, please verify that your Receiving Office accepts PCT-EASY filings.

PCT-EASY SOFTWARE

PCT-EASY is software designed to facilitate the preparation of PCT international patent applications in electronic form and, ultimately, the transfer of such applications by electronic means. It is anticipated that by late 2003, you will be able to file PCT applications online using the PCT-SAFE software that is under development; in the meantime, the online filing functions are limited.

You can download the current software either through the WIPO Web site (http://pcteasy.wipo.int/en). It is updated using a small executable file, called a patch, which modifies the software to reflect any new designations, fee amounts, or other changes. In the future, if you are a registered user of PCT-EASY, you will be able to be notified of patches by e-mail and receive patches as e-mail attachments. You will also be able to check the PCT-EASY Web site periodically to download a new patch. You can check when the software was last updated on the user registration screen (see PCT-EASY registration discussed below).

Currently the use of PCT-EASY software is limited to:

- A Request Form module which provides for the input and validation of data typically included in the PCT Request Form and the attachment of the abstract in electronic form.
- Printout of a computer-generated Request Form, replacing the existing PCT/RO/101 form, for the purposes of PCT-EASY filing.
- Possibility of copying the Request Form data file and attached abstract to diskette for submission with the complete paper filing; and template functionality and an electronic Address Book, both of which facilitate data entry in the Request Form module.

REGISTRATION

The PCT-EASY registration screen (Figure 12.1) is accessed from the Tools menu, Options command in the EASY File Manager. It contains important registration information that is used by the software in many different ways. Select the PCT-EASY application bar to view these details.

Please be sure that your name and address details are current. If you have not yet registered, or in the event of a change in details, update details directly on this screen, print out a registration sheet by selecting the print icon, and forward this information to the PCT-EASY Help Desk (PCT-EASY Help Desk, World Intellectual Property Organization, 34, Chemin des Colombettes, CH-1211 Geneva 20, Switzerland; Phone +41 22 338 9523, fax +41 22 338 8040, and e-mail (scan and attach) pcteasy.help@wipo.int).

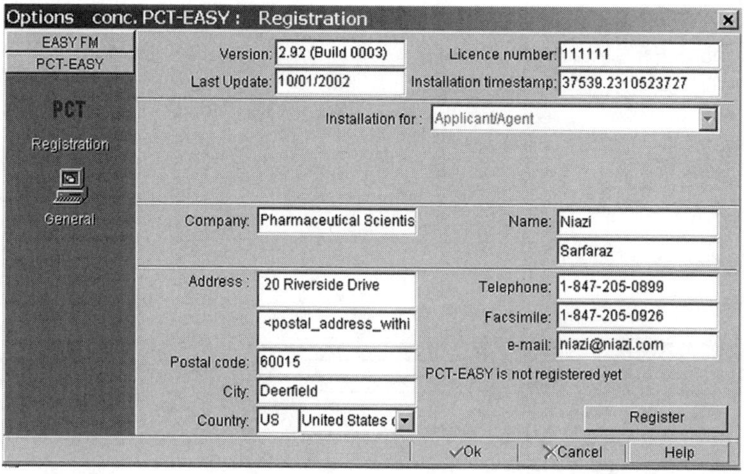

FIGURE 12.1

Soon it will be possible to upload this information online. The applications are not submitted to the Help Desk.

Clicking the Register button on the Registration screen connects you to WIPO to complete the registration process (Figure 12.2).

PCT-EASY INSTALLATION

Routine procedures for installation of new software are followed using either the CD-ROM or the downloaded .exe file. Select the language for installation. Indicate the license number provided with your registration (if you do not have one, indicate 111111) and select OK.

During the installation process you will be prompted to create a password, if you desire. To do so, select the password protection checkbox, enter the password, and then confirm it by entering it a second time. Please take careful note of this password, as it will be needed for accessing PCT-EASY.

There should never be more than one version of PCT-EASY software installed on the same machine. If an earlier version has already been installed, simply follow the instructions for installing PCT-EASY, making sure that the same installation path has been chosen. Existing files will be updated as required and any user templates will be updated accordingly. The Uninstall facility included in this version of PCT-EASY assists the user when removing the software from the hard diskette. In the EASY applications group in the Program Manager, double-click Uninstall.

CREATING A PCT INTERNATIONAL PATENT APPLICATION

Request

The completed form generated using PCT-EASY replaces the standard Request (PCT/RO/101) normally used. This printout contains information entered on the

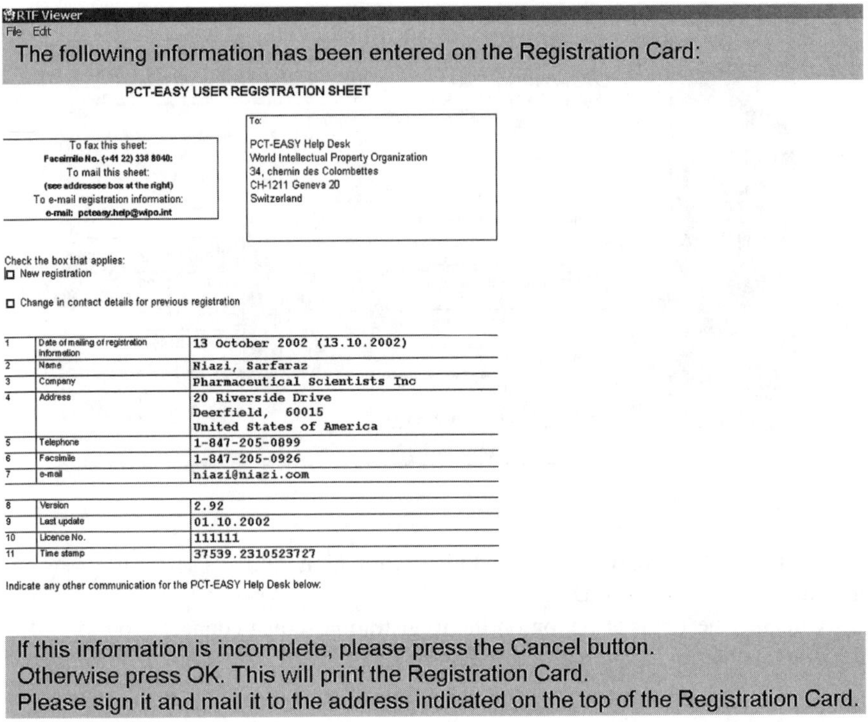

RTF Viewer
File   Edit

The following information has been entered on the Registration Card:

PCT-EASY USER REGISTRATION SHEET

To fax this sheet: **Facsimile No. (+41 22) 338 8040:** To mail this sheet: **(see addressee box at the right)** To e-mail registration information: **e-mail: pcteasy.help@wipo.int**	To: PCT-EASY Help Desk World Intellectual Property Organization 34, chemin des Colombettes CH-1211 Geneva 20 Switzerland

Check the box that applies:
☒ New registration

☐ Change in contact details for previous registration

1	Date of mailing of registration information	13 October 2002 (13.10.2002)
2	Name	Niazi, Sarfaraz
3	Company	Pharmaceutical Scientists Inc
4	Address	20 Riverside Drive Deerfield, 60015 United States of America
5	Telephone	1-847-205-0899
6	Facsimile	1-847-205-0926
7	e-mail	niazi@niazi.com
8	Version	2.92
9	Last update	01.10.2002
10	Licence No.	111111
11	Time stamp	37539.2310523727

Indicate any other communication for the PCT-EASY Help Desk below:

If this information is incomplete, please press the Cancel button.
Otherwise press OK. This will print the Registration Card.
Please sign it and mail it to the address indicated on the top of the Registration Card.

FIGURE 12.2

PCT-EASY screens and should be signed by the applicant or his representative. This printout must accompany the rest of the international application in paper form.

Description, Claims, Abstract, Drawings

Unlike the previous PCT-EASY versions that required that the Abstract text file be created manually in an external program and then attached to the electronic form, PCT-EASY version 2.91 build 0003 includes a built-in editor that allows the Abstract contents to be furnished and saved directly within a form. This allows the software to have better control over the Abstract contents and gives the user the possibility to insert some special characters allowed by the International Bureau's publishing system into the text of the Abstract. The current version 2.91 build 0003 of the PCT-EASY software does not support this functionality for non-Latin applications. Those applications should be handled the same way as they were in the previous versions of the PCT-EASY software, i.e., the Abstract file should be created using an external text editor (e.g., Notepad), converted to ASCII text format and attached to a form or using the editor provided in PCT-EASY.

It is currently not possible to file the description, claims, and drawings of a PCT international patent application in electronic form under the PCT-EASY system. All parts of the international application should be filed in paper form, together with the electronic Request Form and abstract on diskette.

PCT-EASY Diskette

A diskette containing the PCT-EASY Request Form data and the abstract, generated as part of the submission process, should accompany the application in paper form. The diskette should be labeled PCT-EASY with the applicant's or agent's file reference, and the first applicant's name.

Nucleotide and Amino Acid Sequences

If the description of the invention contains a sequence listing, the application documents must be presented as follows:

- A paper copy containing the sequence listing as part of the description.
- A separate machine-readable data carrier containing the file with the sequence listing in the prescribed form (i.e., separate from the diskette used for PCT-EASY data and clearly labeled).

Language

PCT-EASY is available for preparing PCT Request Forms in Chinese, English, French, German, Japanese, Russian, and Spanish. Request Forms prepared using PCT-EASY may be filed in any of those languages provided that the Receiving Office with which the international application is filed accepts that language for the filing of international applications (Rule 12.1(c)).

FILING A PCT INTERNATIONAL PATENT APPLICATION

PCT-EASY leads the user through a system of steps for the creation, management, and preparation for submission of PCT-EASY applications. Its two main features are the EASY File Manager and the PCT-EASY Electronic Request Form module. Request Forms prepared using PCT-EASY may only be filed with those Receiving Offices that are prepared to accept such filings.

The EASY File Manager

The EASY File Manager (Figure 12.3) is the organizing center of the EASY system. You can access all PCT-EASY functions from it. It consists of the following main directories.

1. EASY Central: This directory contains folders where EASY applications that have been previously prepared for submission are kept.
   - Inbox (not yet functional for applicants) where EASY communications from international authorities can be added to the mail manager.
   - Outbox where EASY application forms that have been prepared for submission but are waiting to be sent (i.e., copied to diskette) are kept.
   - Stored Forms where EASY application forms that have been sent are kept.

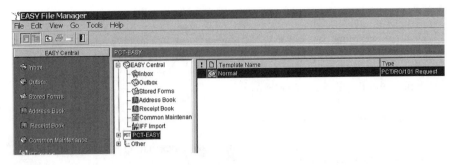

FIGURE 12.3

- Receipt Book where indications relating to a deposited microorganism and/or other biological material can be stored for expedited data entry in PCT-EASY.
- Address Book where applicant, inventor, and agent details can be stored for expedited data entry in PCT-EASY.

2. PCT-EASY Directory: The PCT-EASY directory contains five folders specifically relating to creating new PCT applications:

   New PCT forms: For the creation of new PCT-EASY forms.

   Saved PCT forms: Forms that have been saved in PCT-EASY but have not been prepared for submission are stored in this directory to permit future editing before being prepared for submission.

   PCT Help: Provides online help for PCT-EASY.

   PCT Fees: Fees imported for use on the Fees Notebook page of the Electronic Request Notebook are stored here. This information may be updated and/or completed by the user. Updated files can be obtained from the PCT-EASY Help Desk.

   PCT Maintenance: Provides for the storage of information relating to the PCT-EASY module. The user may not modify this information. Updated files can be obtained from the PCT-EASY Help Desk.

3. Other: Archiving function application files stored in the Stored Forms folder can be copied or moved to an Archive folder.

CREATING NEW PCT FORMS

To create a new PCT/RO/101 Request Form, click the New PCT Forms folder in the PCT-EASY directory (Figure 12.4). Double-click the document NORMAL in the right-hand window. This will open the New Application Reference Information dialog box (Figure 12.5), where the following information is added:

- Indicate the language of the Request.
- Indicate the Agent's or Applicant's File Reference number in the edit field provided. For the purposes of identifying and managing the international application in PCT-EASY, a unique file reference number is mandatory. The file reference cannot exceed 12 characters. It will be shown on the caption of all Request Form notebook pages after entry.

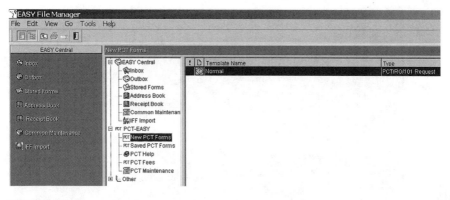

FIGURE 12.4

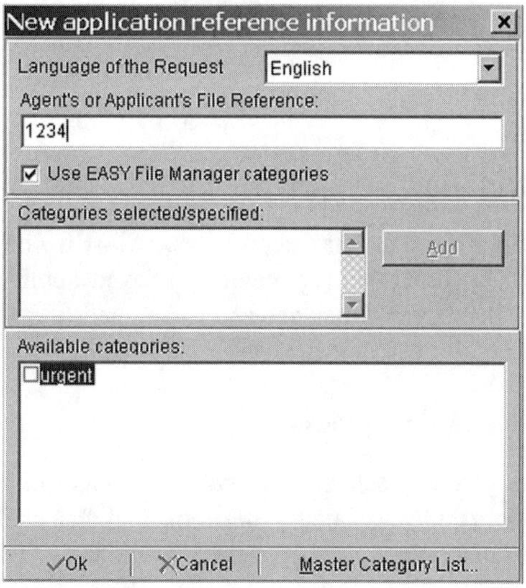

FIGURE 12.5

- Select the Use EASY File Manager categories checkbox if you wish to assign key words used for sorting the application in the EASY File Manager.
- Click OK to open the PCT-EASY electronic request notebook (Figure 12.6) or click Cancel to return to the PCT-EASY Manager.

What Are Categories?

Categories are key words that you assign to PCT-EASY applications so that they are easier to find and to sort within the EASY File Manager. For example, you may wish to create categories to identify the agent or clerk responsible for a given application, and categories relating to subject matter.

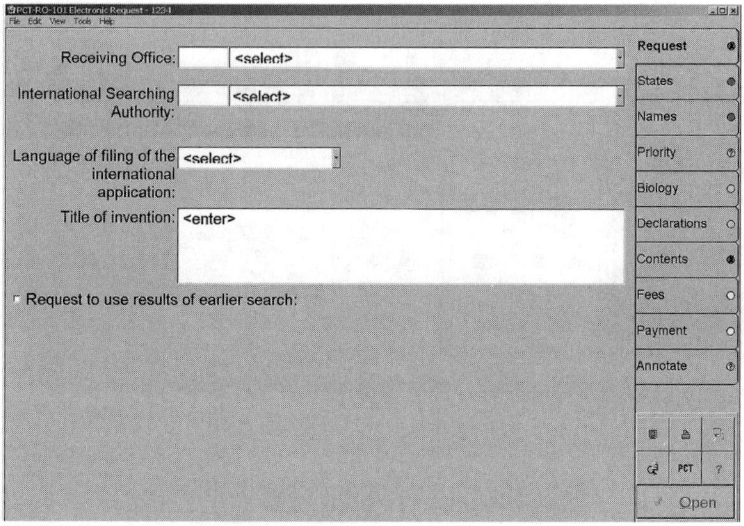

FIGURE 12.6

Accessing Categories Functionality

Select the Use EASY File Manager categories checkbox from the New Application Reference Information screen or, for previously saved applications, highlight the PCT application in the EASY Manager and then select the Categories command from the Edit menu in the EASY Manager.

Creating and Assigning Categories

A category can be created by selecting the Master Category List button, typing the name of the category in the New Category text box, and then clicking the Add button. Categories may be associated to an application by either:

- Entering the name for the new category in the CategoriesSelected/Specified edit field (after which the category is automatically added to the master category list)

OR

- Selecting the boxes from the Available Categories list box, after which selected categories appear in the Categories Selected/Specified edit field.

Disassociating and Deleting Categories

A Category can be disassociated from a saved application by clearing its checkbox from the Available Categories list box. A category can be deleted by selecting the Master Category List button, highlighting the category you wish to delete, and then clicking the Delete button.

SAVED PCT FORMS

PCT applications that have been previously saved (but not prepared for submission) can be accessed from the Saved PCT Forms directory. Double-click the desired application on the Information Viewer. Saved PCT Forms may be listed by file name (Normal), by the applicant's or agent's reference (By Reference) or by category (By Category).

To delete a saved form, Highlight the desired application on the Information Viewer, click the right mouse button and select the delete command.

TEMPLATES

Similar to functionality found in popular word processing programs, PCT-EASY has the capability of generating templates from saved PCT-EASY application data. Any PCT-EASY application file in the Saved PCT Forms folder of the PCT-EASY directory or in the Inbox, Outbox, or Stored Forms directory in the EASY Mail manager can be used to generate a template. This feature can greatly facilitate data entry if you need to input similar data for several applications. Templates can contain as much or as little data as you are likely to reuse. For example, a template could contain agent or applicant information, designations, payment information, etc., so as to avoid repeat entry when creating a new application.

To create a template, locate the PCT-EASY application you want to copy in the EASY Manager. Using your mouse, drag the application to the New PCT Forms folder. A dialog message will ask if the application should be saved as a template. Select Yes to continue. Give the new template a unique file name. The application has been added to the New PCT Forms folder as a template.

You can also generate templates from within the PCT-EASY notebook by creating a new PCT-EASY application, adding the data to be included with the template on the notebook pages, and then selecting the Save as Template command from the File menu. To use a template simply select the desired template file instead of normal.0wo from the New PCT Forms folder when creating a new PCT-EASY application. Attached electronic files (Contents page) and submission details do not save with templates.

PCT-EASY CENTRAL OUTBOX

The Outbox contains PCT application forms that have been prepared for submission but have not yet been copied to diskette for transmittal.

Copying an Application to Diskette

At any time after the submission process, the application file may be copied to diskette from this folder. This is done by inserting a blank formatted diskette in the a:\ drive, then double-clicking on the PCT-EASY application to be copied to diskette from the Outbox folder information viewer. At this point, a Save As dialog box appears. Select Continue, change the drive path if necessary, and then select OK. Select OK again when the dynazip dialog box appears. The zip file will be copied to diskette and saved to the Stored Forms directory in the EASY Manager for later reference.

The diskette containing the zip file should be labeled PCT-EASY; also write the applicant's or agent's file reference, and the first applicant's name on the label. The diskette should be transmitted to the Receiving Office with the international application in paper form.

Viewing an Application in the Outbox

Highlight the desired application from the Outbox folder Information Viewer, click the right mouse button and select the Review command. The locked application will then open for viewing.

Deleting Forms from the Outbox

If it becomes necessary to delete an application prepared for submission, highlight the desired application from the Outbox folder Information Viewer, click the right mouse button and select the delete command.

Correcting an Error or Omission

After the preparation for submission process has been completed it is not possible to modify the application. Accordingly, do not modify any indication on the Request Form printout. If an error or an omission is discovered at this time, the user must copy the submitted application to the New PCT Forms folder as a template and make the change or correction in a new application (using the submitted application as a template).

EASY CENTRAL STORED FORMS

The Stored Forms folder contains PCT application forms that have been prepared for submission previously and have already been copied to diskette.

Viewing an Application in the Stored Forms Folder

Double-click the relevant PCT-EASY application from the Stored Forms folder information viewer. The locked application will then open for viewing.

Adding International Application Number and Date

This information may be added in order to be associated with stored international application forms. It can help identify applications in this folder and will also be useful when PCT-EASY can be used to generate other forms. To add this information, view the Stored application. Go to the Annotate page and select Receive item from the Annotation or Remark menu, then select the Add button. Enter the information in the fields provided.

Recopying an Application to Diskette

If necessary, the application can be recopied to diskette from this directory. This is done by inserting a blank diskette in the a:\ drive, then selecting the PCT-EASY application to be recopied from the Stored Forms folder information viewer. Click the right mouse button and select the Send to diskette command. At this point, a Save As dialog box appears. Select Continue, change the drive path if necessary, and then select OK. Select OK again when the dynazip dialog box appears. The zip file is then recopied to diskette.

Printing Duplicates of the Forms Printed during Submission

If necessary, the forms printed during the submission process can be reprinted. Double-click the relevant PCT-EASY application from the Stored Forms folder information viewer. The locked application will then open for viewing. Select the print speed button or the Print command from the File menu.

The Request Form reprinted after the submission process is identified with the indication Duplicate of Original in the header of each printed page. In the absence of the original printed forms, duplicates from a locked application may be submitted.

Correcting an Error or Omission from an Application Prepared for Submission or Transmitted to the Receiving Office

After the preparation for submission process has been completed it is not possible to modify the application. Accordingly, do not modify any indication on the Request Form printout. If an error or an omission is discovered at this time, the user must copy the submitted application to the New PCT Forms folder as a template and make the change or correction in a new application (using the submitted application as a template).

Archiving Forms from the Stored Forms Folder

For information on copying and moving applications stored in this folder, see Archiving Files from the EASY Mail Directory, Stored Forms Folder.

Deleting Files from the Stored Forms Folder

As a safety precaution, it is not possible to delete files from the Stored Forms folder. To delete files, it is necessary to archive them first and then delete them from the Archive folder. See the section Deleting Archived Forms for further information.

ADDRESS BOOK

The Address Book allows you to import, export and input names and addresses for use in PCT-EASY applications. Display the contents of the address book by selecting the Address Book folder from the EASY Central directory.

Adding an Address to the Address Book

An address may be added directly to the Address Book or from the Names page of the PCT-EASY module. Double-click the Open button to add a new item row from the Address Book folder information viewer. There are three Address Book entry screens:

1. Name/Address: Input relevant data in the fields provided.
2. Other details: Input relevant data in the fields provided, as needed. Use of categories is optional. Specify or select (from available categories) one or more categories by which this entry can be sorted in the EASY Manager after it has been saved. Note that categories are for applicant use only and are not saved with PCT-EASY applications.
3. Registration: Indicate the filing route, role, and registration numbers to be associated with the entry. Note that PCT does not, at the present time, provide for such indications. Consequently, this feature is not presently applicable to PCT-EASY.

Viewing Address Book Contents

Using the View Sorting menu, contents can be viewed according to:

- Normal: By name
- By Preview: Showing full name and address details
- By Categories: By categories assigned to Address Book entries (if any)
- By Registration: By agent or applicant registration number (if any)

Importing and Exporting Entries

It is possible to import and export names to and from the Address Book to the PCT-EASY Names page in several different ways:

A. Directly to the PCT-EASY Names page
   1. Open the PCT-EASY Electronic Request notebook at the Names page.
   2. Click the Address Book button at the bottom of the page.
   3. Highlight the Address Book entry to be copied.
   4. Select the button for the type of entry (Applicant, Inventor, Agent).
   5. Select the OK button.
   6. Add or modify indications as needed directly on the Names page.
B. Directly to the Names page data entry screen
   1. Open the PCT-EASY Electronic Request notebook at the Names page.
   2. Open the type of entry to be created (Applicant, Inventor, Agent) from the Names Master Table.
   3. Enter the name of the entry to be added.
   4. Click the Address Book icon.
   5. The address details corresponding to the name indicated will be imported.

6. Use the Address Book arrows to display additional corresponding Address Book entries, if any.

C. Dragging and dropping entries between the Address Book and the Names page

1. Open the PCT-EASY Electronic Request notebook at the Names page.
2. Using the Alt+Tab keys, switch to the EASY File Manager and select the Address Book folder, then either:

   a. Arrange the Request Notebook and the Address Book so that both can be viewed simultaneously on your screen and, using your mouse, drag the selected entry from the Address Book information viewer and drop to the desired input function row (e.g., +Applicant, +Inventor only, +Agent) of the Names page Master Table; or

   b. Highlight the entry to be imported and select the Copy command using the right mouse button menu. Using the Alt+Tab keys, switch back to the Request Notebook and highlight the desired input function row (e.g., +Applicant, +Inventor only, +Agent). Select the Paste from Address Book command from either the Edit menu or the right mouse button menu.

3. The Names page Master Table detail screen will open with the imported data. Make any modifications or additional indications as needed, then select OK to save or X to cancel.

Archiving Files from the EASY Mail Directory, Stored Forms Folder

Application files in the Stored Forms folder can be copied or moved to an Archive folder, found in the Other directory of the EASY Manager.

Copying an Application from the Stored Forms Folder to the Forms Archive

From the Stored Forms folder select the File, Archive command. This will open the archive screen. Select the date using the calendar or type in the date (day/month/year format). Any files which were stored before that date will be copied to the Forms Archive folder. Select the Use comments to identify the archived application(s) if desired.

Deleting Items from EASY Central Directory after Archiving

If this checkbox is selected, the files that have been copied to the Forms Archive folder will be deleted from the Stored Forms folder. If this checkbox is cleared, a copy of the archived form will remain in the Stored Forms folder. Select OK to copy forms to the Forms Archive folder or Cancel to return to the EASY Manager.

Restoring Archived Forms

It is possible to restore an archived form to the Stored Forms folder. To do this, in the Forms Archive folder, double-click the name of the form to be restored. A dialog box will open with the following message:

Do you wish to restore the selected Archive?

Select OK to restore the archived form back to the Stored Forms folder. Select Cancel to return to the EASY Manager without restoring the archived form.

Deleting Archived Forms

Select the file(s) you wish to delete from the Forms Archive folder and then select the delete command from the right mouse button menu. A dialog box will open with the message:

Do you wish to delete?

Select OK to delete the archived form. WARNING: This function permanently deletes files from this folder.

PCT FEE MAINTENANCE TABLES

Fee amounts saved in the PCT Fees folder may be inserted in the PCT-EASY Fees notebook page by selecting the appropriate currency and fee schedule from the menus on that page. As the applicant may enter and edit fee amounts directly on the PCT-EASY Fees notebook page, use of PCT fee maintenance table functionality is not required. Should there be a fee change, in most cases, users will find it easier to obtain electronic updates of PCT fee amounts from the International Bureau, or simply update the amounts directly on the Fees page, rather than modifying the contents of this folder manually. Consequently, it is only necessary to access this folder to review or modify fee amounts, or to add fees for a Receiving Office not included in the predefined schedules.

Reviewing Amounts

Separate fee schedules are stored in the PCT-EASY folder, classified by Receiving Office, International Searching Authority, currency, and valid date.

For example, if the user wants to access fees applicable for the U.S. Patent and Trademark Office as Receiving Office (RO/US), the European Patent Office as International Searching Authority (ISA/EP) and U.S. dollars as the currency of payment (USD), the user would look for a row on the information viewer of the PCT Fees folder with the codes US EP USD. The date indicates the date from which these fees are valid. Comments can further identify the fees and valid dates.

By double-clicking on the row US EP USD, the user can access details about these fee amounts. (Make sure the EASY Manager, View sorting menu indicates Normal.) The definitions tab of the PCT Fee Schedule Detail screen appears, and contains the following indications:

- Receiving Office (predefined and therefore read-only, see Fee Templates for more information).
- International Searching Authority (predefined and therefore read-only).
- Currency: Describes the currency (or currencies) in which the fee amounts are indicated (predefined and therefore read-only).

- Fee reduction checkboxes: When selected, indicate that the corresponding fee(s)will be reduced by 75% for applicants from certain States, where applicable.
- Comment: Provides for comments that can help identify these particular fee amounts.

The fee details tab of the PCT Fee Schedule Detail screen contains the actual fee amounts themselves.

Using PCT Fees

If it becomes necessary to update current fee amounts indicated in a fee schedule, select the schedule from the PCT Fees information viewer. (Make sure the EASY Manager, View sorting menu indicates Normal.) Select the Fees Detail tab and make the changes to the amounts as needed. Select OK to save or X to cancel. To create a new fee schedule valid at a future date (in order to preserve an existing fee schedule and its amounts), double-click the first line of the PCT Fees information viewer open to add a new fee schedule. (Make sure the EASY Manager, View sorting menu indicates Normal.) From the RO/ISA/Currency menu, select the appropriate combination (if the desired combination cannot be found you will have to create a new fee template before proceeding, see below for more information). Using the date calendar menu, indicate the date on which the fee amounts will be valid. Indicate additional comments in the comment field. Select the checkmark 4 to continue or X to cancel. Select the Fees Detail tab and add the amounts carefully. Select OK to save or X to cancel.

Fee Template

Fee templates provide the structure for the RO/ISA and currency combinations accessed in PCT fees. You would only need to create a new structure when there is no existing combination matching the Receiving Office, International Searching Authority, and currency (currencies) desired.

To create a new template:

1. Ensure that the template you are creating is valid and does not already exist.
2. Change the View sorting menu in the EASY Manager from Normal to Template.
3. Double-click the first row of the PCT Fees Folder information viewer, Add Template.
4. On the Definitions tab, select the Receiving Office.
5. Select the International Searching Authority (only ISAs valid for the RO selected are visible).
6. If all fees are not payable in the same currency select Multiple Currency, otherwise do not modify the radio button selection.
7. Select the currency or currencies.

8. Enter comments, if any.

9. Go directly to Step 11 unless Multiple Currency has been selected in Step 6. In such a case select the fee detail tab.

10. Using the checkboxes, indicate the valid currency in which the corresponding fee is payable. If both currencies are valid, select both checkboxes.

11. Select OK to save or X to cancel.

12. Change the View sorting menu in the EASY Manager back to Normal view.

13. Follow instructions from the paragraph Creating a new fee schedule with amounts valid at a future date to add fee amounts.

OTHER FILE MANAGER FUNCTIONALITY

The EASY Central Options window enables you to change the way in which EASY works. You can change the size and appearance of the main window, default file locations, the default language, and passwords.

To change EASY options:

1. From the Tools menu, select Options (Ctrl+O). The Options window is displayed.

2. From the navigation bar on the left, click the General icon. The General settings are displayed.

3. You can select the default position of the main window, the display resolution of the software, the default locations for the main EASY directories, the default options for sending applications.

4. Click the Setting icon in the navigation bar. This displays the Settings page. These options enable you to select the startup language of the software, the default page margins, the way in which address details (such as city and postal code) are represented, whether to use a mask when creating application numbers for priority claims, whether to use digits after the decimal in fee amounts, whether to display the registration reminder whenever you start the software.

5. Click the Password icon in the navigation bar. This displays the Password page. These options enable you to set a password controlling access to the EASY File Manager and a password controlling write access to the EASY File Manager; for example, you could grant read-only access to the File Manager by clearing the first option and setting a password for the second option.

6. Click OK at any time to save your changes and close the Options window.

PCT-EASY ELECTRONIC REQUEST NOTEBOOK

The PCT-EASY Electronic Request Notebook (Figure 12.6) consists of nine pages. It is assumed that you are fully aware of the PCT regulations regarding the information required to fill out each of these sections, which offer drop-down menus for ease.

- **Request:** For the indication of the Receiving Office the International Searching Authority the language of filing of the international application, the title of the invention, and earlier search (if applicable).
- **States:** For the designation of States for regional and/or national patents, the indication of the kinds of protection desired instead of, or in addition to, patent protection, and a precautionary designation statement.
- **Names:** For the input of information pertaining to applicants and inventors, as well as for the input of information pertaining to agents, a common representative, or a special address for correspondence.
- **Priority:** If the priority of an earlier application is claimed, the details of such earlier application are input here, as well as the request for the Receiving Office to prepare and transmit a copy of a priority document to the International Bureau (where applicable).
- **Biology:** For indications with regard to deposited microorganisms or other biological material which will generate form PCT/RO/134 as part of the submission process. Where applicable, it is also necessary to indicate on this page that the international application contains a nucleotide and/or amino acid sequence listing.
- **Contents:** For the input of details concerning the number of sheets of the request, description (excluding sequence listing part), claims, abstract, drawings (including the figure to be published with the abstract) and sequence listing part of the description (where applicable), and the form in which they are submitted. Any accompanying items (e.g., power of attorney, nucleotide/amino acid sequence listing (diskette)) may also be indicated here.
- **Fees:** For the input and calculation of PCT filing fees. Details concerning the currency of payment and the amounts of fees are indicated here and the total amount is automatically calculated.
- **Payment:** For the indication of the method of payment of fees chosen by the applicant (e.g., authorization to charge deposit account, check, postal money order).
- **Annotate:** For the input of details concerning the signature of the applicant or agent and all further information pertaining to the application which cannot be accommodated on any of the other Notebook pages.

Speed Buttons (Figure 12.7)

Preview Function
You can preview the printout of data entered in the Electronic Request Notebook by selecting the Preview Speed button or the Preview command from the File menu. Use the View menu to preview the different documents and the Zoom pull down menu to adjust the size of the document on your screen.

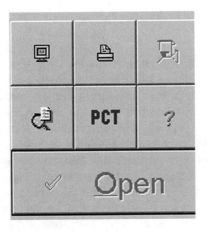

FIGURE 12.7

Print Function

Select the Print Function to print out a draft of selected forms or a duplicate of forms previously printed for submission. *Note:* If the forms to be printed are from an application not yet prepared for submission, forms will be identified with the header, Draft (not for submission). Such printouts are intended for applicant use only and should not be submitted.

If the forms to be printed are from a submitted application, the reprinted forms are identified with the indication Duplicate of Original in the header of each printed page. In the absence of the original printed forms, duplicates from a locked application may be submitted.

Validation Function

Validation is a PCT-EASY feature that allows the user to check and confirm that indications made on the Request Form notebook pages are consistent and meet certain PCT requirements. The validation function works with a system of traffic lights (red, yellow, green), warning symbols (✗, !, ?, ✔) and explanatory text. Each Notebook tab displays a traffic light which changes as data is input on that particular page and a step is made towards correct completion of the application. When a new form is created, these traffic lights are colored only (no warning symbols in them). As data is added to each page, the color will change and validation symbols will appear. For each item that is missing, incomplete, or inconsistent on a particular notebook page, the validation window displays the traffic light color together with any warning symbol and an explanatory text.

The color/symbol combinations on each page have the following meanings:

Plain red: Missing indications mandatory for according an international filing date.
Red with ✗: Incomplete or erroneous indications also mandatory for the according of international filing date or other obvious error.

Plain yellow: Missing indications, the omission of which could prompt further communication from the Receiving Office.

Yellow with !: Incomplete or erroneous indications which could prompt further communication from the Receiving Office.

Plain green: No indication required, but applicant should, all the same, evaluate the need to make such indications.

Green with ?: A reminder questioning the need for indications or verification.

Green with ✔: The indications appear to be in order.

To view more than four lines in the validation message viewer, position your mouse pointer over the validation message viewer. Click the right mouse button and clear the command "Show 4 lines."

To move the validation message viewer to the top of your screen, position your mouse pointer over the validation message viewer. Click the right mouse button and select the command "Move Top."

PCT-EASY Menu Bar Functions

The PCT-EASY menu bar is made up of a title bar that indicates the name of the open form and the following menus:

- **File (Alt+F):** The File menu gives access to the following functions: Save, Save as Template, Preview, Print, Print Setup, Close Form.
- **Edit (Alt+E):** The Edit menu gives access to the following functions: Undo, Cut, Copy, Paste, Move Up, Move Down, Remark, Private Remark.
- **View (Alt+V):** The View menu gives access to the Screen pages as an alternative to clicking on the Screen page tabs: Request, States, Names, Priority, Biology, Contents, Fees, Payment, Annotate.
- **Go (Alt+G):** The Go menu gives access to the following functions: Up One Level, Go to Folder, Inbox, Outbox, Stored Items, Address Book, Go to Group.
- **Tools (Alt+T):** The Tools menu gives access to the following functions: Validation, Submission.
- **Help:** The Help menu gives access to the following Help functions: Contents, Search, What's This?, About PCT....

Online Help is available for most screens and fields but may be incomplete.

PCT-EASY Master Table Functions

Information entered in the details pages appear as entries on the Notebook Master Tables in the same sequence in which they were entered. (For example, Earlier Search: the earlier search input first appears as the first row entry 1, the second 2, etc.) The order of appearance of input of Master Table entries may be changed by highlighting the entry to be moved on the Master Table and then either clicking on the right mouse button or the Edit menu to select the Move up or Move down functions. Repeat use of these functions until the desired position is obtained.

In order to delete an entry on a Notebook Master Table, select the entry to be deleted and then click the right mouse button and select the cut function.

Request (Figure 12.6)

Request consists of the following information:

Receiving Office

The Receiving Office must be selected from the menu. The international application (request, description (excluding sequence listing part), claims, abstract, drawings (if any), and the sequence listing part of the description (where applicable)) must be filed with a competent Receiving Office (Article 11(1)(i)) — that is, subject to any applicable prescriptions concerning national security, at the choice of the applicant, either:

1. The Receiving Office of, or acting for, a PCT Contracting State of which the applicant or, if there are two or more applicants, at least one of them, is a resident or national (Rule 19.1(a)(i) or (ii)); or
2. The International Bureau of WIPO in Geneva, Switzerland, if the applicant or, if there are two or more applicants, at least one of the applicants is a resident or national of any PCT Contracting State (Rule 19.1(a)(iii))

Request Forms prepared using PCT-EASY may only be filed with those Receiving Offices which are prepared to accept such filings.

Note: Do not file PCT-EASY applications with a Receiving Office without first verifying that such Office accepts PCT-EASY. If in doubt contact the PCT-EASY Help Desk or the Receiving Office concerned.

International Searching Authority

The International Searching Authority (ISA) must be selected from the menu. If there is more than one competent ISA for carrying out the international search in relation to the international application — depending on the Receiving Office with which it is filed — the competent authority chosen by the applicant must be selected from the menu (Rules 4.1(b)(vi) and 4.14*bis*).

Language of Filing of the International Application

Where the Receiving Office selected allows the applicant to choose between two or more filing languages, the language of filing of the international application (which may be different from the language in which the PCT-EASY Request Form is prepared) must be selected from the menu (Rule 12.1).

If the language in which the international application is filed is not accepted by the International Searching Authority selected to carry out the international search, the applicant will have to furnish a translation into a language which is all of the following: (1) a language accepted by that authority, and (2) a language of publication, and (3) a language which is accepted by the Receiving Office, unless the international application is filed in a language of publication. This translation must be furnished within 1 month from the date of receipt of the international application by the Receiving Office (Rule 12.3).

Title of Invention

The title must be short (preferably two to seven words when in English or translated into English) and precise. To facilitate the technical preparations for international publication it should be preferably entered in capital letters in the field provided and must be identical to the title heading the description. (Rules 4.3 and 5.1(a))

Request to Use Results of Earlier Search

The earlier search(es), if any, must be identified in such a manner that the ISA can retrieve the results easily. Where those results can be used, the ISA may refund the international search fee or a portion thereof. (Rules 4.11 and 41.1) (Figure 12.8).

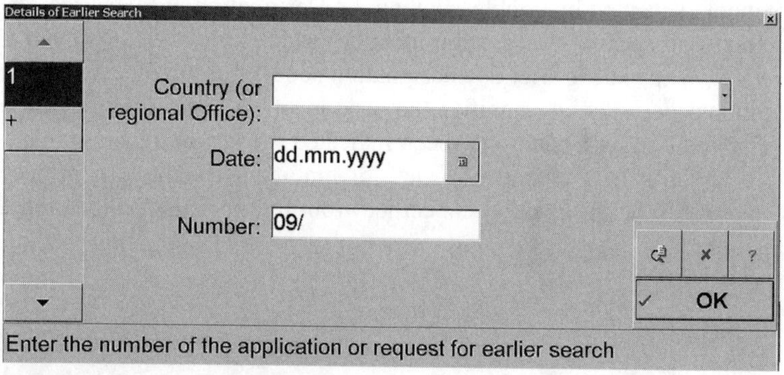

FIGURE 12.8

The Request to use results of earlier search Master Table consists of one function. Double-click the Open to add reference to earlier search row or select this row and click the Open button to add details concerning an earlier search.

Where the earlier search by the International Searching Authority was made in relation to a national, regional or international application, that application (or translation thereof) must be identified in the request by an indication of the country of filing (or the regional Patent Office), and the number and filing date of that application. Where the earlier search was made independently of a patent granting procedure (for instance, a standard search by the European Patent Office), a reference must be made to the date of the request for that search and the number given to the request by the International Searching Authority. This screen is composed of the following fields:

- Country (or regional Office) (menu): Select from the menu the country (or regional Office) where the earlier search was filed. *Note:* This menu defaults to the International Searching Authority indicated by the user and lists other options only where available.

- Date: Enter the date of filing of the earlier application following the prescribed date format provided.
- Number: Enter the filing number, if any, attributed to the earlier search.

After entry, earlier searches appear as entries on the Earlier Search Master Table in the same sequence in which they were entered. (For example, the earlier search input first appears as the first row entry 1, the second 2, etc.)

States (Figures 12.9–12.11)

On this page, the user indicates the PCT Contracting States that are to be designated in the international application. The PCT Contracting States in which protection is desired must be designated under Rule 4.9(a) in PCT-EASY either by using the Select All button or by selecting specific designations on the Designation Details Subnotebook, accessed by double-clicking the Designation of States Master Table.

At least one specific designation must be made (Rules 4.1(a)(iv) and 4.9(a)). An asterisk (*) appearing after any designation code, or group of designation codes for a regional designation, signifies that a kind of protection or treatment other than, or in addition to, a patent has been indicated for that designation (e.g., utility model in addition to a patent). To view or modify such kinds of protection or treatment, select the designation concerned from the relevant Designation Details subnotebook.

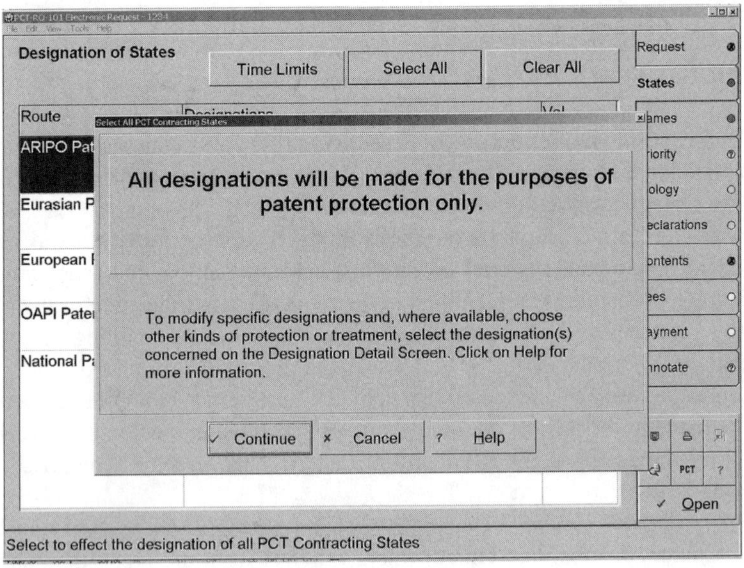

FIGURE 12.9

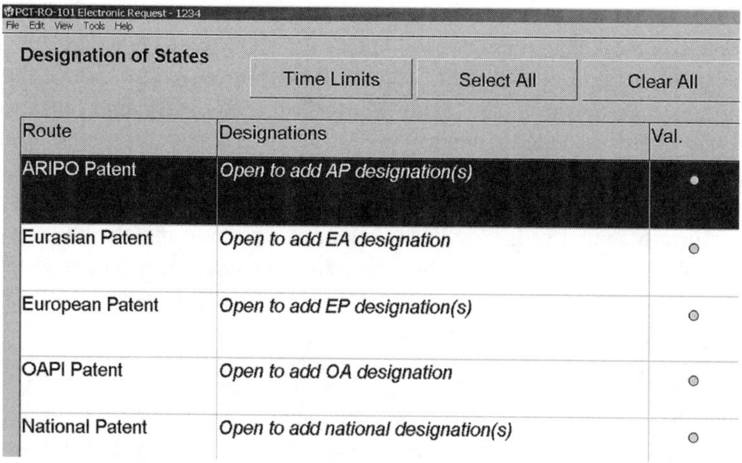
PCT-RO-101 Electronic Request - 1234
File Edit View Tools Help
Designation of States
Time Limits
Select All
Clear All
Route
Designations
Val.
ARIPO Patent
Open to add AP designation(s)
Eurasian Patent
Open to add EA designation
European Patent
Open to add EP designation(s)
OAPI Patent
Open to add OA designation
National Patent
Open to add national designation(s)

FIGURE 12.10

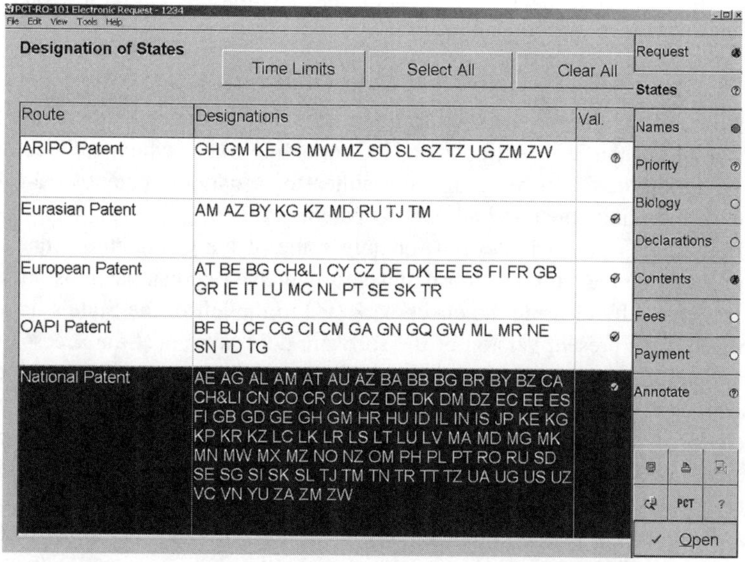
PCT-RO-101 Electronic Request - 1234
File Edit View Tools Help
Designation of States
Time Limits
Select All
Clear All
Route
Designations
Val.
ARIPO Patent
GH GM KE LS MW MZ SD SL SZ TZ UG ZM ZW
Eurasian Patent
AM AZ BY KG KZ MD RU TJ TM
European Patent
AT BE BG CH&LI CY CZ DE DK EE ES FI FR GB GR IE IT LU MC NL PT SE SK TR
OAPI Patent
BF BJ CF CG CI CM GA GN GQ GW ML MR NE SN TD TG
National Patent
AE AG AL AM AT AU AZ BA BB BG BR BY BZ CA CH&LI CN CO CR CU CZ DE DK DM DZ EC EE ES FI GB GD GE GH GM HR HU ID IL IN IS JP KE KG KP KR KZ LC LK LR LS LT LU LV MA MD MG MK MN MW MX MZ NO NZ OM PH PL PT RO RU SD SE SG SI SK SL TJ TM TN TR TT TZ UA UG US UZ VC VN YU ZA ZM ZW
Request
States
Names
Priority
Biology
Declarations
Contents
Fees
Payment
Annotate
PCT
?
Open

FIGURE 12.11

While the general rule is that designations cannot be added after the filing of the international application, it is possible and usual to make a precautionary designation under Rule 4.9(b) covering all other designations which would, as at the international filing date, be permitted under the PCT; see Precautionary Designation of States Subject to Confirmation.

Designation fees must be paid for each State designated up to a maximum of ten. Where regional (ARIPO, Eurasian, European and/or OAPI) patents are desired, only one PCT designation fee must be paid for each regional designation made, independently of how many States are covered by each such designation. Note that

PCT-EASY does not provide for the possibility of marking specific designations with consecutive Arabic numerals to express the applicant's choice of the order of the designations; consequently, the order will be taken as that in which the designations appear on the designated States Master Table, unless the applicant specifying a different order has added a remark. (See the Annotate page for more information on how to make a remark.) This order will only have any significance if the amount received for the designation fees is insufficient to cover all the designations and remains insufficient after the applicant has been invited to pay the balance due; in that case, the amount received will be applied in payment of fees for the designations as instructed by the applicant, or, in the absence of such instruction, following the said order (Rule 16*bis*.1(c) and Section 321).

Designation Details Subnotebook

Clicking the Designation of States Master Table itself also allows access to the Designation Details subnotebook. This is where the user can access details concerning designations, including the full names of PCT Contracting States, kinds of protection or treatment available, and the precautionary designation statement. Any modification, input or deletion of specific designations or kinds of protection or treatment occurs in this subnotebook.

ARIPO Patent (AP)

Select the ARIPO Patent checkbox to designate all Contracting States of the Harare Protocol and of the PCT. All other PCT Contracting States which are also party to the Harare Protocol can be designated either for a national patent or an ARIPO patent, or both a national and an ARIPO patent.

If an ARIPO patent is desired for only some of the Contracting States of the Harare Protocol, the names of those States for which a regional patent is not desired may be deleted by clearing the checkmark (✔) to the left of the State's name.

Because the present version of the software does not reflect the accession to or the ratification of the PCT by States which became bound by it after the date of issuance of the present version of the software, the list of States contains a statement to include any other State which is a Contracting State of the Harare Protocol and of the PCT. When the box corresponding to this statement is selected, any such State will be considered as having been designated for the purposes of an ARIPO patent. If an ARIPO patent is not desired for any such State, this statement may be deleted by clearing the box.

It is recommended that the applicant always designate for the purposes of an ARIPO patent all PCT Contracting States, which are party to the Harare Protocol. A decision to proceed with only some of those designations need not be made until entry into the regional phase, at which stage the corresponding regional designation fees must be paid.

Only one PCT designation fee must be paid for the ARIPO Patent designation, independently of how many States are covered by this designation.

Where any of the States party to the Harare Protocol and the PCT is designated twice, namely both for the purposes of an ARIPO patent and for the purposes of national protection, the applicant must pay one designation fee in respect of the regional patent and as many designation fees as there are national patents or other titles of protection sought (Rule 15.1(ii) and Section 210).

Eurasian Patent (EA)

Select the Eurasian Patent checkbox to designate all Contracting States of the Eurasian Patent Convention and of the PCT. All PCT Contracting States, which are also party to the Eurasian Patent Convention, can be designated either for a national or a Eurasian patent, or both a national and a Eurasian patent. Note, however, that it is not possible to designate only some of these States for a Eurasian patent; any designation of one or more States for a Eurasian patent will be treated as a designation of all the States, which are party to both the Convention and the PCT for a Eurasian patent.

Only one PCT designation fee must be paid for the Eurasian designation, independently of how many States are covered by this designation.

Where any of the States party to the Eurasian Patent Convention and the PCT is designated twice, namely both for the purposes of a Eurasian patent and for the purposes of national protection, the applicant must pay one designation fee in respect of the regional patent and as many designation fees as there are national patents or other titles of protection sought (Rule 15.1(ii) and Section 210).

European Patent (EP)

Select the European Patent checkbox to designate all Contracting States of the European Patent Convention and of the PCT. All other PCT Contracting States which are also party to the European Patent Convention can be designated either for a national or a European patent, or both a national and a European patent.

If a European patent is desired for only some of the Contracting States of the European Patent Convention, the names of those States for which a regional patent is not desired may be deleted by clearing the checkmark (✔) to the left of the State's name.

Because the present version of the software does not reflect the accession to or the ratification of the PCT by States which became bound by it after the date of issuance of the present version of the software, the list of States contains a statement to include any other State which is a Contracting State of the European Patent Convention and of the PCT. When the box corresponding to this statement is selected, any such State will be considered as having been designated for the purposes of a European patent. If a European patent is not desired for any such State, this statement may be deleted by clearing the box.

It is recommended that the applicant always designate for the purposes of a European patent all PCT Contracting States which are party to the European Patent Convention. A decision to proceed with only some of those designations need not be made until entry into the regional phase, at which stage the corresponding regional designation fees must be paid.

Only one PCT designation fee must be paid for the European Patent designation, independently of how many States are covered by this designation.

Where any of the States party to the European Patent Convention and the PCT is designated twice, namely both for the purposes of a European patent and for the purposes of national protection, the applicant must pay one designation fee in respect of the regional patent and as many designation fees as there are national patents or other titles of protection sought (Rule 15.1(ii) and Section 210).

Extension of European Patent (EP) to Certain States

If it is intended, at the time of entry into the European regional phase, to request the extension of the subsequently granted European patent to AL Albania, LT Lithuania, LV Latvia, MK the former Yugoslav Republic of Macedonia, RO Romania, and/or SI Slovenia and/or to any other PCT Contracting State for which, on the date of filing of the international application, an extension agreement with the European Patent Organization is in force, the Designation of States Master Table must contain both a designation of the State concerned for the purposes of a national patent and also a designation, for the purposes of obtaining a European patent, of at least one PCT Contracting State party to the European Patent Convention.

OAPI Patent (OA)

Select the OAPI Patent checkbox to effect the designation of all States that are members of OAPI and party to the PCT. The designation of States members of OAPI and party to the PCT can only be made for the purposes of an OAPI patent (no national protection is available); furthermore, it is not possible to designate only some of them.

Only one PCT designation fee must be paid for the OAPI Patent designation, independently of how many States are covered by this designation.

Where the applicant wishes to designate OAPI for a title of protection other than a patent (e.g., a utility model or certificate of addition), the title of protection should be indicated by selecting it from the Kind of Protection menu. If a certificate of addition is selected, also indicate the number of the parent title or parent application, and the date of grant of the parent title or the date of filing of the parent application in the fields provided (Figures 12.12 and 12.13).

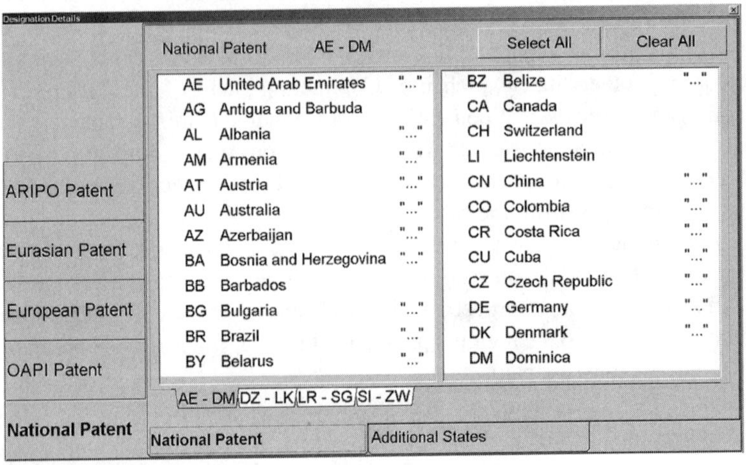

FIGURE 12.12

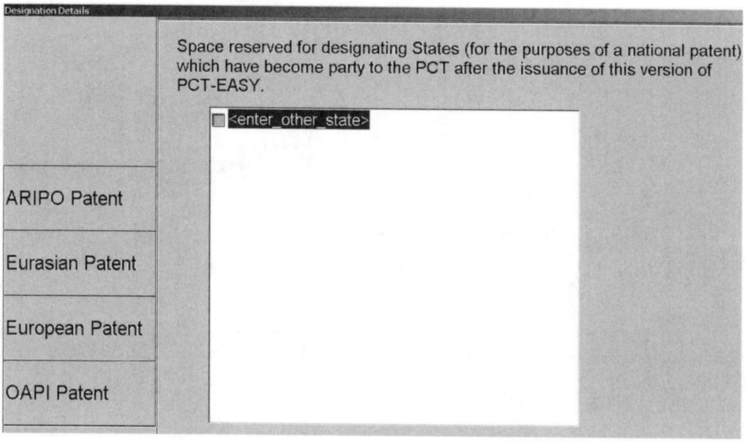

FIGURE 12.13

National Patent

The Contracting States in relation to which national protection is desired must be designated under Rule 4.9(a). A specific designation may be indicated by a check-mark (✔) to the left of the State's name on the National Patent details pages.

- Select the National Patent Select All button to affect the designation of all PCT Contracting States where a national patent is available.
- Select the National Patent Clear All button to clear all designations from the National Patent Designation Detail pages.
- For the designation of a State which has become party to the PCT after the software version release date (the date is displayed on the About PCT-EASY item accessed from the Help menu). The name of the State, preferably preceded by the two-letter country code, must be entered in the space provided on the Additional States designation tab, together with an indication, where applicable, as to whether a special kind of protection or treatment is desired. Only one such designation should be entered per line. Please note, however, that the applicant is strongly urged to obtain an updated version of the software, containing the new designation(s), before attempting to use the Additional States designation field (Figure 12.14).

Choice of Certain Kinds of Protection or Treatment

Where, in respect of any country where it is possible, a national title other than a patent is desired, select the indication "…" after the name of the country on the National Patent Designation Details pages to indicate the Kind of Protection desired from the kind of protection menu appearing in the pop-up window.

An asterisk (*) appearing after any designation code indicates that another kind of protection or treatment selected or group of designation codes for a regional designation signifies that a kind of protection other than, or in addition to, a patent

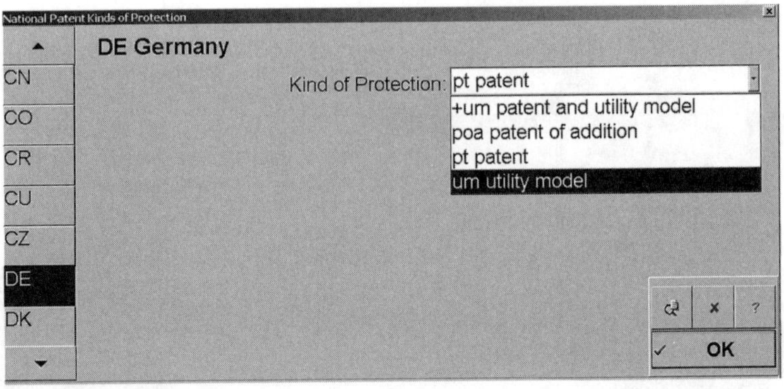

FIGURE 12.14

has been indicated for that designation (e.g., utility model in addition to a patent). On the Designation of States notebook page the following text appears underneath the heading National Patent:

These kinds of protection include:

- Petty patent (pp): Available in AU Australia, YU Yugoslavia
- Provisional patent (pr): Available in AM Armenia, KG Kyrgyzstan, KZ Kazakhstan, TM Turkmenistan, UZ Uzbekistan
- Utility model (um): Available in AL Albania, AM Armenia, AT Austria, BG Bulgaria, BR Brazil, BY Belarus, CN China, CZ Czech Republic, DE Germany, DK Denmark, EE Estonia, ES Spain, FI Finland, GE Georgia, GH Ghana, HU Hungary, JP Japan, KE Kenya, KG Kyrgyzstan, KR Republic of Korea, KZ Kazakhstan, LS Lesotho, MD Republic of Moldova, MX Mexico, PL Poland, PT Portugal, RU Russian Federation, SK Slovakia, TJ Tajikistan, TR Turkey, UA Ukraine, UZ Uzbekistan, VN Viet Nam, OA OAPI
- Utility model in addition to a patent (+um): only Available in AT Austria, CZ Czech Republic, DE Germany, DK Denmark, EE Estonia, FI Finland, SK Slovakia (Rules 4.12 to 4.14 and Section 202)
- Utility certificate (uc): Available in TT Trinidad and Tobago, UG Uganda
- Inventor's certificate (ic): Available in CU Cuba, KP Democratic People's Republic of Korea

Where, in respect of any country where it is possible, it is desired that the international application be treated as an application for a certain title of addition or as an application for a continuation or a continuation-in-part, select the indication "…" after the name of the country on the National Patent Designation Details pages and select the desired protection from the Kind of Protection menu appearing in the pop-up window. If any of these indications is used, also indicate in the fields provided the number of the parent title or parent application, and the date of grant of the parent title or the date of filing of the parent application.

These kinds of treatment include:

- Patent of addition (POA): Available in AT Austria, AU Australia, BA Bosnia and Herzegovina, CU Cuba, DE Germany, ES Spain, GE Georgia, HR Croatia, IL Israel, IN India, MK the former Yugoslav Republic of Macedonia, MW Malawi, NZ New Zealand, SI Slovenia, TR Turkey, YU Yugoslavia, ZW Zimbabwe
- Certificate of addition (COA): Available in BR Brazil, MG Madagascar, OA OAPI
- Inventor's certificate of addition (ICA): Available in CU Cuba
- Continuation (CON) or continuation-in-part (CIP): Both available in US United States of America

Precautionary Designation of States Subject to Confirmation (Rules 4.9(b) and (c) and 15.5)

For the applicant's protection, located below the Designation Details Subnotebook, the Precautionary Designation Statement button reveals a statement indicating the applicant's wish to make, in addition to the specific designations made in the Designation Details Subnotebook (at least one such designation must be made), a precautionary designation of all other PCT Contracting States which are not specifically designated.

If the applicant does not wish to avail himself of this protection and does not wish to make any such precautionary designations, the Precautionary Designation Statement View/Change button must be selected, revealing the precautionary designation statement in a pop-up window (Figure 12.15), at which point the preselected box may then be cleared (Figure 12.16). However, it is strongly recommended that the applicant make the precautionary designations indication, by leaving the Precautionary Designation Statement box selected, unless there is a particular reason for doing otherwise.

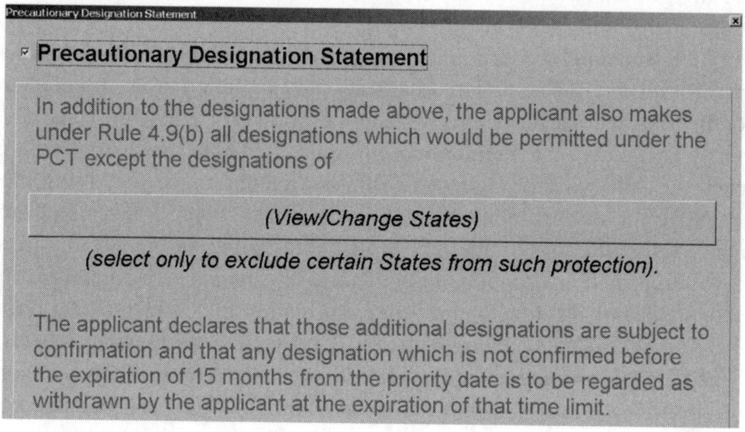

FIGURE 12.15

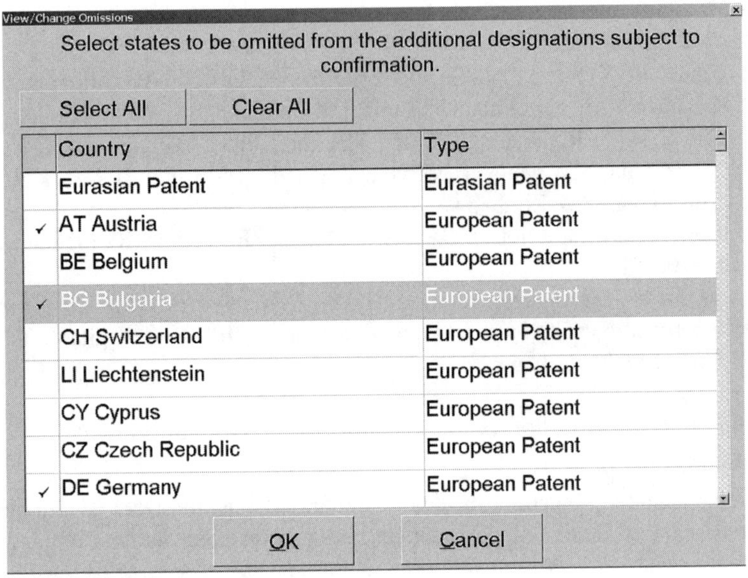

FIGURE 12.16

If the applicant wishes to expressly exclude a certain State from such precautionary designation so that the international application does not have any effect in that State, the Precautionary Designation Statement View/Change button must be selected, after which the button labeled View/Change States must be selected. Selecting this button gives access to a list of States for which a precautionary designation is possible. Click to insert a checkmark (✔) to the left of the State's name to effect the exclusion of that State from such protection. In no other case is it necessary to make use of this list.

If the applicant has made use of the precautionary designation statement, and if, after filing the international application, the applicant notices that there are any omissions and/or mistakes among the specific designations made, it will be possible to rectify the situation by confirming the precautionary designations concerned. The confirmation of any precautionary designation is possible before the expiration of 15 months from the (earliest) priority date indicated on the Priority page or, where no priority is claimed, the international filing date. To effect such confirmation, the applicant must file with the Receiving Office a written notice specifying the name of each State the designation of which is confirmed (with, where applicable, an indication of the kind of treatment or protection desired) and pay to the Receiving Office, for each such designation, a designation fee (even where 10 designation fees have already been paid) together with a confirmation fee corresponding to 50% of the designation fee. The Receiving Office will not send to the applicant any reminder or invitation to confirm precautionary designations. If no precautionary designation is to be confirmed, the applicant requires no action, and the precautionary designations will then be automatically regarded as withdrawn by the applicant at the expiration of 15 months from the priority date.

The Names page is for the input of information pertaining to applicants and inventors, as well as for the input of information pertaining to agents, a common representative, or a special address for correspondence. It consists of the Names Master Table and the Preview Function.

The Names Master Table consists of five input functions:

1. Add Applicant (to indicate an applicant or applicant/inventor)
2. Add Inventor only (to indicate an inventor only)
3. Add Agent (to indicate an agent)
4. Add Common Representative (to select an applicant as common representative)
5. Add Special Address for Correspondence (in the absence of either an agent or a common representative, to indicate a special address to which correspondence should be sent)

After entry, applicants, inventors and agents appear as entries on the Names Master Table in the same sequence they are entered. (For example, the applicant whose name has been input first becomes 1. Applicant, the second 2. Applicant, etc.)

The Preview function permits the user to view details on the Names page formatted to appear as they will when printed on the Request Form printout. Select the Preview checkbox and, using the up/down key or the mouse, click the row containing the details you wish to preview. Simply clear the checkbox to go back to normal view.

Using the Address Book

The names and address of applicants, inventors and agents may be stored in the Address Book. To add an applicant or applicant/inventor, double-click the Add Applicant row or select this row and click the Open button. This screen is composed of the following fields:

Legal entity/Natural person (radio buttons): By selecting one of these two radio buttons the user can identify whether the entry concerns a legal entity or a natural (physical) person.

Name (of legal entity): Names of legal entities must be indicated in this field (preferably in capital letters) by their full, official designations (Rule 4.4(b)).

Name (of natural person): The family name must be indicated in the field (preferably in capital letters) which contains the prompt <last_name>. The given name must be indicated in the field which contains the prompt <first_name>. Titles and academic degrees must be omitted.

This person is also inventor (checkbox): Select this box if the applicant is both applicant and inventor. This box cannot be selected if the applicant is a legal entity. Where the United States of America is one of the designated States, all of the inventors must be named as applicants for the United States of America and the checkbox "This person is also inventor" must be selected.

Names (Figures 12.17 and 12.18)

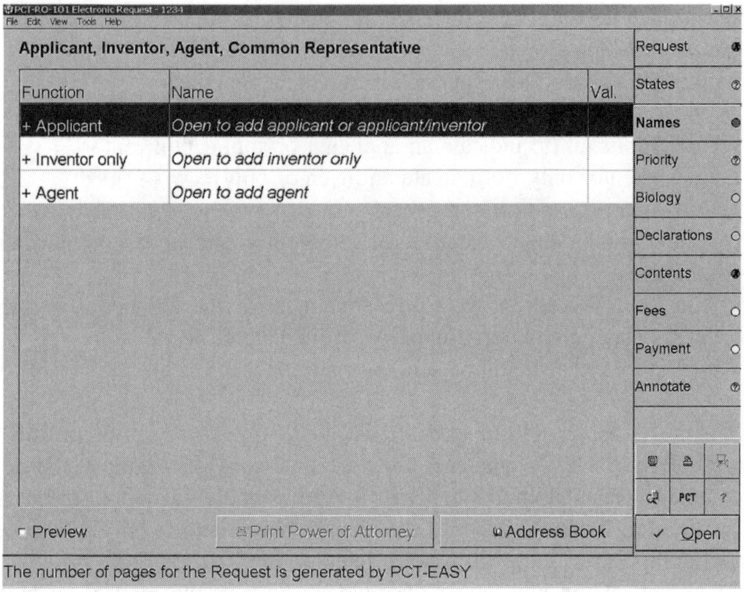

FIGURE 12.17

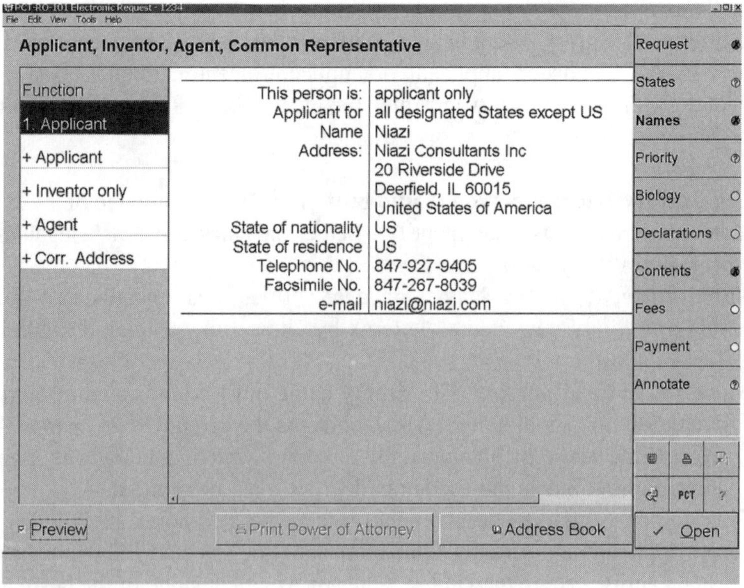

FIGURE 12.18

To indicate an inventor who is not also applicant, use the Add Inventor only function (see the Add Inventor Only section of this chapter).

Country or territory: May be input using the drop-down list, which actually consists of two fields. In the first field, the user can simply input the code for the desired country or territory of the address, after which, the full name of the country or territory is then automatically defaulted into the second field. Alternatively, the user may skip to the second field and select the full name of the country or territory, after which the relevant code for that country or territory is automatically defaulted in the first field.

Address

> **<(optional)_contact,_dept.>/<(optional)_company_c/o> field:** This optional indication can, in the case of a legal entity, be used to identify a contact person, department, etc.. For a natural person it can be used to indicate c/o details or company name.

> **<street_address> field:** The street address is entered here. The address must be indicated in such a way that it allows prompt postal delivery; it must consist of all the relevant administrative units (up to and including the indication of the house number, if any). (Rule 4.4(c))

Only one address may be indicated per person (Rule 4.4(d)). For the indication of a special address for correspondence, see the Add Special Address for Correspondence section.

City: Complete this field with the full city name.

State/County/Province: This field only appears if applicable. Select the State, Province, County, from the list.

Postal code: The address must contain the postal code or zip code (if any). Please do not preface the postal code with the country code.

Telephone: Should be indicated to allow rapid communication with the applicant or agent. Any such number should include the applicable country and area codes.

Facsimile: Should be indicated to allow rapid communication with the applicant or agent. Any such number should include the applicable country and area codes.

E-mail: (Optional indication.) Any such indication should include the full Internet e-mail address. Please note, however, that until further notice, official communications in relation to international applications filed via PCT-EASY will only be sent via paper-based mail service (facsimile, postal or courier service).

Nationality (Rules 4.5(a) and (b) and 18.1): For each applicant, the nationality must be indicated by the name of the State (i.e., country) of which the person is a national. A legal entity constituted according to the national law of a State is considered a national of that State. The indication of the nationality is not required where a person is inventor only.

This indication may be input using the drop-down list, which actually consists of two fields. In the first field, the user can simply input the code for the desired indication, after which the full name of the country or territory is then automatically defaulted into the second field. Alternatively, the user may skip to the second field and select the full name of the country or territory, after which the relevant code for that country or territory is automatically defaulted in the first field.

Residence (Rules 4.5(a) and (c) and 18.1): Each applicant's State (i.e., country) of residence must be indicated. If the State of residence is not indicated, it will be assumed to be the same as the State indicated in the address. Possession of a real and effective industrial or commercial establishment in a State is considered residence in that State. The indication of the residence is not required where a person is inventor only.

This field is automatically populated with the same data as input in the country or territory field, from the address, where possible. It may be altered manually, as required, using the drop-down list, which actually consists of two fields. In the first field, the user can simply input the code for the desired indication, after which, the full name of the country or territory is then automatically defaulted into the second field. Alternatively, the user may skip to the second field and select the full name of the country or territory, after which the relevant code for that country or territory is automatically defaulted in the first field.

Applicant Designations (This person is applicant for the purposes of:): Select the designated States for which the person identified is to be considered applicant by clicking the appropriate radio button:

- All designated States
- All designated States except US
- The United States of America only
- Certain designated States only

Different Applicants for Different Designated States: It is possible to indicate different applicants for the purposes of different designated States. At least one of all the applicants named must be a national or resident of a PCT Contracting State for which the Receiving Office acts, irrespective of the designated State(s) for the purposes of which that applicant is named (Rules 4.5(d), 18.3 and 19.2). If the international application is filed with the International Bureau under Rule 19.1(a)(iii), at least one of the applicants must be a resident or national of any PCT Contracting State. Where the United States of America is one of the designated States, all of the inventors must be named as applicants for the United States of America and the checkbox This person is also inventor must be selected.

All Designated States: This radio button must be selected where the person identified is and qualifies as applicant for all designated States. Where that person is a legal entity or an assignee, this button must not be selected if the United States of America is designated on the Designation of States page. (Except for the purposes of a person named as applicant in a legal capacity for a deceased or incapacitated inventor. See Deceased section for more details.)

All designated States except US: This radio button must be selected where the United States of America is designated on the Designation of

States page and the person identified is not also inventor, since only the inventor can be the applicant for the United States of America.

The United States of America only: This radio button must be selected where the United States of America is designated on the Designation of States page and the person identified is also inventor but is not also applicant for the other designated States. Often the inventor is the applicant only for the United States of America and another person (natural person or legal entity) is the applicant for all other designated States. This radio button must not be marked if the person identified is not also the inventor. (Except for the purposes of a person named as applicant in a legal capacity for a deceased or incapacitated inventor. See Deceased section for more details.)

Certain designated States only: This radio button must be selected only in special cases not covered by the preceding three radio buttons. Where, for example, each of three applicants is applicant for different States, the indication of the States for which each person identified is applicant must be selected for each applicant from their respective applicant details screens. It is possible to make such an indication using the Select/Modify button (appearing only when the Certain designated States only radio button has been selected). Selecting this button gives access to a complete list of designated States. To indicate the designated States for which a person is applicant, click to insert a checkmark (✔) to the left of the State(s) concerned.

Where a particular State has been designated for both a national patent and a regional patent, the same applicant or applicants shall be indicated for both designations. Consequently, for the purposes of the Certain designated States only list, both the national and regional designation for such a State must be selected together.

Add Inventor Only (to indicate an inventor only): *Note:* Where the United States of America is one of the designated States, all of the inventors must be named as applicants for the United States of America and the function Add Applicant or applicant/inventor must be used instead of the Add Inventor only function. Double-click the Add Inventor only row or select this row and click the Open button to add an inventor only (i.e., an inventor who is not also applicant). This screen is composed of fields also found on the Add Applicant screen. Please refer to that part of the Names page for information on their use. It also contains a Deceased field:

Deceased (checkbox): Select this checkbox to indicate that the inventor is deceased. Where the U.S. has not been designated, no further indication (other than the deceased inventor's name) is required.

If the United States of America, which requires that the applicant be the inventor, is designated, the legal representative or the heir(s) of the deceased inventor must be named as the applicant(s) for the United States of America. In such a case complete the following steps:

1. The legal representative must be indicated as applicant for the purposes of the United States of America using the Add Applicant

or applicant/inventor function. The residence, nationality, and address of the legal representative or heir should be indicated rather than those of the deceased inventor.

2. Subsequent to this entry, it is possible to indicate this person as successor to the rights of the deceased inventor for the purposes of the designation of the United States of America from the table appearing on the deceased inventor's details screen. Click to insert a checkmark (✔) to the left of the name of the applicant concerned and select this person's legal capacity from the drop-down menu.

Repeat Steps 1 and 2 where there is more than one legal representative for the deceased inventor.

Naming of Inventor (Rule 4.1(a)(v) and (c)(i)): The inventor's name and address must be indicated where the national law of at least one of the designated States requires that the name of the inventor be furnished at the time of filing. It is strongly recommended to always name the inventor. *Note:* Different persons may be indicated as inventors for different designated States (e.g., in this respect where the requirements of the national laws of the designated States are not the same). However, such an indication may only be made on the Annotate page by selecting the indication Different inventors for different designated States from the drop-down menu. In the absence of any specific indication on that page, it will be assumed that the inventor(s) named is (are) inventor(s) for all designated States (Rule 4.6(c)).

Add Agent (to indicate an agent): Double-click the Add Agent row or select this row and click the Open button to add a person who is (or has been) appointed as agent. This screen is composed of fields found also on the Add Applicant screen. Please refer to that part of the Names page for information on their use. It also contains the following fields:

Same address as first-named agent (checkbox): Select this checkbox only if the agent identified has the same address as the first-named agent. When selected, all agent address fields are removed for this agent.*

Correspondence: Where an agent is appointed, any correspondence intended for the applicant will be sent to the address indicated for that agent (or for the first-mentioned agent, if more than one is appointed). Where several agents are listed, each must be indicated individually and the agent to whom correspondence should be addressed is to be listed first (Rule 4.4(d) and Section 108).

---

* Manner of appointment of agent: Any such appointment may be made by designating the agent(s) in the request or in one or more separate powers of attorney. Each applicant must sign either the request or a separate power of attorney. Where the international application is filed with reference to a general power of attorney, a copy thereof must be attached to the request. Any applicant who did not sign the general power of attorney must sign either the request or a separate power of attorney (Rules 90.4, 90.5, and Section 106).

Add Common Representative (to select an applicant as a common representative): Double-click the Add Common Representative row or select this row and click the Open button to open the Common Representative Details screen where one of the applicants can be indicated as common representative. Election of a common representative by the other applicants is only possible where more than one applicant or applicant/inventor has been indicated on the Applicant screen. The common representative must be one of the applicants who is a national or resident of a PCT Contracting State entitled to file an international application (Rule 90.2(a)). This screen is composed of fields also found on the Add Applicant screen. Please refer to that part of the Names page for information on their use. It also contains the following fields:

Name of Common Representative (drop-down menu): Select the name of one of the applicants to indicate this person as common representative. *Note:* Where an applicant has been selected as common representative, the address indicated for this person as applicant is automatically copied to the common representative address fields. This address may be modified or changed should the applicant have a different address for the purposes of his election as common representative.*

Correspondence: Any correspondence intended for the applicant will be sent to the address indicated for the common representative (Rule 4.4(d) and Section 108).

If a common representative is not appointed, the applicant first named in the request who is entitled to file an international application with the Receiving Office concerned will automatically be considered to be the common representative (the deemed common representative) (Rule 90.2(b)) and any correspondence will be sent to his address.

Add Special Address for Correspondence: Where no agent or common representative is appointed, any correspondence will be sent to the address indicated on the Names Master Table for the applicant (if only one person is named as applicant) or of the applicant who is considered to be common representative (if there are two or more persons named as applicants).

However, if correspondence is to be sent to a different address, that address may be indicated by using the Add Special Address for Correspondence function. In this case, and only in this case, should the Add Special Address for Correspondence function be used. This screen is composed entirely of fields also found on the Add Applicant screen. Please refer to that part of the Names page for information on their use.

---

* Manner of appointment of common representative: Any such appointment may be made by designating the common representative in the request or in one or more separate powers of attorney. Each applicant must sign either the request or a separate power of attorney. Where the international application is filed with reference to a general power of attorney, a copy thereof must be attached to the request. Any applicant who did not sign the general power of attorney must sign either the request or a separate power of attorney (Rules 90.4, 90.5, and Section 106).

Priority

General Information on Priority Claims

If the priority of an earlier application is claimed, the declaration containing the priority claim must be made in the request (Rule 4.10).

The request must indicate the date on which the earlier application was filed and the number it was assigned. *Note:* The date must fall within the period of 12 months preceding the international filing date.

Where the earlier application is an international application, the Receiving Office with which that earlier application was filed must be indicated.

Where the earlier application is a regional application (other than an ARIPO application), or an international application, the priority claim may also, if the applicant so wishes, indicate one or more countries party to the Paris Convention for which that application was filed (Rule 4.10(b)(i)); such an indication is not, however, mandatory. Where the earlier application is an ARIPO application, at least one country party to the Paris Convention for which that earlier application was filed must be indicated.

Certified Copy of Earlier Application (Rule 17.1)

A certified copy of each earlier application the priority of which is claimed (priority document) must be submitted by the applicant, irrespective of whether that earlier application is a national, regional, or international application. The priority document must be submitted to the Receiving Office or to the International Bureau before the expiration of 16 months from the (earliest) priority date or, where an early start of the national phase is requested, not later than at the time such a request is made. Any priority document received by the International Bureau after the expiration of the 16-month time limit but before the date of international publication shall be considered to have been received on the last day of that time limit (Rule 17.1(a)).

Where the priority document is issued by the Receiving Office, the applicant may, instead of submitting the priority document, request the Receiving Office (not later than 16 months after the priority date) to prepare and transmit the priority document to the International Bureau. Such request may be made by selecting the applicable checkbox on the Details of Priority Claim of Earlier Application screen. *Note:* Where such a request is made, the applicant must pay to the Receiving Office the applicable fee for priority document; otherwise, the request will be considered not to have been made.

The Priority Notebook Page

The Priority notebook page contains a Priority Claim master table where the priority claims of such earlier applications can be indicated. The Priority Claim master table consists of one input function: Open to add priority claim. Selecting this row opens up the Details of Priority Claim of Earlier Application screen where indications concerning the priority can be made. Only one priority claim should be entered per screen.

After entry, priority claims appear on the Priority Claim master table as entries in the same sequence in which they were entered. (For example, the priority claim input first becomes 1, priority claim input second becomes 2, etc.) It is recommended, but not mandatory, that the earliest priority be entered first.

It is also possible to sort the priority claims chronologically. To do so, click the right mouse button and select the Sort Priority Claims Chronologically function.

Details of Priority Claim of Earlier Application

The content of this screen depends on the Filing Route selected:

National: Select this radio button if the earlier application is a national application.

Regional: Select this radio button if the earlier application is a regional application.

International (PCT): Select this radio button if the earlier application is an international (PCT) application.

Details of Priority Claim of Earlier Application (National)

This screen is composed of the following fields when National has been selected from the Filing Route radio button group:

Country: By entering the country code, or selecting the country from the drop-down menu, indicate the country party to the Paris Convention in which the earlier national application was filed (Rule 4.10(a)(iii)).

Filing Date: The date on which the earlier application, for which priority is claimed, was filed must be entered in this field (Rule 4.10(a)(i)). The filing date of the earlier application must be entered in the format specified in the edit field. For the purposes of the PCT Request Form printout, all dates will automatically be formatted to PCT standards.

Number: The number assigned to the earlier application for which priority is claimed must be indicated in this field (Rule 4.10(a)(ii)).

Request Copy of Priority Document from RO: Where the priority document is issued by the Receiving Office, the applicant may, instead of submitting the priority document, request the Receiving Office (not later than 16 months after the (earliest) priority date) to prepare and transmit the priority document to the International Bureau. Such request may be made by selecting the corresponding checkbox on the Details of Priority Claim of Earlier Application screen for each earlier application for which the priority document is requested. *Note:* Where such a request is made, the applicant must pay to the Receiving Office the applicable fee for priority document, otherwise, the request will be considered not to have been made (Rule 17.1(b)).

Details of Priority Claim of Earlier Application (Regional)

This screen is composed of the following fields when Regional has been selected from the Filing Route radio button group:

Regional Office: Select the appropriate regional office from the drop-down menu to indicate the Office with which the regional application was filed (Rule 4.10(a)(iv)).

Filing Date: The date on which the earlier application, for which priority is claimed, was filed must be entered in this field (Rule 4.10(a)(ii)). The filing date of the earlier application must be entered in the format specified in the edit field. For the purposes of the PCT Request Form printout, all dates will automatically be formatted to PCT standards.

Number: The number assigned to the earlier application for which priority is claimed must be indicated in this field.

Country party to the Paris Convention for the Protection of Industrial Property for which the Earlier Application Was Filed (ARIPO application): Where the earlier application is an ARIPO application, at least one country party to the Paris Convention for which that earlier application was filed must be indicated (Rule 4.10(b)(i) and (ii)). By entering the country code, or selecting the country from the drop-down menu, enter the country or one of the countries party to the Paris Convention for which the earlier ARIPO application was filed (i.e., the country or one of the countries designated for protection in the ARIPO application).

Request Copy of Priority Document from RO: Where the priority document is issued by the Receiving Office the applicant may, instead of submitting the priority document, request the Receiving Office (not later than 16 months after the (earliest) priority date) to prepare and transmit the priority document to the International Bureau. Such request may be made by selecting the corresponding checkbox on the Details of Priority Claim of Earlier Application screen for each earlier application for which the priority document is requested. *Note:* Where such a request is made, the applicant must pay to the Receiving Office the applicable fee for priority document; otherwise, the request will be considered not to have been made (Rule 17.1(b)).

Details of Priority Claim of Earlier Application (International (PCT))

This screen is composed of the following fields when International (PCT) has been selected from the Filing Route radio button group:

Receiving Office: By entering the country or office code, or selecting the country or office from the drop-down menu, indicate the Office with which the international application was filed (i.e., the Receiving Office) (Rule 4.10(a)(v)).

Filing Date: The date on which the earlier application, for which priority is claimed, was filed must be entered in this field (Rule 4.10(a)(ii)). The filing date of the earlier application must be entered in the format specified in the edit field. For the purposes of the PCT Request Form printout, all dates will automatically be formatted to PCT standards.

Number: The number assigned to the earlier application for which priority is claimed must be indicated in this field.

Request Copy of Priority Document from RO: Where the priority document is issued by the Receiving Office the applicant may, instead of submitting the priority document, request the Receiving Office (not later than 16 months after the (earliest) priority date) to prepare and transmit the priority document to the International Bureau. Such request may be made by selecting the corresponding checkbox on the Details of Priority Claim of Earlier Application screen for each earlier application for which the priority document is requested. *Note:* Where such a request is made, the applicant must pay to the Receiving Office the applicable fee for priority document, otherwise, the request will be considered not to have been made (Rule 17.1(b)).

Biology (Indications Relating to Deposited Microorganism and Other Biological Material)

The Biology master table consists of one function. Double-click the Open to add new item row or select this row and click the Open button to add details concerning indications relating to a deposited microorganism and/or other biological material.

Under PCT Rule 13*bis*.3 the applicant is required to give the following indications with regard to deposited biological material:

1. The name and address of the depositary institution with which the deposit was made
2. The date of deposit of the biological material with that institution
3. The accession number given to the deposit by that institution

Certain designated Offices require that the indications relating to the deposit of biological material must be included in the description at the time of filing otherwise such indications will not be taken into account by those Offices in the national phase.

To the extent that indications relating to the deposit of biological material are not given in the description, they may be furnished on Form PCT/RO/134. If this form is submitted when the international application is filed, a reference to it should be made in the checklist. A printout containing the information found on Form PCT/RO/134 will be generated by PCT-EASY at the same time as the Request Form.

Where the international application contains disclosure of one or more nucleotide and/or amino acid sequences these should be contained in a separate part of the description (Rule 5.2(a)). In such a case the checkbox The description contains a sequence listing should be selected.

Details Concerning Indications Relating to a Deposited Microorganism and Other Biological Material

Information entered in the Biology Details subnotebook will be used to generate Form PCT/RO/134.

Indications in the Description: Where the indications relating to the deposit of biological material have been included in the description, the page and line numbers of where such indications have been made should be entered in the appropriate fields.

Depositary Institution: Select the name of the depositary institution with which the biological material was deposited from the drop-down menu. The depositary institutions are listed by alphabetical order of their acronym followed by the name of the institution.

Address: The address of the depositary institution will be automatically generated when selecting the name of the depositary institution concerned from the drop-down menu.

Accession Number: The first of the two fields under the heading Accession Number will show the acronym of the depositary institution with which the biological material was deposited. This information will be automatically generated when selecting the name of the depositary institution concerned from the drop-down menu. Enter the accession number attributed to the deposit in the <no.> field.

Date of Deposit: Enter the date of deposit of the microorganism following the date format provided.

Additional Indications: The national laws of some designated Offices require that, besides indications concerning the deposit of biological material, an indication be given concerning the biological material itself, for example, a short description of its characteristics, at least to the extent that this information is available to the applicant. These requirements must be met, provided that the requirements have been notified to the International Bureau and published in the PCT Gazette. Annex L of Volume I/B of the PCT Applicant's Guide indicates, for each of the designated Offices, the requirements (if any) of this kind which have been so notified and published (Rules 13*bis*.3(a)(iv) and 13*bis*.7(a)).

If additional indications are given, enter them in the field entitled Additional Indications.

Separate Furnishing of Indications: If any indication is not included in a reference to deposited biological material contained in the international application as filed, it may be furnished to the International Bureau within 16 months from the priority date unless the International Bureau has been notified (and, at least 2 months prior to the filing of the international application, has published in the PCT Gazette) that the national law requires the indication to be furnished earlier. However, if the applicant makes a request for early publication, all indications should be furnished by the time the request is made, since any designated Office may regard any indication not furnished when the request is made as not having been furnished in time. Annex L of Volume I/B of the PCT Applicant's Guide specifies, for each designated Office whose national law requires a reference to deposited biological material to be furnished earlier than 16 months after the priority date, the applicable time limit(s) for furnishing such indications (Rules 13*bis*.3(b), 13*bis*.4, and 48.2(a)(viii)).

If indications will be made separately from the filing of the international application, enter the appropriate information in the field entitled Separate Furnishing of Indications.

Designated States for which Indications Are Made: A reference to deposited biological material may be made for the purposes of all designated States or for one or only some of the designated States. A reference is considered to be made for the purpose of all designated States unless it is expressly made for certain designated States only. References to different deposits may be made for the purposes of different designated States (Rule 13*bis*.5).

  All Designated States: Click the All Designated States button if the indications relating to a deposited microorganism apply to all designated States.

  Certain Designated States Only: Click the Certain Designated States Only button if the indications relating to deposited biological material apply to one or only some of the designated States. Click the Select/Modify button to access a list of the States designated in the application. The designated States for which the indications relating to deposited biological material apply should be indicated by a checkmark (✔) to the left of the State's name on the View/Change States details page.

Contents

The Contents page contains indications relating to various items that are part of, or accompany, the international application. This page comprises two master tables, identified by the following notebook tabs:

- International Application master table (where indications relating to the contents of the international application itself are entered)
- Accompanying Items master table (where indications relating to items which accompany the international application are entered)

Both master tables contain a detail table where details concerning attached paper documents and electronic files can be specified.

Please note that for this version of PCT-EASY only paper documents can be attached to the international application with the exception of the Abstract, in which case a file in plain text (.txt) format may be attached in electronic form in addition to the paper document. This is the only circumstance where electronic file attachments should be used for the time being. (For information on creating and saving these types of file formats, see your word processor documentation.)

International Application Master Table (Checklist)

This master table contains the following items:

- Request
- Description/Description (excluding sequence listing part) (as applicable)
- Claims
- Abstract
- Drawings
- Sequence listing part of description (where applicable); this item will only appear where the checkbox on the Biology page has been selected

Double-click a row, or select a row and click the Open button, to indicate the number of pages for the paper document, and any electronic file attached, for each item. (Only the Abstract should be attached in electronic form at this time and submitted with the request on diskette.)

Completion Tips

Indication of the number of sheets comprising the description and claims is mandatory. The user must complete these fields.

The total number of pages comprising the international application appears just below the Drawing or Sequence listing part of description item, as applicable, on this master table, in the field marked total.

The Calculate Button

Once the International Application checklist has been completed, select this button to generate a page total. This is a mandatory operation as the total number of pages of the Request form is generated by PCT-EASY at this point, and the total number of pages of the international application is used to determine the calculation of the International Fee. You should select the button a second time after having either added or deleted information from notebook pages. When the preparation for submission procedure is invoked, the page count will automatically be recalculated.

International Application Content Details

The user may scroll through items on the Content Details screen using the navigation bar on the left-hand side of the screen:

Request
 Paper document: The Request form is automatically generated by PCT-EASY as is the page count for the request. This number appears in the Pages column.
 Electronic file: Not applicable.
Description/Description (excluding sequence listing part)
 Paper document: To indicate the number of pages of the description/description (excluding sequence listing part), select the Is Enclosed radio button and enter the number in the edit field.
 Electronic file: It is not possible to attach an electronic file for this item using this version of PCT-EASY.

Claims

Paper document: To indicate the number of pages of the claims, select the Is Enclosed radio button and enter the number in the edit field.

Electronic file: It is not possible to attach an electronic file for this item using this version of PCT-EASY.

Abstract

Paper document: To indicate the number of pages of the abstract, select the Is Enclosed radio button and enter the number in the edit field.

Electronic file: The abstract may be attached in .txt format (Plain Text Format). To attach the file, select the Is Copied radio button, then select the file's location and name from the Windows File Manager menu and click the OK button.

Drawings: Where the international application contains drawings, the applicant must indicate in the edit field provided the number of the figure of the drawings which the applicant believes best characterizes the invention. Only one figure should be indicated, if useful for the understanding of the abstract. If none of the figures is useful for the understanding of the abstract, no figure need be indicated (Rules 3.3(a)(iii) and 8.2).

Paper document: To indicate the number of pages of the drawings, select the Is Enclosed radio button and enter the number in the edit field.

Electronic file: It is not possible to attach an electronic file for this item using this version of PCT-EASY.

Sequence listing part of description: Where the application contains disclosure of one or more nucleotide and/or amino acid sequences, such sequences must be presented as a separate part of the description (Sequence listing part of description) in accordance with the standard provided in Annex C of the Administrative Instructions. This item will only become available where the checkbox on the Biology page has been selected.

Paper document: To indicate the number of pages of the sequence listing part of the description, select the Is Enclosed radio button and enter the number in the edit field.

Electronic file: The electronic file containing the sequence listing part of the description in the prescribed format should be submitted on a separate diskette and this should be added as an item on the Accompanying Items Checklist.

Accompanying Items Master Table (Checklist)

Double-click a row, or select a row and click the Open button, to indicate that items have been attached. This master table may contain the following automatically generated items:

Fee Calculation Sheet

Paper document: Should accompany the Request form printout, even if fees are not paid at the time of filing, and is therefore automatically attached in paper form.

Electronic file: Not applicable.

Priority Document (Contents page) (multiple instance): As a reminder, a priority document item is automatically added as a row on the Accompanying Items master table for each national, regional priority and international claim indicated on the Priority notebook page when a copy of that document has not been requested to be prepared and transmitted to the International Bureau by the Receiving Office. Please note, however, that such a document is only indicated as attached when such an indication has been made under Paper document below.

> **Paper document:** To indicate that this priority document accompanies the international application, select the Is Enclosed radio button.
>
> **Electronic file:** It is not possible to attach an electronic file for this item using this version of PCT-EASY.

This master table can also contain the following items which can be added by selecting the desired item from the drop-down menu and then selecting the Add button. Once added, double-click a row, or select a row and click the Open button, to indicate that the item has been attached:

Separate Signed Power of Attorney

> **Paper document:** To indicate that this item accompanies the international application, select the Is Enclosed radio button.
>
> **Electronic file:** It is not possible to attach an electronic file for this item using this version of PCT-EASY.

Copy of General Power of Attorney

> **Paper document:** To indicate that a copy of a general power of attorney, the original of which has been previously deposited with the Receiving Office according to Rule 90.5, accompanies the international application, select the Is Enclosed radio button. If the Receiving Office has accorded a reference number to the deposited general power of attorney, that number may be indicated.
>
> **Electronic file:** It is not possible to attach an electronic file for this item using this version of PCT-EASY.

Statement Explaining Lack of Signature

> **Paper document:** To indicate that this item accompanies the international application, select the Is Enclosed radio button.
>
> **Electronic file:** It is not possible to attach an electronic file for this item using this version of PCT-EASY.

Separate Indications Concerning Deposited Microorganisms and/or Other Biological Material

> **Paper document:** Indicate a paper document is attached by selecting the Is Enclosed radio button where a filled-in Form PCT/RO/134 or any separate sheet containing indications concerning deposited biological material is filed with the international application. For certain States, Form PCT/RO/134 or any other sheet containing the said indications must be included as one of the sheets of the description. If the relevant indications (which may be contained on a separate sheet or on Form

PCT/RO/134) form part of the international application, do not make an indication for this item. For further information, see Rule 13*bis* and Section 209.

Electronic file: It is not possible to attach an electronic file for this item using this version of PCT-EASY.

Nucleotide and/or Amino Acid Sequence Listing (diskette)

Paper document: The number of pages of the sequence listing part of the description should be entered on the International Application checklist.

Electronic file: Where the description of the international application contains disclosure of a nucleotide and/or amino acid sequence, and a copy of the sequence listing is required in computer readable form by the ISA, the applicant may furnish the listing in computer readable form to the Receiving Office with the International application. In such a case, select the Is Copied radio button on separate diskette (Rule 5.2).

Translation of International Application Into …: Where a translation of the international application for the purposes of international search (Rule 12.3) is filed together with the international application, indicate the language of translation in the <language> field.

Paper document: To indicate that this item accompanies the international application, select the Is Enclosed radio button.

Electronic file: It is not possible to attach an electronic file for this item using this version of PCT-EASY.

Other (specify) (multiple instance): Enter the details of this item in the drop-down menu when the <specify> prompt appears. Select the Add button and this other item will be added to the list of accompanying items.

Paper document: To indicate that this item accompanies the international application, select the Is Enclosed radio button.

Electronic file: It is not possible to attach the electronic file for this item using this version of PCT-EASY.

Fees

The purpose of the Fee Calculation page is to help the applicant identify the prescribed fees and to calculate the amounts to be paid. It is strongly recommended that the applicant use the PCT-EASY fee calculation functionality either by manually entering the appropriate amounts in the fields provided or by importing these amounts from a supplied, or user saved, fee table (see Fee Schedule). Use of this page will help the Receiving Office verify fee amounts and help eliminate calculation errors.

Information about the applicable fees payable can be obtained from the Receiving Office. The amounts of the international and search fees may change due to currency fluctuations. Applicants are advised to check which are the latest applicable amounts. All fees, except in some cases the designation fee, must be paid within 1 month from the date of receipt of the international application. See Designation Fees for further details concerning the possibility of later payment of the designation fee.

The Fee Calculation page consists of the following items:

Currency
If there is more than one acceptable currency for payment of the international fees (which depends upon the choice of Receiving Office and International Searching Authority indicated on the Request page), the desired currency for payment may be chosen by the user from the drop-down menu.

Fee Schedule (Drop-Down Menu and Memo Field)
Selection of a fee schedule from the drop-down menu effects the importation of corresponding fee amounts valid from the date indicated. (Use of this functionality is optional.)

Fee Calculation Table
Fee information is displayed directly on this table. Fee multipliers are automatically calculated from data input on other notebook pages. Using the Currency and Fee Schedule drop-down menus, the fee amounts themselves are automatically imported from fee data stored in the Maintenance section of the software. The fee amounts do not include digits after the decimal. If these digits need to be displayed it is possible to change the display settings from the EASY File Manager. Fee amounts can also be input or modified directly on this table by the user. Total amounts are automatically generated. This table consists of the following items:

Transmittal Fee: This fee is for the benefit of the Receiving Office (Rule 14.1). The amount of the transmittal fee, if any, shall be fixed by the Receiving Office, and shall be paid within 1 month from the date of receipt of the international application.

Search Fee: This fee is for the benefit of the International Searching Authority (ISA) (Rule 16.1). The amount of the search fee is fixed by the ISA and must be paid within 1 month from the date of receipt of the international application by the Receiving Office.

Where two or more ISAs are competent, the applicant must indicate his choice on the Request notebook page and pay the amount of the international search fee fixed by the ISA chosen.

Please note that where the US has been indicated as the International Searching Authority, and an earlier search has been indicated on the Request page (corresponding to a prior US national application under 35 USC 111(a) that has been filed and the basic fee paid), the search fee will reflect the reduced amount.

International Fee. Basic Fee: The amount of the basic fee depends on the total number of sheets of the international application, which appears in the Total field below the International Application master table on the Contents notebook page. This fee must be paid within 1 month from the date of receipt of the international application by the Receiving Office.

International Fee. Supplement per Sheet over 30: The amount of this fee depends on the total number of sheets of the international application, which appears under in the Total field below the International Application master table on the Contents notebook page. If the international application consists of 30 sheets or less no supplemental fee is charged.

If the international application consists of more than 30 sheets a supplement fee per sheet over 30 is charged. If this is the case, the total number of sheets over 30 will automatically appear as the multiplier for this fee. This fee must be paid within 1 month from the date of receipt of the international application by the Receiving Office.

International Fee. Designation Fee: The number of designation fees due corresponds to the number of national and regional designations made on the Designation of States page. PCT-EASY calculates this number and it is automatically inserted as the multiplier for the purposes of calculating the total of the designation fee.

The number of designation fees which are due is the same as the number of national patents and regional patents in respect of which specific designations under Rule 4.9(a) are made. Only one designation fee is due for the designation AP, the designation EA, the designation EP, or the designation OA, irrespective of the number of States for which an ARIPO patent, a Eurasian patent, a European patent, or an OAPI patent, respectively, is sought.

Where any State is designated twice (once for the purposes of an ARIPO patent, a Eurasian patent or a European patent and once for the purposes of national protection), the applicant must pay one designation fee in respect of the ARIPO patent, the Eurasian patent, or the European patent and a further designation fee in respect of each national patent or other title of protection sought (Rule 15.1(ii) and Section 210).

Any designation, in excess of 10 designations for which the fee is due, is free of charge. Therefore, the maximum amount to be indicated as a multiplier for the designation fee is 10 times the amount of the designation fee. If, for example, 15 national patents and four regional patents (an ARIPO patent, a Eurasian patent, a European patent, and an OAPI patent) are sought (totaling 19 designations), the figure to be indicated as multiplier is 10 times the amount of the designation fee.

The designation fees must be paid within 1 month from the date of receipt of the international application by the Receiving Office, or 12 months from the priority date, whichever time limit expires later.

International Fee. PCT-EASY Reduction: A reduction of 200 Swiss francs of the international fee (or the equivalent in the currency in which the international fee is paid to the Receiving Office) is available if the following two conditions are met: (1) the international application must be filed with a Receiving Office which is prepared to accept the filing of international applications containing requests in PCT-EASY format together with PCT-EASY diskettes; and (2) the request must be presented as a computer print-out prepared using PCT-EASY and filed together with a computer diskette, prepared using PCT-EASY, containing a copy in electronic form of the data contained in the request and of the abstract as a text (.txt) file.

Where the abstract has been added in electronic format on the Contents page, the amount of the fee reduction will appear as a negative amount in red. Where the abstract has not been attached in electronic form, the amount of the fee reduction will appear as 0.

Fee for Priority Document: Where the authority with which the earlier application was filed is the same office as the Receiving Office, the applicant may, instead of submitting the priority document, request the Receiving Office to prepare and transmit the priority document to the International Bureau. Such request may be made by marking the applicable checkbox on the Priority notebook pages where the applicant identifies such document. Where such a request is made, the applicant must pay to the Receiving Office the applicable priority document fee which may be entered here (Rule 17.1(b)). The multiplier for the priority document fee corresponds to the number of requests for such documents that have been made on the Priority notebook pages.

If that fee is not paid at the latest before the expiration of 16 months from the priority date, the Receiving Office may consider the request under Rule 17.1(b) as not having been made.

If the Receiving Office does not have a flat fee per priority document requested (e.g., amount depends on number of pages) this field will also contain the indication (total amount). In such a case, the priority document multiplier will be disabled (always indicating one irrespective of the number of priority documents requested). The user should calculate the total fee amount for all priority documents requested and enter the total in the Amount column.

Reduction of Fees for Applicants from Certain States: PCT-EASY performs a validation to assess if all applicants indicated have the right to claim the fee reduction according to the conditions indicated below.

Where a fee schedule has been selected on the Fees page, reductions will automatically be calculated where applicable. In such a case the multiplier column (X) on the Fees page will indicate the reduction applied between brackets in red. Where the amounts in the fee schedule have not be predetermined (due to local currency fluctuations) the correct amounts should be confirmed with the Receiving Office and the full (nonreduced) amount should be indicated in the Amount column.

Where no fee schedule has been selected, the user should input the reduced amounts of the fees manually (PCT-EASY will not calculate the fee reduction). Please note that the international fee for the PCT-EASY reduction should also be reduced accordingly.

Reduction of the International Fee for Applicants from Certain States: An applicant who is a natural person and who is a national of and resides in a State whose per capita national income is below 3000 US dollars (according to the average per capita national income figures used by the United Nations for determining its scale of assessments for the contributions payable for the years 1995, 1996, and 1997) is entitled, in accordance with the Schedule of Fees, to a reduction of 75% of certain PCT fees including the international fee. If there are several applicants, each must satisfy the above-mentioned criteria. The reduction of the international fee (basic fee and designation fees) is automatically available to any applicant (or applicants) who is (or are) so entitled on the basis of the indications of name, nationality and residence given on the Request page.

The fee reduction is available even if one or more of the applicants are not from PCT Contracting States, provided that each of them is a national and resident of a State that meets the above-mentioned requirements and that at least one of the applicants is a national or resident of a PCT Contracting State and thus is entitled to file an international application.

Natural persons who are nationals of and reside in the following PCT Contracting States are eligible: AL Albania, AM Armenia, AZ Azerbaijan, BA Bosnia and Herzegovina, BF Burkina Faso, BG Bulgaria, BJ Benin, BR Brazil, BY Belarus, CF Central African Republic, CG Congo, CI Côte d'Ivoire, CM Cameroon, CN China, CU Cuba, CZ Czech Republic, EE Estonia, GA Gabon, GD Grenada, GE Georgia, GH Ghana, GM Gambia, GN Guinea, GW Guinea-Bissau, HR Croatia, HU Hungary, ID Indonesia, IN India, KE Kenya, KG Kyrgyzstan, KP Democratic People's Republic of Korea, KZ Kazakhstan, LC Saint Lucia, LK Sri Lanka, LR Liberia, LS Lesotho, LT Lithuania, LV Latvia, MD Republic of Moldova, MG Madagascar, MK The former Yugoslav Republic of Macedonia, ML Mali, MN Mongolia, MR Mauritania, MW Malawi, MX Mexico, NE Niger, PL Poland, RO Romania, RU Russian Federation, SD Sudan, SK Slovakia, SL Sierra Leone, SN Senegal, SZ Swaziland, TD Chad, TG Togo, TJ Tajikistan, TM Turkmenistan, TR Turkey, UA Ukraine, UG Uganda, UZ Uzbekistan, VN Viet Nam, YU Yugoslavia and ZW Zimbabwe. As far as other States are concerned, inquiries should be addressed to the International Bureau.

Other fee reductions may also be available for applicants from Certain States. Please check with the Receiving Office to see which other reductions may apply. In such cases, the applicant should indicate the reduced fee amount, where applicable, on the Fee Calculation Page.

Designation Fees not Paid at this Time (checkbox): Where the time limit of 12 months from the priority date expires later than 1 month from the date of receipt of the international application by the Receiving Office, and the applicant wishes to delay the payment of the designation fees, it is recommended that the corresponding checkbox be selected. In such a case, the designation fee total is calculated as 0 on the Fee Calculation Table and the designation fees due, but not paid, will appear below this checkbox.

Payment

This page allows the applicant to indicate the mode of payment of the prescribed fees, which can be selected from the drop-down menu. Not all modes of payment may be available at all Receiving Offices. *Note concerning authorization to charge deposit accounts:* The Receiving Office will not charge fees to deposit accounts unless the deposit account authorization is signed (on the Request Form printout) and indicates the deposit account number (in the edit field provided when this mode of payment has been selected).

In addition, Indicate Deposit Account Authorization: If the user wishes to indicate a deposit account authorization in addition to another mode of payment as a precaution, select this box and indicate the deposit account number in the field provided.

More than One Mode of Payment: Where the applicant has the possibility of paying different fees by different modes of payment the mode of payment more than one mode of payment should be selected from the drop-down menu. A details table will then appear. For each type of fee payable a drop-down menu appears in the right-hand column. The users should select from this menu the applicable mode of payment for each of type of fee.

Annotate

The Annotate master table contains the Signature of Applicant or Agent function, used to create a list of signatories, and the Validation Log, which allows the user to view all outstanding validation messages for this international application.

This table may also be used to include additional indications, if any, relating to the international application, and consists of the following functions:

- Inventor for certain designated States only
- Statement concerning nonprejudicial disclosures or lack of novelty
- Remarks
- Private remarks

When selected from the drop-down menu, items appear as entries on the Annotation master table. Select the item to view or edit.

Signature of Applicant or Agent: Here the user can create a list of persons who will sign the Request Form printout. To create such a list, select the person (or persons) from the upper list — in the case of a legal entity also enter the name of the person signing and the capacity in which the person signs (if such capacity is not obvious from reading the request) — in the fields provided. Select the Insert button and repeat this process for each person signing the Request Form printout. Selected persons are added to the list at the bottom of the table. Where there are several entities on the list, the Move Up button can be used to rearrange the order. The Delete button can be used to delete an entity which has been selected.

The signature must be that of the applicant (if there are several applicants, all must sign); however, the signature may be that of the agent or common representative where a separate power of attorney appointing the agent or common representative, or a copy of a general power of attorney already in the possession of the Receiving Office, is furnished. If the power is not attached to the request, the Receiving Office will invite the applicant to furnish it subsequently.

If the United States of America is designated and an inventor/applicant for that State refused to sign the request or could not be found or reached after diligent effort, a statement explaining the lack of signature may be furnished. It should be noted that this applies only where there are two or more applicants and the international application has been signed by at least one applicant. The statement must satisfy the requirements of the Receiving Office. If such a statement is filed with the international application, the item Statement explaining lack of signature should be selected from the Accompanying Items master table (Contents page) (Rules 4.1(d) and 4.15).

If deposit account has been selected as the Mode of Payment from the Payment page, an additional signature field will appear where the name of the first selected signatory will default as the Name of Person Signing the Deposit Account Authorization. This indication may be modified by the user.

Inventor for Certain Designated States Only: Different persons may be indicated as inventors for different designated States (e.g., where, in this respect, the requirements of the national laws of the designated States are not the same); in such a case, this item should be selected. Upon selection, a table containing a list of all inventors indicated on the Names page appears. Click the indication all designated States to the right of the person's name and indicate those States for which this person is to be considered inventor by selecting them from the complete list of designated States that appears. In the absence of any indication, it will be assumed that the inventor(s) named is (are) inventor(s) for all designated States (Rule 4.6(c)).

Statement Concerning Nonprejudicial Disclosures or Lack of Novelty: A statement concerning nonprejudicial disclosures or exceptions to lack of novelty, unless contained in the description, may be given in this edit field after this item has been added from the Annotate drop-down menu. It should comply with the provisions of the national law applicable by the designated Office(s) to which the statement is addressed.

Remarks: This item is for the input of remarks which the user wishes to communicate to the Receiving Office when submitting the international application. This information is downloaded to a diskette with all other information during the preparation for submission process and is included as part of the printout of the Annex to the Request Form (Fee Calculation Sheet).

Remarks can also be made from, and associated with, any notebook page by selecting the Remarks command from the Edit menu.

Private Remarks: This item is for the input of remarks which the user does not wish to communicate to the Receiving Office when submitting the international application. These remarks may serve as a reminder to the user when returning to an incomplete application or as a communication to another user involved at a different stage of the preparation. This information is not copied to diskette during the submission process.

Private remarks can also be made from any notebook page by selecting Private remarks from the Edit menu.

ABSTRACT EDITOR GUIDELINES

Unlike the previous PCT-EASY versions that required that the Abstract text file be created manually in an external program and then attached to the electronic form, PCT-EASY version 2.91 build 0003 includes a built-in editor that allows the Abstract contents to be furnished and saved directly within a form. This allows the software to have a better control over the Abstract contents and gives the user the possibility to insert some special characters allowed by the International Bureau's publishing system into the text of the Abstract. Please note the following requirements that the Abstract should meet:

- The Abstract should not contain any title, names of applicants, file references, figure of drawings etc. Please fill in the body of the Abstract only.
- No hard returns should be contained within the text of the Abstract.
- The length of the Abstract text should preferably be between 50 and 150 words in English or after translated into English.

Note: The current version 2.91 build 0003 of PCT-EASY does not support this functionality for non-Latin applications. Those applications should be handled the same way as they were in the previous versions of PCT-EASY, i.e., the Abstract file should be created using an external text editor (e.g., Notepad), converted to the plain ASCII text format and attached to a form. Future versions might make this step redundant. Check your current version features.

FURNISHING AN ABSTRACT

1. Start a PCT-EASY Request Form in the usual way, go to the Contents page within the form and double-click the Abstract line within the table (Figure 12.19). The Content details dialog box appears (Figure 12.20). The Electronic file radio group indicates whether the Abstract file was attached. This radio group is controlled by the software and cannot be changed by the user. Click the Edit Abstract File button to start the Abstract Editor.
2. *Important note:* If the form was prepared using a previous version of PCT-EASY, the Abstract Editor is unable to convert the old Abstract contents to the new format, therefore it can be neither viewed nor edited. In that case starting the Abstract Editor drops the contents of the previous Abstract and requires that the Abstract be furnished anew. However, an old form that already has the Abstract file attached can be submitted as is, without the possibility to preview the Abstract file. Start the Abstract Editor and thereby drop the previous contents of the Abstract file unless you are absolutely sure that the old Abstract file is correct and is in the proper format.
3. The text of the Abstract can be filled into the Abstract Editor using common formatting functions available to most word processors (Figure 12.21):

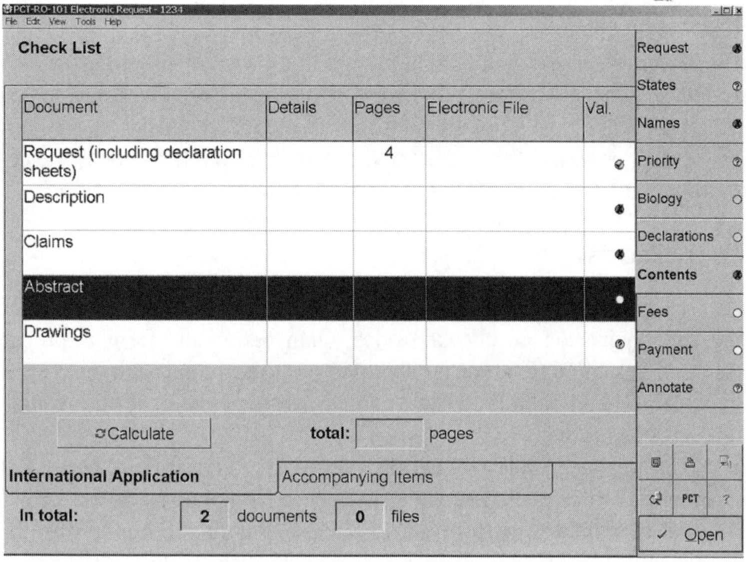

FIGURE 12.19

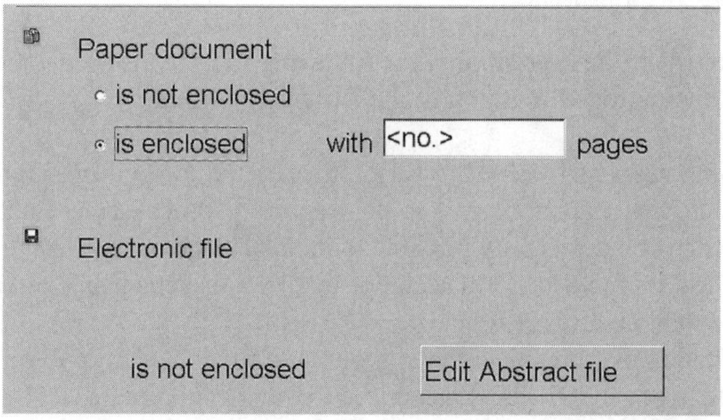

FIGURE 12.20

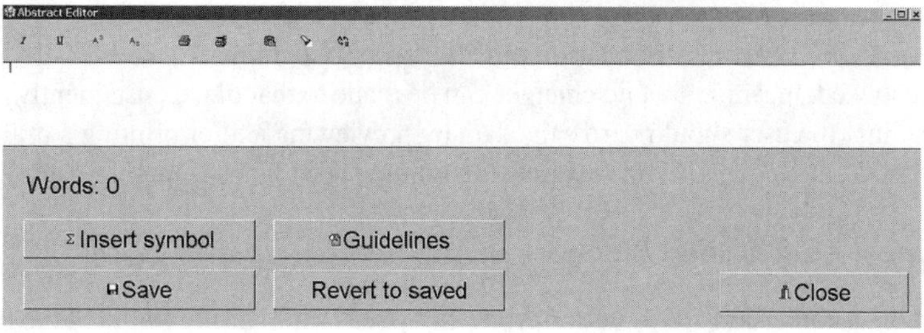

FIGURE 12.21

FILLING IN THE TEXT OF THE ABSTRACT FROM AN EXTERNAL SOURCE

You can, if you wish, use an external text editing program like Microsoft Word to prepare the text of the Abstract. After the text has been prepared it has to be copied to the Clipboard using the Copy functionality of the external editor and inserted into the Abstract Editor window by means of the Paste button (alternatively the keyboard key combination Ctrl+V can be used):

SUBMISSION PROCESS

When the user starts the submission process, the Abstract is previewed, so that its contents and layout can be checked once again before the form is prepared for submission. Click the OK button to continue with the submission process or press the Cancel button and open the abstract in the Abstract Editor if you would like to make any changes to it.

Note: The Abstract file is an essential part of the Request Form and is delivered to the Receiving Office packaged along with other components of the form. Therefore, it is not permitted to perform any manual manipulation on the resulting submission diskette as it can result in the included Abstract and other parts of the electronic form being inaccessible for the target system.

Preparation for Submission

This function takes the user through the following steps in the preparation of a PCT-EASY application for submission to the Receiving Office:

1. Submission log (where the user indicates the method of submission of the international application to the Receiving Office). Please note that for the time being it is only possible to indicate paper with diskette (i.e., full application in paper form accompanied by a diskette generated as part of the submission process).
2. Indication of who will sign the printout of the PCT-EASY Request Form.
3. Printout of the PCT-EASY generated Request Form suitable for submission.
4. Creation and copying of a zip file to diskette (containing a Request Form data file as well as any files attached on the contents page) for transmittal to the Receiving Office.

Important: Once the submission process has been completed, the PCT-EASY file will be locked, meaning that no changes can be made to that file. Consequently, before proceeding, the user should verify the data by previewing and/or printing a draft copy of the filled-in Request Form (accessed from the speed buttons or File menu).

Starting the Submission Process

Select the Submission speed button from the speed button group found at the bottom right-hand corner of the Request Form notebook or, alternatively, select the Submission command from the Tools menu.

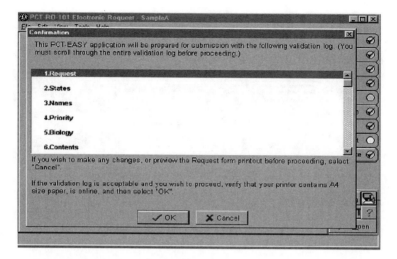

FIGURE 12.22

Please note that the Submission speed button and command can only be selected when all red validation messages relating to the data entered for this international application have been cleared.

Confirmation

Before proceeding, carefully review the validation log (Figure 12.22), which contains important information about your PCT-EASY filing. This is the last opportunity you will have to make modifications. Select Cancel to correct any errors or make any changes before proceeding. If the validation log is acceptable, select Continue.

Submission Log

The Submission Log (Figure 12.23) displays the progress of the submission process. It also indicates the date of preparation, the submission file name, and the method of submission.

Signature

As part of the submission process, the Signature table is displayed (Figure 12.24). The user can create a list of persons who will sign the Request Form printout by using the Signature of Applicant or Agent function on the Annotate page. If such a list has not been created using this function it may be created during the submission process. It is also possible at this point to modify the details of the Signature of the Applicant or Agent that my have been made earlier. Select OK to continue with the submission process.

PCT-EASY Generated Request Form and Other Forms (Figure 12.25)

The Print dialog box appears as part of the submission process. Before selecting the OK button to print, verify that your printer is online and loaded with A4 size paper

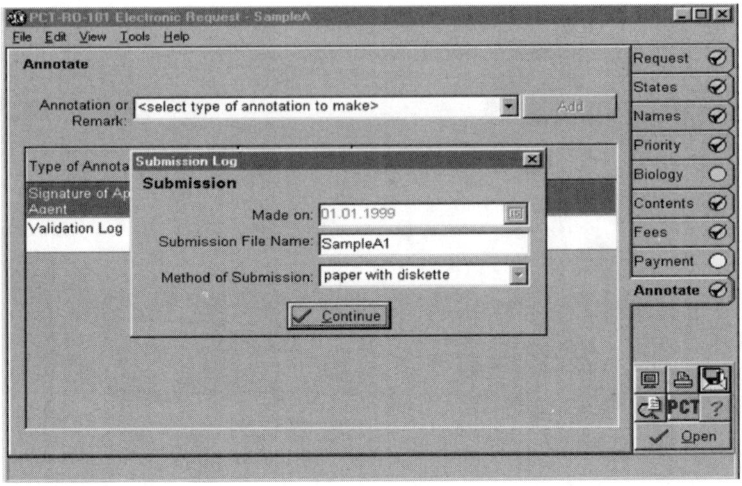

FIGURE 12.23

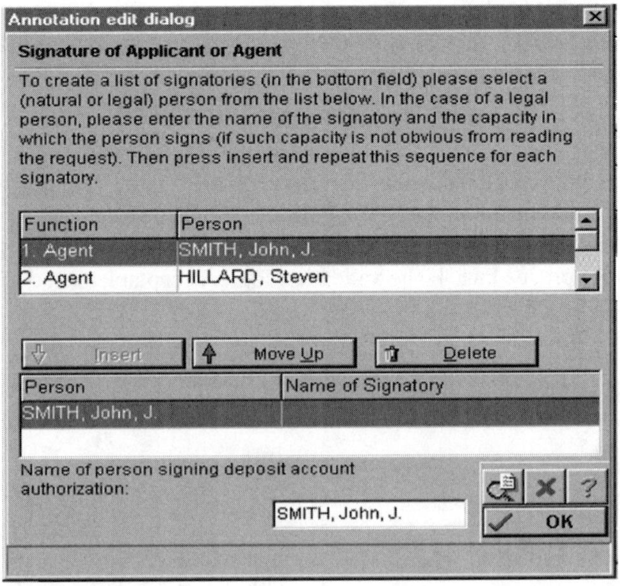

FIGURE 12.24

(different from $8^1/_2 \times 11$ or letter size). Also verify that the correct paper size is indicated in your print setup (accessed by selecting the Setup... button from the Print dialog box).

The Request Form printout generated as part of the submission process is identified with the indication Original (for submission) in the header of each printed page. (This printout differs from the one generated using the Print speed button or

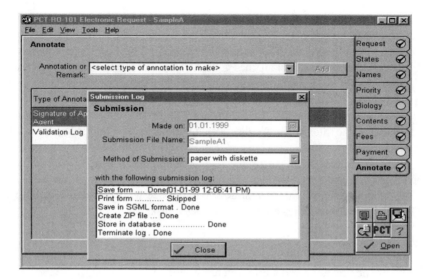

FIGURE 12.25

File menu command in that the latter is identified with the indication Draft (not for submission).)

A PCT-EASY Information Sheet is also printed. It contains a log of outstanding validation messages and should be reviewed carefully. The information sheet also contains information about other items that should be checked carefully before submitting the international application. (This sheet is intended for applicant use only and should not be submitted with the international application.)

If the user has made indications relating to a deposited microorganism and/or other biological material on the Biology page, a printout of form PCT/RO/134 indications will also be included.

Creation and Copying of the PCT-EASY Generated Zip File to Diskette

After closing the Submission Log, an Information dialog box appears indicating that the PCT-EASY application may now be copied to diskette for submission. Insert a blank formatted diskette in the a:\ drive and select Continue (change the drive path if necessary in the Save As dialog box that appears) and then select OK. Select OK again when the dialog box appears. The zip file will be copied to diskette and saved to the Stored Forms folder in the EASY File Manager, EASY Central directory for later reference.

Copying to Diskette Later

After closing the Submission Log, when the Information dialog box appears indicating that the PCT-EASY application may now be copied to diskette for submission, select Exit if you do not wish to copy to diskette now. The zip file will be saved in the Outbox folder in the EASY File Manager, EASY Central directory for copying to diskette later. At any time after the submission process, the zip file may be copied to diskette from this folder. This is done by inserting a blank formatted diskette in the a:\ drive, then double-clicking the PCT-EASY application to be copied to diskette from the Outbox folder information viewer. At this point a Save As dialog box appears. Select Continue, change the drive path if necessary, and then select OK. Select OK again when the dialog box appears. The zip file will be copied to diskette and saved to the Stored Forms directory in the EASY File Manager for later reference.

The diskette containing the zip file should be labeled PCT-EASY, also write the applicant's or agent's file reference, and the first applicant's name on the label. The diskette should be transmitted to the Receiving Office with the international application in paper form. Indicate on all PCT-EASY diskettes:

1. PCT-EASY
2. First Applicant's Name
3. Agent's or Applicant's File Reference No.

Correcting an Error or Omission from an Application Prepared for Submission

After the preparation for submission process has been completed it is not possible to modify the application. Accordingly, do not modify any indication on the Request Form printout. If an error or an omission is discovered at this time, the user must copy the submitted application to the New PCT Forms folder as a template and make the change or correction in a new application (created from the application file).

STORED FORMS

At the completion of the preparation for submission process, the completed electronic form will be stored in the EASY File Manager Stored Forms folder (Figure 12.26). Double-click the relevant PCT-EASY application from the Stored Forms folder information viewer. The locked application will then open for viewing. If necessary, the application can be recopied to diskette from this directory. This is done by inserting a blank diskette in the a:\ drive, and selecting the PCT-EASY application to be recopied from the Stored Forms folder information viewer. Click the right mouse button and select the Send to diskette command. At this point a Save As dialog box appears. Select Continue, change the drive path if necessary, and then select OK. Select OK again when the dialog box appears. The zip file is then recopied to diskette.

If necessary, the forms printed during the submission process can be reprinted. Double-click the relevant PCT-EASY application from the Stored Forms folder information viewer. The locked application will then open for viewing. Select the Print speed button or the Print command from the File menu.

The Request Form reprinted after the submission process is identified with the indication "Duplicate of Original" in the header of each printed page. In the absence of the original printed forms, duplicates from a locked application may be submitted.

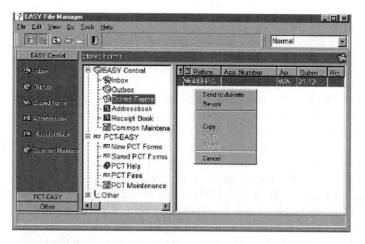

FIGURE 12.26

As a safety precaution, it is not possible to delete files from the Stored Forms folder. To delete files it is necessary to archive them first and then delete them from the Archive folder.

EXTENDED EXPORT/IMPORT FUNCTIONALITY

The current version of PCT-EASY is for local use only and cannot be installed on a network. Until version 2.90 build 0003 it was only possible to exchange EASY data with other EASY systems by means of the Intermediate File Format (IFF). However, the IFF approach is oriented more toward the exchange of EASY Form data with external systems, its use for data exchange between EASY systems being limited. Therefore, it has been necessary to develop a temporary approach which allows for PCT-EASY data sharing. This approach also provides the possibility for creating backup files of essential PCT-EASY data, facilitating recovery in the event of data loss.

The new functionality also allows for the transfer of data, in the case of the Address Book, not only between two EASY systems but also between EASY and an external program (for example, Excel, Outlook) which supports the export/import of data from a text file in the comma separated values (.csv) format. The .csv file is in a format commonly used for this purpose.

To summarize, the objective of the Export/Import functionality is

- To allow PCT-EASY form and Address Book data transfer between two local PCT-EASY systems installed on two different computers;
- To allow bidirectional Address Book data transfer between EASY and an external program (e.g., Excel, Outlook); and
- To allow for the creation of a backup copy of essential PCT-EASY data (Forms, Templates and Address Book contents) on an external media and its recovery in the event of data loss.

Essentially, the export of EASY forms consists of two functions:

1. Selection of particular forms or folders to be exported to a file.
2. Creation of a file containing the complete information about the items.

For the Address Book, however, it is only possible to export the entire Address Book, without the choice of selecting particular address records. An export file can be created on a network or local drive from where it can be copied to another local computer. This allows the exported data to be incorporated into another PCT-EASY system, or allows for centralized backup storage, providing the possibility of data recovery later on. The import (recovery) process is the opposite to the export, i.e., the data contained in the export file becomes an input which is processed into the PCT-EASY system. Please note that after being created, an export file is independent of the source EASY system and its improper use can cause a data security hazard or ambiguity (mishmash) in the internal record keeping. The proper use of export files should be ensured by organizational means.

DATA FORMATS

The export file for EASY forms and templates is represented in an internal format and includes information not only about the contents of forms, but also about their status (i.e., about which EASY Form folder each form belongs to). It can only be read and processed by the EASY File Manager. Please use the IFF function if you would like to transfer your EASY form data to/from an external system. The EASY forms export file has an extension .ezf. The resulting file for the Address Book Export is represented as a flat text file in the .csv format and can be imported both into another PCT-EASY system and into a third-party software product that supports the CSV format. In the case of Address Book data transfer from or to a third party software the user should associate each field within the .csv file with the corresponding field in the receiving system. In the case of Address Book data transfer between two EASY systems the fields within the .csv file are already mapped to the corresponding fields within the destination EASY system by default.

EASY FORMS AND TEMPLATES EXPORT

When the Export -> Forms option is selected from the File menu in the EASY File Manager, the Forms Export dialog box appears, which allows the selection of forms or folders to be exported to an arbitrary external destination. The Forms Export dialog box represents the tree of the EASY Forms folders in the left panel and the list of forms in the selected folder in the right panel. The user can select one, several or all folders to be copied into the export file by selecting the corresponding checkbox. Where an upper level node in the folder tree is selected, all subfolders and their contents are included in the export list. Therefore, in order to export the entire contents of all Forms folders the user can simply select the upper level EASY folder. Please note that as long as one or more folders are selected for the export, the entire contents of the selected folders are exported. Alternatively, the user can choose one or more individual forms to be exported, but only from within the same folder. In this case no multiple folder selection is possible. Please do the following to select one or more forms for export:

- Clear all of the EASY Folders combo boxes in the left panel.
- Go to the desired lowest level EASY Folder containing forms to be exported. The entire contents of the selected folder will be listed in the right panel.
- Select the form to be exported. If you would like to select multiple forms within the right panel, press the Ctrl key while selecting all desired forms with the mouse.

Additionally, it is possible to add a comment to the resulting export file in the upper edit field. By selecting the checkbox Delete items ... after export, it is possible to request the EASY File Manager to delete all exported forms after the export is complete. *Warning:* Use this delete option with care, especially if the entire contents are to be exported. A safer alternative is to create an export file and then delete the corresponding forms manually. After all necessary selections have been made; click the OK button in order to proceed. The Save File dialog box appears. Choose the destination of the resulting Export file and provide the file with a name (the file name by default is the creation timestamp of the format YYYYMMDD_HHMMSS). The extension .ezf cannot be changed. *Note:* This functionality allows the export of user defined Templates along with Forms. However, it is impossible to export predefined Templates like the Normal Template from the New PCT Forms folder.

The user is only able to export forms to which he has full access (see the User Management section for further information). All forms having read-only accesses are skipped from the export process.

USER MANAGEMENT

User management has been implemented in EASY 2.90 in order to provide the possibility of data sharing in the forthcoming networking version of the EASY software. It also provides a unified approach to secure access to the software and to maintenance information both for the single user version (which uses an internal database engine) and for the real database version working via full database servers. The main reason for user management is that the software needs to distinguish between different users in order to provide mechanisms for data sharing. The User Management option can be switched off (default in the single user version) or on via the EASY File Manager Tools -> Options dialog box. There are five possible groups of users:

1. Default User
2. Administrators
3. Power Users
4. Maintenance Users
5. Users

Ownership of a form is attributed to the user who creates the form. Users have unrestricted access to forms, which they own. Access to items such as forms created by other users or maintenance information depends on one's group.

Default User: The Default User access level is activated whenever the User Management is disabled (this is the default state for the single user version right after the installation). It allows anonymous access to the system. The Default user has the same rights as an Administrator does (i.e., there are no restrictions) except maintenance tables are not accessible.

Administrators: The highest level of accessibility within the EASY system. Every user who gets membership of this group has full access rights. There is one special user within this group, set by default the first time User Management is activated. The name of this user is Administrator but this can be changed later via Users Management. There can be more than one member of the Administrators group. With the exception of the predefined default Administrator; users can also be removed from this group. If a user is deleted, forms, which he owned, are reassigned to the pre-defined Administrator.

Power Users: Compared to the Administrators group members of this group are not allowed to update software, activate and deactivate the User Management, or edit the properties of other users.

Maintenance Users: Members of this group have restricted (read only) access to forms owned (created) by other users, and to maintenance and fees tables. They are not allowed to update the software or change other user's access rights.

Users: Members of this group, compared to the group of Maintenance Users, are not allowed to view the contents of maintenance tables.

If it is necessary to restrict access to forms, to the software, and/or to maintenance information, then User Management has to be activated. To do so, start EASY File Manager; go to the Tools menu, Options item, General group; select the User Management Enabled checkbox; close the Options dialog box and the EASY File Manager; start the File Manager again. The log-in window will appear. EASY is delivered with a predefined means of administering access rights. It does this via the special user name Administrator, which is not password protected. To login via this name: Enter Administrator in the Name field; leave the Password filed empty. Click OK. The program will log you into the File Manager as an Administrator.

Note: Administrator is a predefined user name. This user name cannot be removed from the system, but it can be changed. Moreover, the default Administrator becomes owner of any forms which had been created by other users if the user is deleted. The Administrator can create users and add them to the Administrators group. Any user with Administrator privileges can log into the system and perform all Administrator tasks, including the removal of other users. It should be noted however, that one is not allowed to remove oneself from the system, nor can the Administrator user be removed. It is recommended to assign a password to the Administrator, as it is initially not password protected. Assigning a password helps to keep your EASY software and data secure. After you have activated User Management and logged into the File Manager as Administrator you can create new users, define passwords for them, and delete or disable existing users accounts as well as move existing users from one group to another. The normal users can only change their password and description. Users who are not Administrators are not allowed to change the properties other users nor can they deactivate User Management.

EASY ADDRESS BOOK EXPORT

The EASY Address Book can only be exported as a whole. When the Export -> Address Book option from the File menu in the EASY File Manager is selected the Save File dialog box appears. The user needs to specify the destination and the name of the export file. After the Save button is clicked, the Address Book export is performed.

EASY Forms Import

As the first step in the forms import process the user should choose the file from where the forms are to be imported. The selected .ezf file is then read by the EASY File Manager, and the following Forms Import dialog box, similar to the Forms Export dialog box, appears. In the same way as the Form Export dialog box, this dialog box allows the selection of one or more folders or one or more forms within one folder for import. It is not possible to make multiple form selections within different folders simultaneously. Select the top-most EASY combo box to import the entire contents of the export file into the EASY system. Should a form being imported have the same Agent's or Applicant's File Reference as a form which already exists in the destination EASY folder (there can be only one form having the same reference number within one folder), the following message appears:

> The user should choose whether to skip the import of the form or to overwrite the existing form.

Note: From the point of view of the EASY File Manager and the EASY database, the forms contained in the Outbox folder and in the Stored Forms folder have the same status, i.e., regarding their identity they are handled as though they belong to the same folder. In other words, there can be two different forms having the same File Reference, e.g., one in the Saved PCT-Forms folder and one in the Stored Forms folder, at the same time. However, it is not possible to have two forms with the same File Reference, one in the Outbox and the other in the Stored Forms folder. As a result, if the export file contains, for example, an Outbox Form having a certain File Reference, and a form having the same File Reference is already present in the EASY Stored Forms folder, an ID collision is detected and the above dialog box appears. If the Overwrite option is selected the old stored form is overwritten. The new form with the same File Reference is placed in the Stored Forms folder, and, although initially (at the time of export and within the Export file) it was an Outbox form, the actual state of the exported form is changed by the import routine.

There is no owner information stored in the import file. The user who is uploading forms from the import file automatically becomes the owner of all forms he uploads. Should a File Reference No./Folder conflict occur between an uploaded form and a form the user does not have full access rights to, the corresponding form is skipped from being uploaded.

Address Book Import

When the Import -> Address Book option from the File menu in the EASY File Manager is selected, a Select file dialog box appears to select the CSV source file. Once the source file has been selected the CSV Import dialog box appears where the left static column lists all internal fields of the EASY Address Book, and the right column defines which field of the input .csv file should be mapped to each particular internal EASY Address Book field.

The Address Book import routine tries to bind corresponding fields automatically. For this purpose, it goes through the .csv file and searches for all CSV fields the names of which are the same as internal EASY Address Book fields. Should such a name be found, it is mapped automatically to the corresponding field in the left column. Obviously, in the case when the .csv file was created by an EASY Program, all fields will be mapped properly by default.

If the import routine is unable to find a field within the .csv file having the same name as an internal EASY Address Book field, it sets the default mapping value to None, which means that this field is omitted by the CSV data import. For all fields that do not comply with any Address Book field by their name, and for all fields that accidentally have the same name but a different meaning, the user should perform mapping manually, by selecting each field and choosing an appropriate CSV field name from the combo box.

Please note that at least the Last Name or the Last Name (National) field should be filled for the successful addition of a new entry into the Address Book. Therefore at least one of these fields should be mapped to enable the Address Book import. Furthermore, during the import all records that do not have at least one of these two fields filled in cannot be processed and are skipped from the import process. The First String Is Data checkbox option is present in the dialog box for CSV-compatibility to some external programs and means that the first string that usually represents names of CSV fields should be imported as data. This option should usually be cleared. The .csv file is imported after the OK button is clicked. If a record being imported has the same name and type (legal or natural person) as a record already present in the Address Book, the user is given the option to skip the record, to overwrite the existing one, or to add the record along with the existing one.

Note: In the event that the input .csv file was produced by a third party software (such as Microsoft Outlook), it is very likely that some essential EASY information (e.g., the indication whether the person is a legal entity or a natural person) will not be present or will be present in an inappropriate form. The EASY CSV import routine makes some assumptions based on contents of other fields to fill in missing information. As these assumptions can occasionally be incorrect, it is recommended to go through all newly imported Address Book contents and to make any necessary corrections after the CSV import has been performed.

PCT-EASY IFF Functionality

The IFF (Intermediate File Format) is a flat text tag file format designed to facilitate the exchange of data between the EASY software and third-party patent management system databases. Data in IFF files are the same as those found on the EASY Request Form and can be imported and exported easily. Although the IFF is a flat text format it should rarely be viewed and/or edited manually using a text editor. The IFF serves to exchange information between EASY software and third-party systems, so the export to and the import from an IFF file should happen by electronic means.

The EASY software includes functionality to export form data from the EASY application to an IFF file and to import data from an IFF file to the EASY application. The IFF export and import routines on a third-party side should be created extra using a corresponding EASY form specification for IFF. The following IFF-related functions are provided from within the PCT-EASY software:

- Import from an existing IFF file into a new Request Form
- Export from the existing EASY application (stored or saved) into an IFF file

There are two ways the IFF file can be processed within the PCT-EASY software: (1) through mouse activation and (2) EASY File Manager activation.

Activation from Mouse
The .iff file extension is registered within the Windows system when the PCT-EASY software (Version 2.90 or later) is installed on your PC. Consequently, when you double-click an IFF file, the EASY File Manager is activated (if it is not already running) (Figure 12.27).

Activation from within the EASY File Manager
An IFF import folder exists within the EASY File Manager and displays all IFF files placed in a predefined subdirectory of the EASY directory (the same subdirectory is the default destination directory for the export of IFF files). It is possible to activate the Request Form Application importing the contents of the IFF file by double-clicking an IFF file from this folder.

After the .iff file has been selected, the New application reference information dialog box appears (Figure 12.28), which defines the route of the new application (PCT-EASY, EPO, etc.), the language of the request and the application file reference. Once these indications have been made and the OK button has been selected, the Request Form starts within EASY, and fields of the newly created Request Form are filled with the data contained in the IFF file.

Note: If the route selected differs from the one that the .iff file was created with, only a restricted set of fields is imported into the new Request Form (i.e., fields which are common for both routes). Entities, which are not applicable for the route, are ignored.

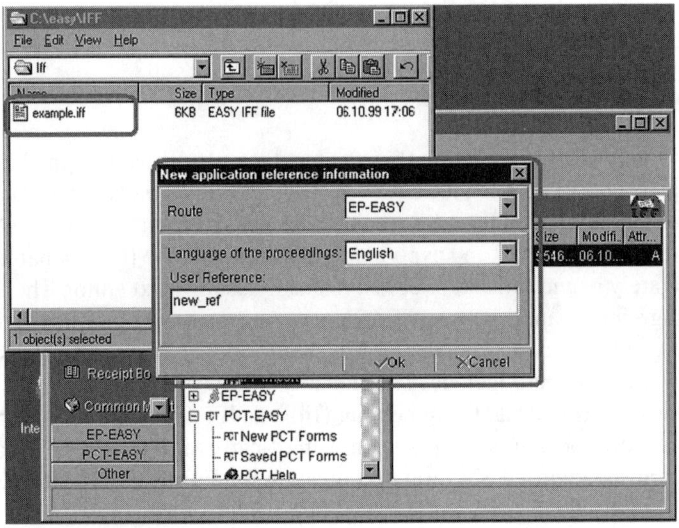

FIGURE 12.27

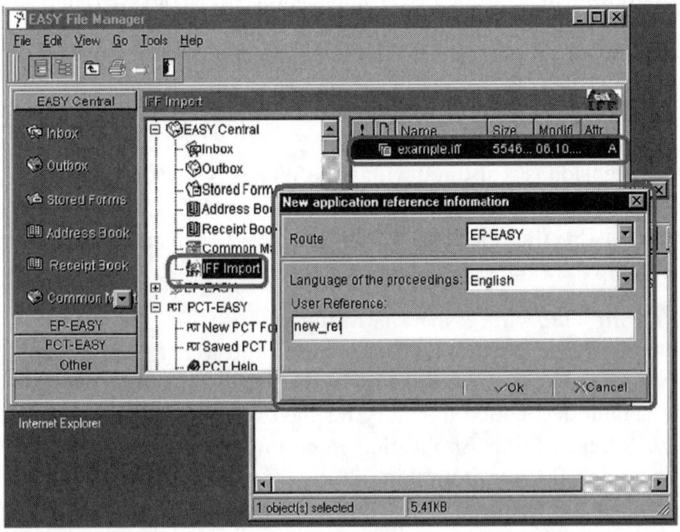

FIGURE 12.28

Exporting Data to an IFF File

The export function is available via the Export to IFF file function on the File menu of the Request Form. After clicking the menu item the user is given the Save as IFF dialog box, where the destination folder can be selected and the name of the IFF file to be created can be assigned. As a result of this operation, a flat text IFF file is created, including all data that has been filled in on the Notebook pages of the active Request Form. The resulting IFF file can be read electronically either by the PCT-EASY software (using Import from the IFF file functionality) or by a third-party product which supports the IFF import-export functionality (in which case corresponding routines should be implemented on the side of this third-party product).

IFF File Structure

An IFF file consists of tags and their contents. Each tag consists of the start tag and the end tag. A start tag begins with the tag name and can include attributes. IFF tags build a three-level hierarchy:

1. Level: Form
2. Level: Entities
3. Level: Fields

The Form tag is the overall bracket for all other tags. Entity tags bracket corresponding fields tags and group them corresponding to the structure of the form template for which the IFF file is created. Field tags include the form specific information for each field of the corresponding template. Generally the IFF tag structure is derived from the internal form structure rather than from the EASY database, i.e., all entity and field tag names appear in the IFF file as they appear in the corresponding EASY form, and field contents represent the data structure found there. The name of every tag is the same as the name of a corresponding field or entity. A tag of the end of the entity has a /:

<...> — beginning of tag
</...> — end of tag

Note: Strings can have some special characters. In this case they are replaced according to the following substitution:

- "&": "&amp"
- "<": "&lt"
- ">": "&gt"
- " ": "&quot"
- CrLf: "<BR>"

Each template supports only those fields that are needed for this procedure. The IFF on the other hand is a common format for all procedures. Therefore it acts as an envelope, i.e., it comprises all fields from all templates.

Additionally, shared fields should only appear once in the IFF (with the same name and type). For example, all entity and field tags within the Request Form templates for PCT and EP have already been given an unique name, the uniqueness of which is guaranteed by prefixing of every entity and field name by the route indicator (Pct- for the PCT RO 101 form and Ep- for the EP form) and for field tags, an indicator of the entity the field belongs to (e.g., PctARIPOCodes field of the entity PctARIPOEnt). Entity and field names, which are common for all templates, are not prefixed in this way (e.g., field TitleInvention of the entity TitleEnt). While uploading the IFF file into a new form the program goes through all IFF tags picking up, parsing, and putting into the form those data which are suitable for the current form and ignoring the others.

An IFF file has the following structure:

```
<FORM VER = [version number] APP = [procedure ID] APPREF = [appli-
  cation reference]>
  <Entity1 ID = [entity ID]>
    <Field1 {Attribute1 = [attribute 1 value]} {...} {AttributeN = [attribute
      N value]}>[field 1 value]</Field1>
      ...
    <FieldN {Attribute1 = [attribute 1 value]} {...} {AttributeN = [at-
      tribute Nvalue]}>[field N value]</Field1>
  </Entity1>
  ...
  <EntityN ID = [entity ID]}>
    <Field1 {Attribute1 = [attribute 1 value]} {...} {AttributeN = [attribute
      N value]}>[field 1 value]</Field1>
      ...
    <FieldN {Attribute1 = [attribute 1 value]} {...} {AttributeN = [at-
      tribute Nvalue]}>[field N value]</Field1>
  </EntityN>
</FORM>
```

13 WIPO PCT-SAFE

INTRODUCTION

Whereas the current PCT filing is limited to electronic writing and media submission, it is anticipated that in the second quarter of 2003, PCT applications may be filed online, first with the International Bureau (IB) and then gradually at other patent offices. The World Intellectual Property Organization (WIPO), which manages PCT filings, has established the procedures that will be used in this filing. It is expected that no major changes will be made to the system described below but you are advised to consult with the WIPO Web site (http://www.wipo.int/pct/en/index.html) to learn about the current status of filing software.

The Patent Cooperation Treaty (PCT) Electronic Filing Project adopted a new name at the end of February 2002: the PCT-SAFE (Secure Applications Filed Electronically) Project. Electronic filing software being developed by the International Bureau as an extension of the PCT-EASY software will be made available to applicants and Receiving Offices. That software will support all of the requirements of the basic common standard and certain alternatives as described below. Use of that software is not mandatory but any applicant may choose to use it, in which case the Receiving Office (RO) must accept the filed international application. Any RO may also specify other filing software acceptable to it.

It is noteworthy that because of the differences in how the ROs handle applications, PCT-SAFE offers several options, several levels of authentication, and a complex system of handling of application between the applicant and the office, and between offices. The PCT-SAFE software is expected to automate many functions; however, the information given here should be thoroughly examined to understand how this system will work to make sure the applicant chooses the best method filing an electronic PCT application.

TERMINOLOGY

Basic electronic signature is an electronic signature which can be:

- A particular string of text entered by a user
- A facsimile image of the handwritten signature
- A click-wrap signature

Enhanced electronic signature is an electronic signature in respect of which it can be shown, through the use of a security procedure, that the signature:

- Is unique to the signature holder within the context in which it is used.
- Was created and attached to or logically associated with the electronic document by the signature holder or using a means under the sole control of the signature holder and not by any other person.
- Was created and is linked to the electronic document to which it relates in a manner which provides reliable assurance as to the integrity of the document; one implementation of an enhanced electronic signature is a digital signature which is produced using a PKI-generated certificate and corresponding private key.

Digital certificate is a record issued by a certification authority and which identifies a person or entity who holds a particular key pair, in the context of public key infrastructure; for example, a digital certificate shall, among other requirements, identify the certification authority issuing it, identify its subscriber, contain the subscriber's public key, identify its period of validity, and be digitally signed by the certification authority issuing it.

Certification authority is an entity which issues digital certificates and provides other services related to electronic signatures, such as managing digital certificates and keys and maintaining a register of them.

Low-level certificate is a digital certificate which has been issued to the applicant, e.g., as part of the registration of the online filing client or obtained from a certification authority, and which identifies the applicant without prior verification of the applicant's identity.

High-level certificate is a digital certificate which has been issued to the applicant by a trusted party and which identifies the applicant with prior verification of the applicant's identity.

SUMMARY STANDARDS

The basic common standard contains certain options for the Receiving Office to specify its requirements for such applications, in relation to physical requirements and in relation to signature. The Receiving Office must accept an international application filed with it if the application meets those requirements, which include:

- **As to electronic document format**
  The international application documents are encoded in XML format, using either of the following, as specified by the Receiving Office:
  - The Unicode 3.0 (International Standard ISO/IEC 10646:2000) coded character set with UTF-8 character encoding scheme; or
  - A coded character set confined within the repertoire of Unicode 3.0 with encoding scheme specified by the Receiving Office
  Any sequence listing complies with the Administrative Instructions (WI-PO Standard ST.25).

Any drawings are in TIFF format, as specified by the Receiving Office.

• **As to means of transmittal**

If the Receiving Office accepts the filing of international applications on-line and the international application is transmitted using the E-Filing Interoperability Protocol.

If the Receiving Office accepts the filing of applications by physical means and the international application is stored on 3.5 inch diskette or CD-R, as specified by the Receiving Office.

• **As to electronic packaging**

The international application is packaged as a wrapped and signed package (WASP) prepared using a low-level digital certificate issued by the Receiving Office or the International Bureau.

• **As to electronic filing software**

The international application is prepared and filed using software made available for that purpose by the International Bureau.

• **As to viruses, etc.**

The international application is free of viruses and other forms of malicious logic.

• **As to signature**

The international application is signed with any basic electronic signature.

• **As to fee**

Where an international application is filed in electronic form, the basic fee shall be calculated on the basis of the number of sheets that the application would contain if presented as a printout on paper complying with the physical requirements prescribed.

• **As to physical media**

It complies with the requirements of the Receiving Office regarding the physical media types and electronic document formats acceptable to it, and whether it will accept a filing where the application is partly on physical media.

It must conform to the relevant standards and the contents of each physical medium must be encoded in an electronic document format as specified:

- ISO/IEC 9529, double-sided, high-density, 135 TPI, 80 track, 3.5 inch diskette. 1.44 MB IBM PC compatible DOS format
- ISO/IEC 10149:1995, 120 mm CD-ROM ISO 9660, 650 MB S-04/2001 (E)
- 120 mm CD-Recordable Disk ISO 9660, 650 MB
- ISO/IEC 16448:1999, 120 mm DVD Read-Only Disk 4.7GB, conforming to either ISO 9660 or OSTA UDF (1.02 and higher)
- Standard ECMA-279, 120 mm (3.95 GB per side) DVD-Recordable Disk (DVD-R) 3.95 GB, conforming to either ISO 9660 or OSTA UD F(1.02 and higher)
- Iomega zip disk 100 or 250 MB, Iomega format
- Imation SuperDisk diskette 120 MB, PC (IBM) format

The content is in the form of a package type (wrapped package, wrapped and signed package or signed and encrypted package).

The package must take the form of a single logical file and be located in the root directory of the physical media.

It is within the size limits imposed by the Receiving Office, which may limit the files written on the physical medium to be no larger than 15 MB each. If a single document needs to be divided into multiple files to comply with this requirement, then the file names must indicate the sequence of the files in relation to the document (e.g., Sequence Listing XXX part 4 of 17.txt).

It must be enclosed in a hard case within an unsealed padded and protective mailing envelope and accompanied by a transmittal letter on paper. The transmittal letter must list for each physical medium the machine format (e.g., IBM PC), the operating system compatibility (e.g., MS-DOS, Windows, UNIX), a list of the files contained on the physical medium including their names, sizes in bytes, and dates of creation, plus any other special information that is necessary to identify, maintain, and interpret the information on the physical medium. Physical media submitted to the Office will not be returned to the applicant. If the physical medium has been sent as a backup copy to an international application filed in electronic form, then the transmittal letter must state that it is a backup copy, that the contents of that copy are identical to that of the application as filed in electronic form.

It is submitted in duplicate, on request of the Office. The physical medium and duplicate copy must be labeled Copy 1 and Copy 2, respectively. The transmittal letter that accompanies the physical media must include a statement that the two physical media are identical. In the event that the two physical media are not identical, the Office will use the physical medium labeled Copy 1 for further processing.

Any amendment to the information on a physical medium must be by way of a replacement physical medium containing the original text and incorporating the substitute information, and must be accompanied by a statement that the replacement physical medium contains no new matter. The physical medium and copy must be labeled COPY 1 REPLACEMENT YYYY/MM/DD (with the month, day, and year of creation indicated), and COPY 2 REPLACEMENT YYYY/MM/DD, respectively.

The application must contain an incorporation-by-reference of the material on the physical medium in a separate paragraph identifying each physical medium by the names of the files contained on each of the physical media, their date of creation, and their sizes in bytes. One example of this is a reference to a large sequence listing contained on a CD-ROM or CD-R separate from the application.

Must be physically labeled with the following information:
- The name of each applicant (if known)
- Title of the invention

- The docket number, or application number if known, used by the person filing the application to identify the application
- Creation date of the physical medium
- If multiple physical media are submitted, the label shall indicate their order (e.g., 1 of X); an indication that the disk is Copy 1 or Copy 2 of the submission.
- **As to backup and substitution**

Where an international application was filed in electronic form, the applicant may, if the Receiving Office so permits and within 16 months from the priority date, file a backup copy of the application on paper or on a physical medium, provided that the backup copy shall be identified as such and shall be accompanied by a statement by the applicant that the content of the backup copy is identical to that of the application as filed in electronic form.

Where an international application was filed in electronic form, the Receiving Office may, of its own volition or at the request of the applicant, prepare a backup copy of the application on paper or on a physical medium, provided that the content of the backup copy shall be identical to that of the application as filed in electronic form. The Office shall, upon request by the applicant and subject to the payment of a fee, send to the applicant a copy of such a backup copy.

E-PCT FORMAT AND SUBMISSION STRUCTURE

TYPES OF FILES

Electronic international application submissions contain many different types of documents and information. Text, images, and sequence listings can all be printed on paper, but each of these requires a different electronic representation. For example, text can be stored in character codes, while images can be stored in grids of picture elements called bitmaps. The concept is further complicated by the fact that most information can be stored in multiple electronic formats. Sequence lists can be stored as plain text. Printed text can be optically scanned and stored as an image. In addition to format, the structure (or lack of structure) of information can have a large impact on the ability of automated systems to facilitate processing of the information. Images of typed pages of text have no electronic text structure and must be electronically recognized or hand-keyed by a human operator before they can be searched for meaningful words and symbols. On the other hand, text and other information can be structured to enforce business rules and associate information with meaningful business identifiers. The format specified by this standard for such structured text is called XML (Extensible Markup Language). Using XML, computer systems can identify specific pieces of business information and reach new levels of capability. For example, if an international application document has been structured in XML according to the E-PCT standard, a computer system could automatically display the first claim; it could link figure references to the actual figure (within drawings); it could hyperlink patent and other citations to the actual documents cited. Publication and information retrieval systems also gain significant capabilities from structured documents. In addition to structured information within an electronic format, international application submissions may contain documents that are composed of multiple types of information stored in multiple electronic formats. This collection of documents must have an overall structure that allows computer systems to identify the type of document and each of its components.

XML

All XML documents must conform to one of the specified DTDs (document type definitions). Applicants will be able to create XML documents conforming to this standard by using the extended PCT-EASY software (the new version that supports this standard). The coded character set for all XML documents must be confined within that specified by International Standard ISO/IEC 10646:2000 (Unicode 3.0). The standard character encoding scheme for XML documents is UTF-8. Any document created using the WIPO Standard ST.25 (Standard for the Presentation of Nucleotide and Amino Acid Sequence Listings in Patent Applications) must be included as a referenced document. For the Applicant-Office (international phase) PCT communications sector, a Receiving Office must accept this format per the basic common standard. For the Office-Office sector, Offices must be able to transmit and receive this format.

ASCII

Any file in this format must be included as a referenced document. For the Applicant-Office (international phase) PCT communications sector, a Receiving Office shall notify the IB whether it will accept documents in this format, which documents it will accept in this format, and whether it will accept seven-bit and eight-bit ASCII. For the Office-Office sector, this format may not be included in document packages, except when included in the original wrapped application documents filed by the applicant, as part of the record copy.

PDF

Any file in this format must be included as a referenced document. All documents in Portable Documents Format (PDF) must meet the following requirements:

- Adobe Acrobat 3.0 compatible
- Noncompressed text to facilitate searching
- Unencrypted text
- No digital signatures
- No embedded OLE objects
- All fonts must either be embedded, standard PS17 or built from Adobe Multiple Master (MM) fonts

For the Applicant-Office (international phase) PCT communications sector, a Receiving Office shall notify the IB whether it will accept documents in this format.

In order to accommodate Offices that do not accept PDF documents, any Office that chooses to accept documents in this format must also convert the document text to XML and drawings to TIFF images and transmit the document in both formats to the IB. For the Office-Office sector, Offices shall notify the IB whether they will transmit or accept documents in this format. For documents originally submitted in PDF format, Offices may request transmission of the original PDF documents in addition to the converted XML and TIFF format.

Image Formats

Images may be used for drawings, figures, equations or other illustrations. This format is not intended to be used as a replacement for character-coded document formats, except in the Office-Office PCT communications sector when sending scanned paper documents between Offices. In exceptional cases, a Receiving Office may choose to allow applicants to submit all or part of the description or claims in image format where the applicant does not have access to character coded versions of the documents.

Tagged Image File Format (TIFF)

Any file in this format must be included as a referenced document. TIFF facsimile (black and white) images for use in IA document exchange must meet the following requirements: TIFF V6.0 with Group 4 compression, single strip, Intel encoded; resolution of either 200, 300, or 400 dpi; maximum size: whole pages should be either A47 or Letter8 size; however, the recommended maximum size is 255×170 mm.

For the Applicant-Office (international phase) PCT communication sector, a Receiving Office must accept this format per the basic common standard. Images may be used for drawings, figures, equations or other illustrations. This format is not intended to be used as a replacement for character-coded document formats. For the Office-Office sector, Offices must be able to transmit and receive this format. Images may be used for drawings, figures, equations, or other illustrations. This format may also be used to transmit scanned documents between offices in the form of page images.

JPEG File Interchange Format (JFIF)

Any file in this format must be included as a referenced document. JFIF images for use in IA document exchange must meet the following requirements: resolution of either 200, 300, or 400 dpi; maximum size of 255×170 mm.

For the Applicant-Office (international phase) sector, a Receiving Office shall notify the IB whether it will accept images in this format. Images may be used for drawings, figures, equations or other illustrations. This format is not intended to be used as a replacement for character-coded document formats. For the Office-Office sector, an Office shall notify the IB whether it will transmit or accept images in this format.

The electronic filing software (PCT-SAFE) being developed by the International Bureau as an extension of the PCT-EASY software will be made available to applicants and Receiving Offices. That software will support all of the requirements of the basic common standard and certain alternatives available under Annex F. Use of that software is not mandatory but any applicant may choose to use it, in which case the Receiving Office must accept the international application concerned. Any Receiving Office may also specify other filing software acceptable to it.

SUBMISSION STRUCTURE

In order to accommodate the need for multiple documents and electronic information formats while preserving structure that a computer system can understand, an E-PCT submission and its documents must conform to a specific structure. Each electronic IA submission contains an XML package data file that explicitly references the submission documents, and must conform to the package-data DTD (document type definition). The referenced documents (e.g., the request and the new patent application) are logically part of the submission as shown in Figure 13.1.

The referenced documents (external entities) are typically request, application, priority documents, etc., which in turn may contain images, tables, and drawings which are separate but related objects that may be encoded as either XML, PDF, ST.25, ASCII, or image types TIFF or JFIF. Each XML document shall conform to one of the DTDs specified, except for referenced other documents, where a Receiving Office may choose to accept XML documents conforming to DTDs not specified.

ELECTRONIC SIGNATURE

For IA document exchange, a number of electronic signature types are permitted. Each Receiving Office shall notify the IB which types of signature it will accept. The sections below describe these signature types, categorized as basic and enhanced

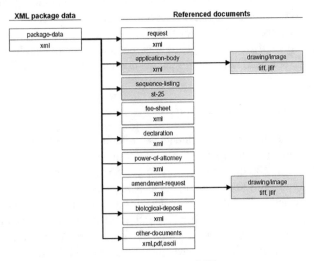

Note: All referenced XML documents may point to other documents formatted in PDF.

FIGURE 13.1

electronic signatures. At this time, this standard does not support the use of multiple enhanced electronic signatures but it does support the use of multiple basic electronic signatures.

Facsimile Signature

To create this type of signature, an XML file (e.g., the request) must include the <fax> element and an external entity reference set in the File attribute that points to a TIFF file containing a bitmap of the signature. The TIFF file must meet the requirements as described earlier.

Text String Signature

To create this type of signature, an XML file must include the <text-string> element containing a text string that represents your wet (ink) signature, enclosed in slash / characters (e.g., /janedoe/). The text-string must be a string of characters, not including the forward slash / character, chosen by you as your electronic signature. Valid examples include:

- /John Smith/
- /Tobeornottobe/
- /1345728625235/
- /Günter François/

Click-Wrap Signature

To create this type of signature, typically you click on a button labeled I Accept in a user interface. This is indicated in an XML file by the presence of a <click-wrap/> empty element.

Enhanced Electronic Signature

An enhanced electronic signature relies on the use of a PKI and a PKCS #7 digital signature data type.

DOCUMENTS PACKAGING

Because an IA document will generally consist of several files, it is useful to assemble these files together into a single electronic package for transmission. Two IA package types are included under this standard: non-PKI and PKI-based packages. The wrapped application documents file (WAD) is a non-PKI package. The two forms of PKI-based packages are a wrapped and signed package (WASP) and a signed and encrypted package (SEP). All electronic document exchange files under this standard first must be packaged as a WAD. WAD, WASP, and SEP package types are permitted in the Applicant-to-Office (international phase) sector while only WASP or SEP data types are permitted in the Office-Office sector.

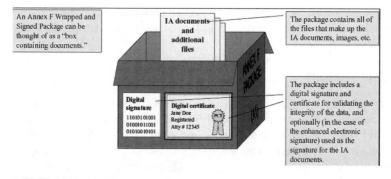

FIGURE 13.2

NON-PKI-BASED PACKAGE

This standard includes only one non-PKI based package: the WAD. The IA submission along with any referenced documents are wrapped and treated as one data block. This data block is called the wrapped application documents package (WAD) and is created using the wrapping standard, zip. The software used to create the zip file must conform to the zip file format specification as published in the PKWARE PKZIP. All zip files must have a flat directory structure. The zip standard allows the compression software to select from among a number of compression algorithms. The compression method must be deflation with the normal compression option.

PKI PACKAGE TYPES

The WASP and the SEP rely on the use of a PKI. The digital signature for the WASP may be produced either by the applicant or the applicant's representative. If an enhanced electronic signature is chosen by the applicant (or the applicant's representative), it is the signature in the WASP that is used for this purpose. Figure 13.2 is a simplified anatomy of the WASP.

SIGNED AND ENCRYPTED PACKAGE (SEP)

An SEP, which provides a secure container, is required in those cases where a package is sent over a nonsecure network such as the Internet (without channel encryption). Prior to creating a SEP, a WASP must be created as indicated above. The SEP contains additional data items to the WASP that are wrapped together using zip into a Wrapped Transmission Package (WTP) (Figure 13.3).

TRANSMISSION

The IA package can be transmitted over secure or nonsecure channels depending on the package type. This protocol to be followed as well as the package/transmission combinations that are permitted in the Applicant-Office (international phase), Office-Office, and designated Office communication sectors include HTTP and SSL. IA documents may be filed by online means (using PKI) over the public Internet, over

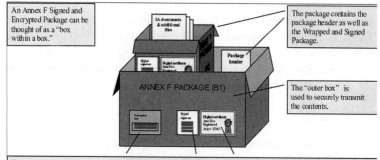

The package includes an encrypted key that the recipient (for example, the receiving Office) uses to 'open' the package and read the contents. The package also includes a digital signature and certificate for validating the integrity of the data.

FIGURE 13.3

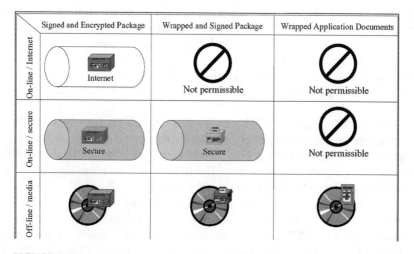

FIGURE 13.4

a private network, or transmitted offline (using PKI or non-PKI) on physical media. The option of online filing of an IA utilizing a non-PKI method is not presently permitted, except under possible transitional situations. Figure 13.4 shows the various combinations possible.

All Office-Office sector data exchange must be conducted utilizing PKI-based data exchange. IA documents may be exchanged by online means over the public Internet or over a private network (such as Tri-Net or WIPONET), or transported on physical media. The SEP, WASP, or WAD package may be used when exchanging IA documents under the designated Office sector.

Public Key Infrastructure (PKI)

The objectives for the use of PKI are to provide adequate security for sensitive information throughout the PCT process, provide the necessary services to enable the business processes of the PCT to become part of a system of secure electronic records and provide, through cryptographic mechanisms, four basic security services for PCT Offices and authorities and for PCT applicants which include authentication (validating identity of filer), integrity (that data was not modified during transmission), nonrepudiation (that data has been delivered), and confidentiality (that it is read only by authorized entities).

PCT PKI Standards

The E-PCT trust model is based on the software itself (e.g., PCT E-filing software) to utilize a trust list of CAs (certification authorities).

A Certification Authority (CA) is a trusted party that issues and revokes public key certificates for a user community. The CA is responsible for verifying the information appearing on the public key certificates. A CA is supported by CA servers, or computer systems, and the policies and procedures surrounding the operation of these servers. The term server refers specifically to the hardware and software that actually generates certificates and CRLs. The E-PCT permits two types of CAs, an Office CA and a Public CA. An Office CA is defined as a CA that issues certificates bearing the name of that Office (whether internal or outsourced). A public CA is defined as a CA that issues certificates that do not bear the Office's name, but that CA is recognized by certain Offices as being suitable for issuing certificates for E-PCT transactions.

A Registration Authority (RA) is an entity responsible for identification and authentication of certificate subjects, but not for signing or issuing certificates (i.e., a registration authority, or RA is delegated certain tasks related to identity-proofing on behalf of a certification authority). The RA may delegate functions and corresponding authority to local registration authorities.

PKI client software will process certificates issued by one of the trusted CAs to determine whether the public key certificate of a user in another community should be trusted. In the E-PCT environment, each Office will maintain a trust list of recognized CAs. Under this architecture, all entities in the trust list and their subordinates would be trusted equally by E-PCT software. Each Receiving Office will specify the certification authorities that are recognized by that Office to issue certificates for purposes of the E-PCT. The list may include Office CAs or public CAs. This list of recognized CAs will be published by the International Bureau including a link to the published policy of those certification authorities. A recognized certification authority is responsible for maintaining the accuracy of the electronic certificates that prove a party is who he says he is. In addition, the certification authority publishes certificate revocation information. Whenever a certificate is used to authenticate an individual, the certification authority that maintains certificate revocation information is consulted by the Office to ensure that the certificate has not been revoked. In order to support nonrepudiation, the system ensures that the subscriber generates his or her signing key pair on that subscriber's own system and only transferring his public verification key to others (e.g., public verification key is sent to the CA during the registration process).

Digital Certificates

Two classes of certificates have been defined, low-level and high-level certificates. Certificates issued by a recognized CA may be used for digital signature and data encryption purposes. Each certificate has a set life span before it expires and needs to be renewed. A subscriber's certificate may be revoked for several reasons by the subscriber, the Registration Authority (RA) or Local Registration Authority (LRA), and authorized management.

The low-level certification process does not require pre-registration. However, the subscriber states, at a minimum, his name and a verifiable e-mail address. Additional proof of identity is not required. The subscriber uses online software (e.g., a future version of PCT-EASY or PCT-SAFE) or a Web-based facility to obtain an instant low-level certificate from the IB or recognized CA. This operation is envisioned to be available only online. The International Bureau will publish a list of recognized CAs for low-level certificates acceptable to each Office. The subscribers to low-level certificates will only include PCT applicants, assignees, and their representatives. The certification process may vary due to implementation details and certificate policy, but generally will involve the following steps:

- In the software provided by the International Bureau or Receiving Office, the applicant/agent selects the option to request a low-level certificate.
- The applicant/agent enters the following information: name, e-mail address, challenge phrase, selected recognized certification authority (CA).
- The applicant/agent's computer generates public/private key pairs for a signing certificate and encryption certificate.
- The applicant/agent's computer generates a PKCS #10 certification request and sends it to the selected CA.
- The CA performs basic validation on the data submitted (Name given must be unique, challenge phrase must meet security policy criteria, etc.) and either generates the certificate or an error response.
- In the case of an error response, the applicant/agent is prompted to correct information and retry. Otherwise, the applicant/agent is sent a message (e-mail address indicated during the application process) to retrieve the new certificate. The message will include an authorization code that is generated by the CA.
- The applicant retrieves the new certificate (via secure channel, e.g., SSL) after the authorization code and challenge phrase is validated.

A high-level certificate means a digital certificate which has been issued to the subscriber by a trusted party and which identifies the subscriber with prior verification of the subscriber's identity. Offices and Authorities within the PCT system are required to obtain and utilize high-level certificates issued by the International Bureau for Office-to-Office data exchange. Applicants may obtain and utilize a low-level certificate for E-filing purposes. However, Offices may require that applicants obtain and use a high-level certificate after the initial filing. The International Bureau will handle applications for and issuance of certificates on an individual basis. The registration process may vary depending on the Office or on the chosen CA, but generally includes the following steps:

- The applicant/agent completes and signs a paper application.
- The applicant/agent sends the paper application to the Registration Authority (RA) for review.
- If approved, the applicant is typically sent a confirmation of registration via physical mail containing information required to proceed with the certification process.

The RA may require that the applicant/agent appear in person with identifying documents.

The certification process may vary due to implementation details, but generally will involve a similar process as described for the low-level certificate. The major differences in the high-level certification process are

- The applicant provides information from the confirmation of registration (rather than name, e-mail address, etc.).
- The generation and storage of private keys may vary depending on the chosen CA's policy. For example, smart cards may be used to generate and/or store the key pairs.
- The CA may require that the private key used for encryption be backed up.

A subscriber's certificate may be revoked for several reasons. Certificate revocation may be initiated by the subscriber, the RA or LRA, and authorized management. Subscribers should advise the cognizant RA or LRA if they:

- No longer require use of the certificate (e.g., termination of employment, change of job responsibilities)
- Know of or suspect a compromise of their private key
- Have changed their name

In the absence of a request by the subscriber, the cognizant RA or LRA should request revocation of a subscriber's certificate for any of the above reasons. The cognizant RA or LRA should also initiate revocation of a subscriber's certificate if there is a material breach of the subscriber agreement. The CAs may optionally provide the capability for key recovery of subscriber decryption keys. However, if key recovery is made available, it will only apply to decryption keys. Nonrepudiation is supported by having the subscriber generate his signing key pair on that subscriber's own system and only transferring his public verification key to the CA during the registration process.

INSPECTION

The international application transmitted to the Receiving Office in electronic form, shall be legible and appear to have been fully received and without any virus infection. If all or part of the international application is illegible or that part of the application appears not to have been received, the international application shall be treated as not having been received to the extent that it is illegible or, where transmitted by electronic means, that the attempted transmission failed, and the Office shall, if practicable having regard to the indications furnished by the applicant, promptly notify the applicant accordingly.

The electronic application shall be free of infection by viruses and other forms of malicious logic. Where the Office finds that the purported application is so infected, the Office is not required to disinfect the purported application and may, under Section 703(e), refuse to receive it; or disinfect it and make a backup copy. If the Office finds that it is able to read and store the purported application, it shall determine whether an international filing date should be accorded. If the Office accords an international filing date to the application, it shall, if possible having regard to the indications furnished by the applicant, promptly notify the applicant and, if necessary, invite the applicant to submit a substitute copy of the application free of infection.

If the Office accords an international filing date to the application, it shall prepare the home copy, the record copy and the search copy on the basis of the disinfected application, the backup copy or the substitute copy provided that the application shall be stored by the Office for the purposes of Rule 93.1.

COMMUNICATION

Unlike the filing of online applications to a designated office such as USPTO or EPO, the online filing of PCT undergoes a routing process as shown in Figure 13.5.

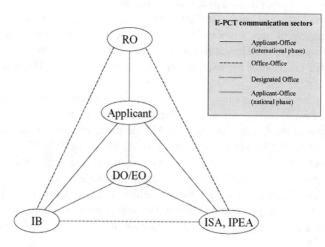

FIGURE 13.5

APPLICANT-OFFICE (INTERNATIONAL PHASE) SECTOR

The Applicant-Office (international phase) sector includes all communications between applicants and Offices in the international phase and is of most relevance to the reader. The initial filing is included along with subsequent exchanges between the applicant and the RO, IB, International Searching Authority (ISA), and International Preliminary Examining Authority (IPEA).

Some of the PCT workflow transactions included in this sector are

- Applicant files IA with RO
- Applicant sends amendments to the IB or IPEA
- Applicant sends request for changes to IB (PCT Rule 92)
- Applicant sends demand to IPEA
- Applicant furnishes power of attorney
- Applicant withdraws IA
- IB sends copy of pamphlet to applicant
- IB sends forms to applicant
- IB sends translation of international preliminary examination report (IPER) to applicant

ISA SENDS INTERNATIONAL SEARCH REPORT (ISR) WITH CITED DOCUMENTS TO APPLICANT

This is the first step in the electronic processing of PCT documents. An applicant who files an international application with a RO would have to obtain, at minimum, a low-level digital certificate to enable communications in electronic form between the applicant and the International Bureau, the International Searching Authority, or the International Preliminary Examining Authority. If the applicant does not obtain a low-level digital certificate, communication with other Offices would be accomplished through conventional (paper-based) means.

The applicant/agent obtains a digital certificate from the IB or a recognized CA. The applicant/agent uses software provided by the IB or RO to package and send the IA documents to the chosen RO. It is expected that the software will handle the details of this process for the user, which are summarized here. The software:

1. Validates the applicant/agent's certificate, and the certificate of the chosen RO. Invalid certificates must be replaced before the process can continue.
2. Packages the documents into a WAD file using zip compression.
3. Creates a WASP file by signing the WAD file in a PKCS #7 signed data object using the applicant/agent's private key and signing certificate
4. Creates a second WASP that contains the package header.
5. Optionally, creates the SEP file by signing and encrypting the ZIP file in a PKCS #7 signed and encrypted data object using the applicant/agent's private key to sign the data and the chosen RO's public key to encrypt the data.

6. For online transmission, in the case of transmission using WASP packages, the client initiates an SSL session and sends the WASP containing the package header. In the case of SEP transmittals, a SSL session may optionally be initiated by the client.
7. The SEP, or the package data WASP is then sent using the protocol specified above.
8. The client requests the receipt.
9. Receives a transmission receipt object from the Office's server to conclude the transaction.
10. Displays the validated transmission receipt to the applicant/agent.

RO Receives WASP or SEP

The RO accepts a new electronic IA as a WASP or SEP package. Upon receiving an inbound SEP package, the RO system must first decrypt and validate the SEP package, resulting in a zip file. The WASP package is then extracted from this zip. All attempts are made by the server to properly extract these data. However, if this or any further operation fails due to unrecognizable format, unrecoverable data, invalid certificate, etc., a transmission receipt is returned to the applicant containing error information describing the failure.

RO Validates Certificate and Signature

The WASP package certificate and digital signature are validated. At this stage, a recognized certificate type is accepted. If an invalid digital signature is detected, this information is included on the transmission receipt.

RO Performs Automated Formalities Examination on Purported Application

In order to grant the date of receipt, the purported application is examined for the minimum required information content. The WAD file is extracted from the WASP. The application files are extracted from the WAD file and scanned for virus infection. The file format and structure is examined for compliance with the format described above. The information provided is examined, to the extent practicable, by machine (e.g., whether in the XML document structure there is a portion of the document entitled Claims and Description, if an applicant is indicated, if the application contains a designation and whether there is an indication that the application is intended as an IA, these being five content-based requirements under PCT Article 11(1)(iii) for an international filing date).

RO Time-Stamps Application

If all of the above conditions are met, and if the other requirements under PCT Article 11(1) (right to file with the RO, and prescribed language) are met, a date of receipt is established and the WASP files are time-stamped. A numbered transmission receipt is created and returned to the applicant containing information describing the successful application.

RO Stores Application

The original WASP file, along with the associated RO-request-receiving-info, will be stored in the RO's internal system. Furthermore, the transmission-receipt to which the enhanced electronic signature of a receiving office was given is also stored in the RO's internal system.

Offline Transaction Using SEP, WASP, or WAD Packaging on Physical Media

Applicant Sends Documents to RO

The software performs the Steps 1 and 2, as above. If transmitting WASP or SEP packages over physical media, the software also performs Steps 3 and 4 to create the WASP files, or Steps 3 through 5 to create SEP packages, as above. For transmission on physical media:

1. The software initiates the offline send transaction by saving the SEP, WASP or WAD package files (created in the same manner as described above) for subsequent copying to physical media.
2. Depending on implementation, the software may allow the applicant/agent to import and view/validate an electronic confirmation package received at a later date from the RO; alternatively, the software may perform some other action (such as print out an instruction sheet) to refer the applicant/agent to information regarding confirmation of filing.

Filing Amendments

The applicant/agent may send amended claims to the IB (PCT Article 19) or IPEA (PCT Article 34). In this workflow transaction, the process involves the applicant/agent making changes to the claims and/or (in the case of PCT Article 34) description and figures, and then sending these to the IB or IPEA in the form of a changes document (a letter with attached amended claims and optionally a statement).

The applicant/agent sends WASP or SEP containing the changes document to the IB and a WASP or SEP containing the Demand form to the IPEA.

Additional workflow transactions include:

- Applicant withdraws IA
- Applicant furnishes power of attorney
- IB sends copy of pamphlet to applicant
- IB sends forms to applicant
- IB sends translation of IPER to applicant
- ISA sends ISR with cited documents to applicant

APPLICANT-OFFICE (NATIONAL PHASE) SECTOR

In order to proceed with the national phase examination, the applicant may be required by the DO to submit a national phase document to that DO. The security technology, packaging and transmission may vary among DOs. However, any DO may need to authenticate the applicant as the same applicant that submitted the first filing to the RO. For example, depending on national law, the electronic version of a national phase document may require an enhanced electronic signature. However, there may be differences between the type of electronic signature, certificate and/or packaging protocol used during the international phase and that required by the DO. The DO may require a different type of authentication of the applicant before proceeding. The differences between the signature or authentication methods must be resolved in order to correctly identify the international phase applicant. This can be accomplished using the applicant's name and e-mail address used in the international phase.

OFFICE TO OFFICE COMMUNICATION

Document exchanges and communications taking place in the Office to Office sector generally involve one PCT Office sending documents and data to another Office during the international phase. The designated Office sector includes communications between the Designated/Elected Offices (DO/EOs), and the IB. Document exchanges and communications include priority documents and publication data.

14 EPO *epoline*®

INTRODUCTION

The *epoline*® Online Filing product enables you to submit patent applications to the European Patent Office electronically. To use *epoline* Online Filing, you must first register and receive the software and validating device by mail from the European Patent Office. Unlike the current system of the USPTO and PCT, this is a rather long procedure that may take weeks and months before you can be ready to use the system. The EPO processes the requests on a batch basis, meaning you have to wait until enough requests have been made for the EPO to assemble the package for you.

The application for registration is available at http://www.*epoline*.org/onlinefilingdocs/enrolmentEN.doc (Figure 14.1). Complete the enrollment form as follows:

1. *epoline* ID: This field is to be completed by the EPO.
2. Ensure that all mandatory fields are completed (shown in bold, italic, small caps).
3. For the purpose of issue of a Smart Card for access to the secure areas of the *epoline* server, you are required to authenticate your identity either by means of your passport details or by means of your EPO number (representative number, general authorization number, or applicant number).
4. Indicate your role before the EPO and take note of the asterisked note at the end of the form, requiring persons not authorized to act before the EPO to have their enrollment form countersigned by a representative (or authorized employee) known to the EPO.

Then proceed in one of the following ways:

1. Print the PDF Enrollment Form, sign and send to European Patent Office, *epoline* Customer Services, P.O. Box 5818, Patentlaan 2, 2280 HV Rijswijk (Z-H), The Netherlands. Fax number: 00 31 70 340 4600.
2. Fill in the Online Enrollment Form, add your bitmap or JPEG signature and send the document online to *epoline* Customer Services using the SEND function.

Your application will then be processed by the EPO. Once you have successfully registered, the following items will be sent to you free of charge to enable you to

Europäisches Patentamt | European Patent Office | Office européen des brevets

epo line

epoline® Enrolment Form

Personal details

epoline® ID ______ (office use only)

Title: (Mr/Mrs/Ms/Dr/Other): ______

FIRST NAME(S): ______

LAST NAME: ______

Authentication by:

O Passport details / Other official ID
- Date of birth: ______
- Place of birth: ______
- Nationality: ______
- Passport: No. ______
- ID No. ______
- Place of issue: ______
- Date of issue: ______

O EPO Number
- O Representative No.: ______
- O Gen. Auth. No. ______
- O Applicant No: ______

ADDRESS TYPE O Business O Private

Organisation: ______

Department: ______

STREET: ______ NUMBER: ______

CITY: ______ POSTCODE: ______

STATE/COUNTY: ______

COUNTRY: ______

Phone: ______

E-Mail: ______

Fax.: ______

Mobile: ______

URL: ______

PREFERRED LANGUAGE: O English O French O German

*ROLE: O Attorney O Applicant O Authorised employee O Administrative staff

* Please note that administrative staff applying for a smart card must have this form duly countersigned by a representative known to the EPO.

Hardware, O/S etc.

Type of PC used: ______ Operating System ______

If Windows: O 95 O 98 O ME O NT O 2000 O XP

Communication Ports: O Serial only O USB only O Both

Web Browser: ______

Please check that all details are correct and append your signature.

Signed.............................. Date..............................

*Countersigned by:.............................. Date..............................

Name in print:..............................

Please return to: *epoline*® Customer Services
P.O. Box 5818
Patentlaan 2
2280 HV Rijswijk (Z-H).
The Netherlands Fax number: 00 31 70 340 4600.

D:\Abelle\web site\enrolment.doc

FIGURE 14.1

make use of *epoline* Online Filing and further *epoline* secure services as they become available (Figure 14.2):

1. Online Filing CD-ROM with the relevant software needed for online filing
2. Smart Card reader
3. Smart Card (separate mailing): Smart Card contains certificates, provides unique identification of individuals, and is issued by a Certification Authority (CA)
   a. Banks
   b. Governments (Finland as of 12/99)
   c. Post offices
   d. EPO will initially act as the *epoline* CA
4. Pin code (separate mailing)
5. Documentation

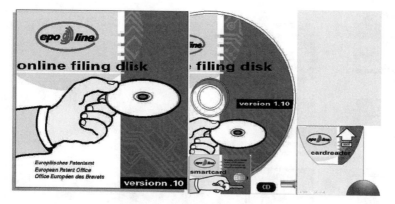

FIGURE 14.2

These will enable you to use not only *epoline* Online Filing, but also other secure *epoline* services as they become available.

FILING ONLINE

The process of filing a patent application online is divided into the following steps:

- Complete the bibliographic data using *epoline* Online Filing.
- Attach existing electronic files (made with word processor or scanned) containing technical specifications.
- Submit and file application from *epoline* Online Filing (encryption and online dispatch); the required filing format is PDF (Portable Document Format).
- During the online session, application is digitally signed and encrypted.
- Application is then sent to the Receiving Office.
- An electronic receipt is returned to the sender.

The following security features are built into *epoline* Online Filing:

- Authentication of users: Each party knows who the other is.
- Confidentiality: No one else can see the data that is submitted.
- Integrity: Data transmitted and received are identical.
- Accountability: Both parties can prove receipt of data.

OVERVIEW

The process of sending a patent application online consists of the steps shown in Figure 14.3.

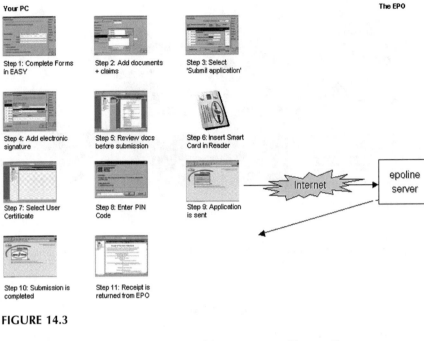

FIGURE 14.3

STEP 1: CREATE PATENT APPLICATION USING *EPOLINE* ONLINE FILING

Prepare the patent application using your national language version of *epoline* Online Application Filing Software (Figures 14.4 and 14.5).

STEP 2: ADD ALL REQUIRED DOCUMENTS

Add all the required documents to the application (description, claims, drawings, abstracts) (Figures 14.6 and 14.7). Note that when you select the documents to add to the application, documents are not automatically converted to PDF. You have to do this yourself. The blob (whole application comprising bibliographic data and technical documents) is subsequently converted to PDF using the Amyuni® Converter provided with the Online Filing software. The Amyuni Converter can be used to convert existing technical documents into PDF prior to attaching them to the application. Applying a common format to all documents provides the following benefits:

- It speeds up the process of sending the files to the EPO.
- It simplifies the process of extracting the data from them.

STEP 3: SELECT "SUBMIT APPLICATION"

When all required fields have been completed within *epoline* Online Filing, select the Submit Application button in the main menu tab. The Submission window appears, as shown in Figure 14.8. Check that the file name is correct. Make sure that the Method of Submission is *epoline*. To begin the *epoline* Online Filing process, select Continue.

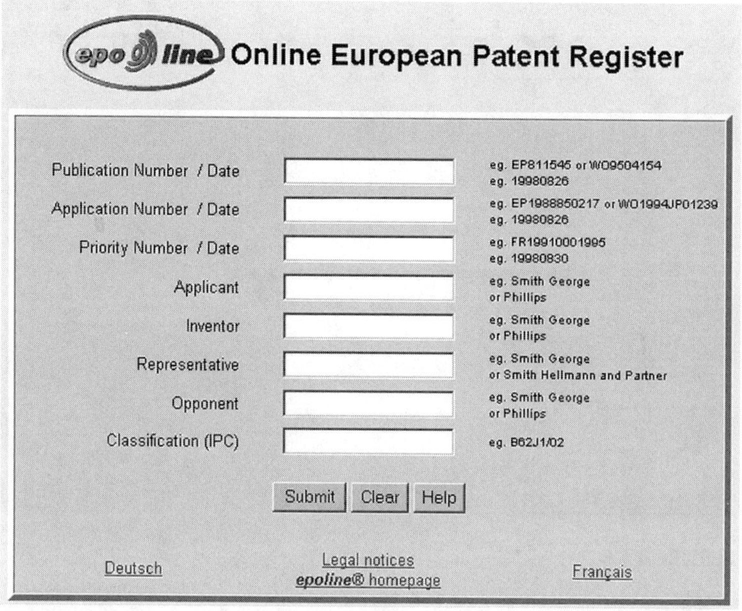

FIGURE 14.4

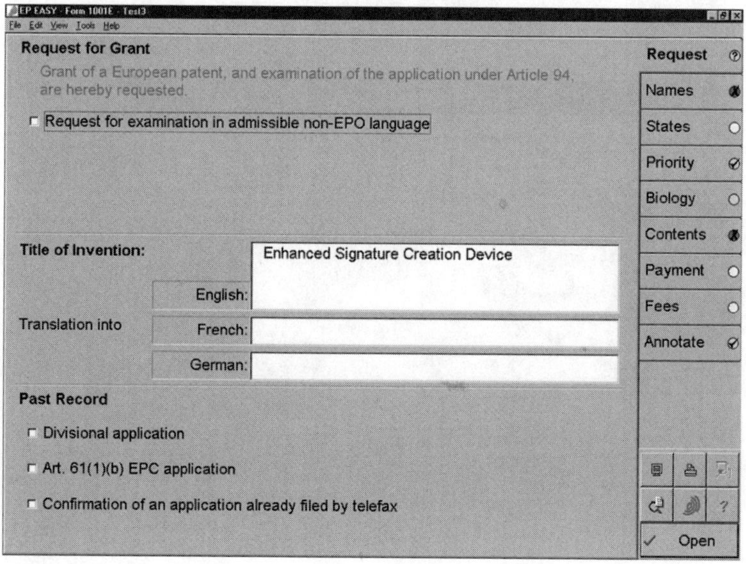

FIGURE 14.5

Step 4: Complete the List of Signatories

The List of Signatories window appears. Each name in the list has an electronic signature associated with it. This is assigned to the person or organization by a

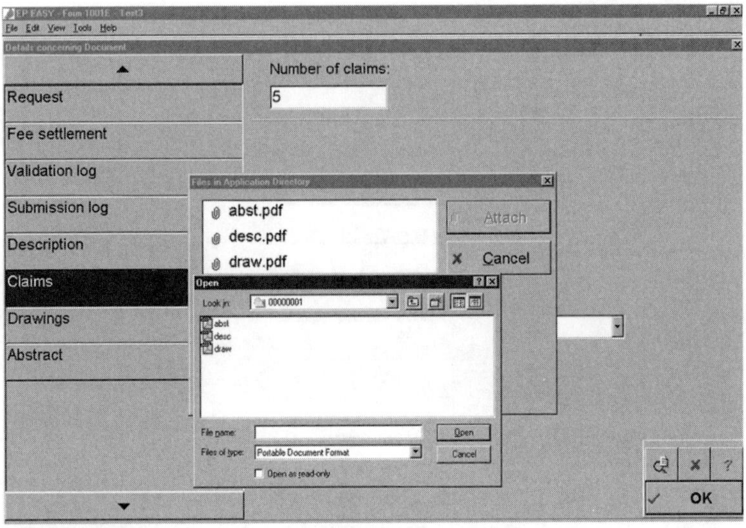

FIGURE 14.6

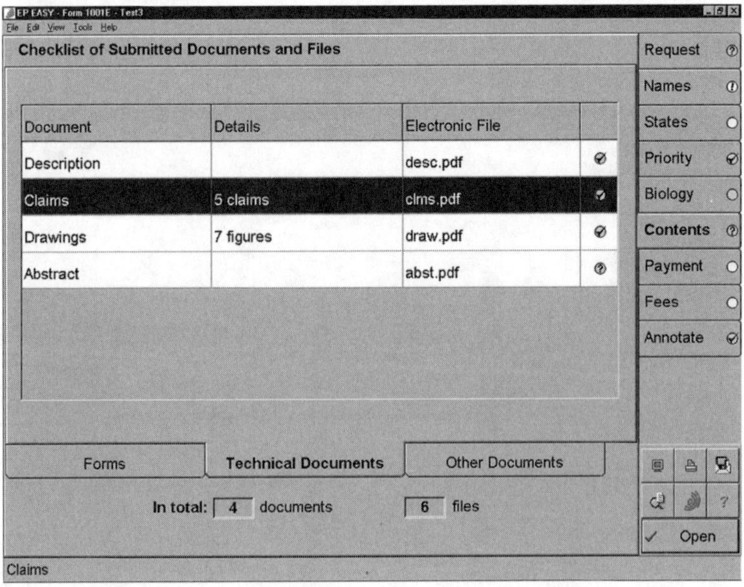

FIGURE 14.7

recognized Certification Authority, and it is used to validate the information that is sent to the EPO (Figure 14.9). To add a name to the list:

1. Select a name from the list of Applicants and Representatives.
2. Click the Add button.
3. When you have completed the list of signatories, click the OK button.

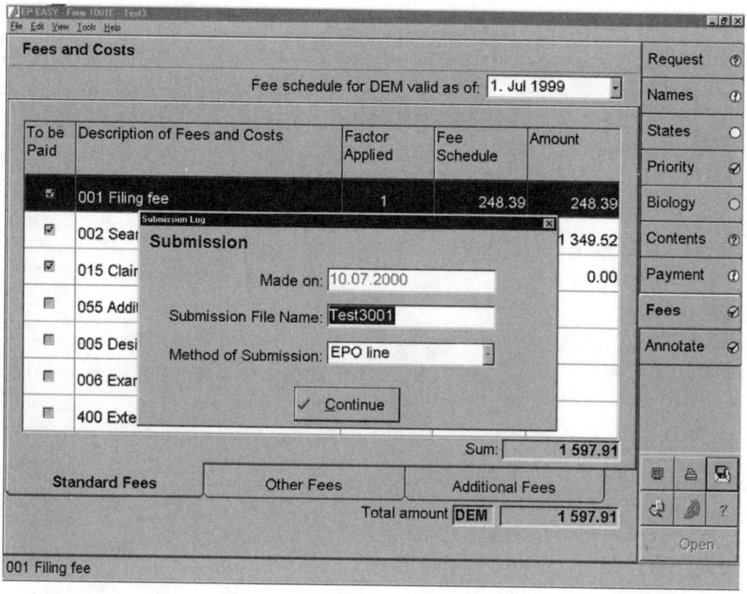

FIGURE 14.8

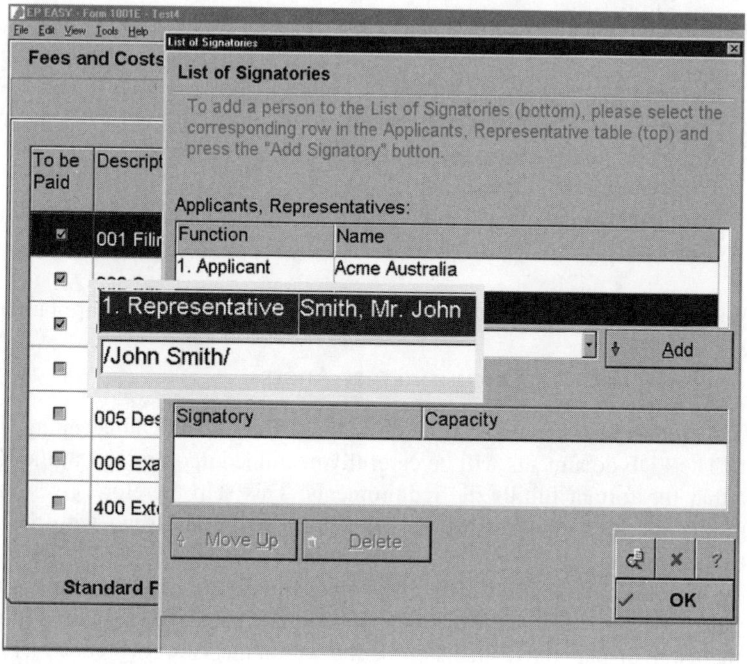

FIGURE 14.9

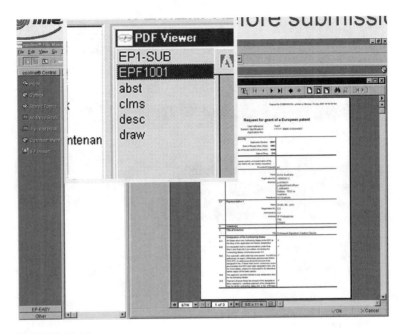

FIGURE 14.10

There are three legally permitted signature types (Figure 14.13).

1. Alphabetical, e.g., /A. N. Other/
2. Facsimile (graphical image of handwritten signature); normally in .jpeg or .jpg format; click on the button to the right of the Facsimile field to insert your graphic file.
3. Advanced Digital; uses Smart Card owner's name, requires inserted Smart Card.

Use any of the three signature types and click the Apply Signature button.

Step 5: Check that All Documents Are Added

The PDF Viewer appears within the File Manager of *epoline* Online Filing (Figure 14.10). The PDF documents will be carefully examined upon receipt at the EPO to verify that the format fulfills the requirements. This step therefore gives you the opportunity to check the documents that you will sign and send with the patent application.

The list of files to the left of the PDF Viewer viewing window displays all the documents contained within the patent application (Figure 14.11). Select a file name from the list to display the contents of the file within the Viewer (Figure 14.12). The toolbars at the top and bottom of the Viewer provide standard Adobe® Acrobat commands for moving through the document, zooming in and out, etc. If an incorrect document is attached to the application, click the Cancel button. You can then return

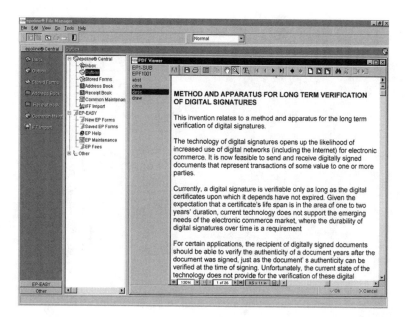

FIGURE 14.11

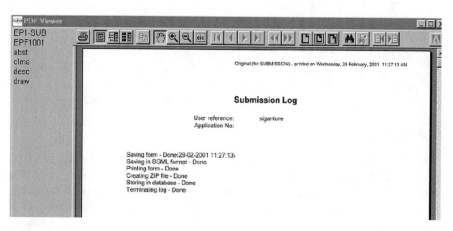

FIGURE 14.12

to the entry form and attach the correct document. When you are satisfied that the correct documents are attached, proceed to the next step.

STEP 6: INSERT SMART CARD IN THE CARD READER

Make sure that the card reader is switched on and working properly (the light on the side of the reader will be steady once the Smart Card has been inserted, otherwise it will blink). The only exception is with Windows® 2000, where the light continues blinking when the card is in the card reader.

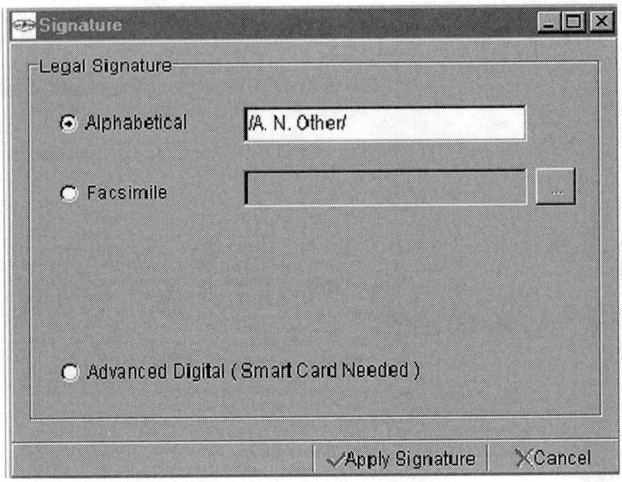

FIGURE 14.13

The Smart Card is created by a Certification Agency, and it contains:

- The private key of the user.
- The public key of the user.
- A certificate, which testifies that this public key has been allocated to this user.

Each user should have one Smart Card.* If there are several people within a company with the right to submit patents, there should be one Smart Card for each of them. Click the Sign Now button. The Signature window appears (Figure 14.13).

STEP 7: SELECT A USER CERTIFICATE

When you apply the chosen signature, the User Certificate Selection window (Figure 14.14) appears on your screen. It is a display of the User Certificate, which consists of information that identifies you as a valid, unique user of the system. The information displayed in this screen is taken from the Smart Card, and consists of the following:

- Your name
- Serial number of the Smart Card
- The code of the authority that issued the electronic certificate

---

* The card needs only to be inserted before the actual submission process begins. To verify that the Smart Card reader and the Smart Card have been properly installed and are recognized by the PC, use the supplied iD2 personal software (Start\Programs\iD2 Personal\Administration Utility). The green light should go from blinking to steady after the card is inserted (except in Windows 2000). When inserting, make sure that the side of the card with the element (metal maze) shown in Figure 14.19 is inserted head down and is facing the Gem Plus logo in a vertical SCR or up in a horizontal SCR.

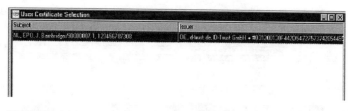

FIGURE 14.14

To proceed:

1. Select your name from the list.
2. Click the OK button (bottom right-hand side, not shown).

STEP 8: ENTER A PIN CODE

This is a final security check to authenticate the card. When you have entered the PIN code, click the OK button from the main menu (Figure 14.15). This launches your Web browser. A Certificate Name Check window appears.

Click Continue. You are then asked to reenter your PIN code. Enter your PIN code, and click OK. This opens the SSL

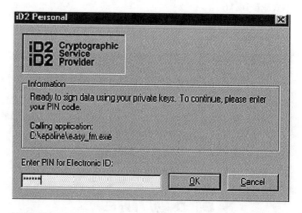

FIGURE 14.15

connection to the EPO. (Please note that we have used the same PIN codes for this test session only. In the future, two different PIN codes will be necessary.)

STEP 9: SEND APPLICATION ONLINE

The application is then sent online to the EPO. The progress of the submission is displayed within the browser window (Figure 14.16). You need not do anything while this is happening unless an error occurs during the submission. Error messages are displayed below the Progress window, along with suggestions for what to do next.*

---

* Netscape Communicator and Internet Explorer are supported for online filing. The current encryption used for online file is 128 bits. During submission, if you get a "No class deffounderror: org/*epoline*/olf/gui/Applet comm" or "Load: class org.*epoline*.olf.gui EPO client not found" error in the Web browser, it means that the Java software and class modules have either not been installed properly or the class path for these modules have not been set up correctly.

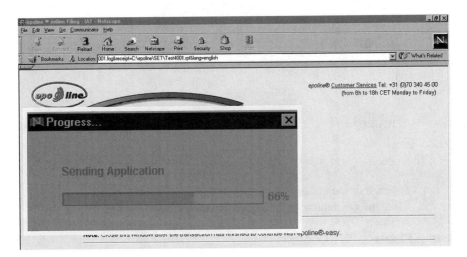

FIGURE 14.16

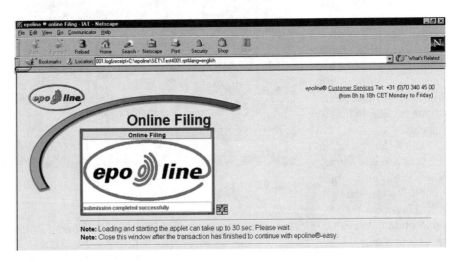

FIGURE 14.17

STEP 10: SUBMISSION IS COMPLETED

When the application has been submitted successfully to the EPO, a message to that effect appears in the browser (Figure 14.17). To proceed, close the browser window. To know exactly what has been received at the EPO as a result of your filing, sort the sent zip files under stored forms by zip folder using the browser, and you will be able to see the contents of the received zip files by clicking on the required application. You do not have to prepare an application again if submission fails. An

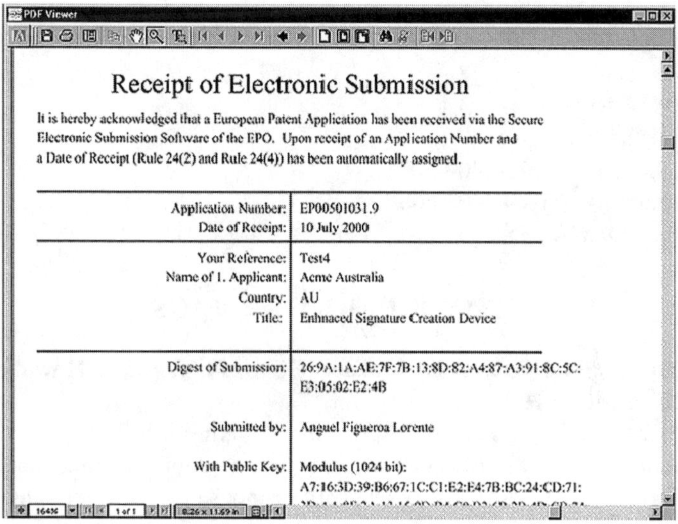

FIGURE 14.18

application remains in the Outbox until it is successfully sent. It can be resent from the Outbox in case of submission failure.

STEP 11: RECEIPT IS RETURNED FROM THE EPO

When you close the browser, the following message is displayed:

Filing Complete. Do you wish to view the Receipt?

Click Yes. The receipt is then displayed in the PDF viewer (Figure 14.18). The Application Number and Date of Receipt are shown on the receipt.

RESENDING A PATENT APPLICATION

If you cannot send an application because, for example, an error occurred during submission:

- Within the entry form (1000E), select the Submit Application button. This begins the process from Step 3.
- In the File Manager of *epoline* Online Filing, open the Outbox folder, then double-click on the name of the stored application.

CONTACTING *EPOLINE* CUSTOMER SERVICES

For all questions on *epoline* products in general and the *epoline* Online Filing software in particular, contact:

epoline Customer Services
European Patent Office
Patentlaan 2
2280 HV Rijswijk (Z-H)
The Netherlands
Telephone 011-3170-340-4500
Facsimile 011 31 70 340 4600
e-mail *epoline*@epo.org

TROUBLESHOOTING FAQS

1. **My GemPlus Smart Card reader (SCR) is plugged in. How do I turn the power on?**
   Make sure that the green light on top is blinking, which means the power is on. If it is not blinking, insert the power cord into any functioning PS/2 port (keyboard or mouse). Keyboard or mouse can be safely plugged on top of the card reader power plug. Do all the plugging/unplugging with your computer off to avoid port damage.

2. **I have plugged the SCR power cord in. Why is the light not blinking?**
   Try changing the power cord to any other PS/2 port you might have. If none of them work, check your SCR on a different computer. In case your SCR works on other machines, consult your computer dealer; if it does not, ask for an SCR replacement.

3. **The green light on my SCR is blinking. How do I know that the Smart Card Reader recognizes my card?**
   The green light should go from blinking to steady after the card is inserted. When inserting, make sure that the side of the card with the element shown in Figure 14.19 is inserted head down and is facing the GemPlus logo in a vertical SCR or up in a horizontal SCR.

FIGURE 14.19

4. **Is there any way to check that my SCR is installed correctly?**
   For a Windows NT workstation, go to Start\Settings\Control Panel\GemPlus Smart Card Reader and click the icon shown in Figure 14.20. A window appears, similar to Figure 14.21. Click the Check button to run a check. If you do not find the icon in your Control Panel, or if you are using a Windows 95 or 98 workstation,   go to <CDROM:>\GemPlus\Installer_August_ 2000\Drivers and run the GemCheck.exe program.

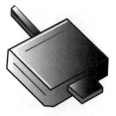

Gemplus Smart
Card Reader

FIGURE 14.20

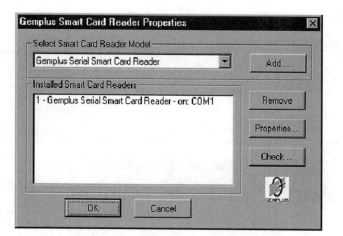

FIGURE 14.21

5. What if I insert my card correctly and the light continues to blink?

For a Windows NT workstation, go to Start\ Settings\Control Panel\Services and click the icon shown in Figure 14.22. A window appears, similar to Figure 14.23. Make sure that Smart Card Resource Manager is set to Automatic and Started. Use the Startup... button to make it Automatic and the Start button to start it. If an error occurs, try reinstalling Microsoft®

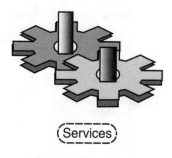

FIGURE 14.22

Smart Card Base components or you can get help from Microsoft's Web site (http://www.microsoft.com/security/tech/smartcards/components.asp) or the GemPlus documentation (<CDROM:>\GemPlus\Installer_August_2000\Gemrdr.hlp) and Web site (http://www.gemplus.com/products/hardware/index.htm).

You can also go to Start\Settings\Control Panel\Devices to open a window similar to Figure 14.24. Make sure that Serial is set to Automatic and Started. Use the Startup... button to make it Automatic and the Start button to start it. If an error occurs, consult your hardware specialist or computer dealer. Also check that GrSerial exists on this list and is set to Automatic and Started (Figure 14.25). If it does not start, try to start it manually. If that results in an error message, refer to the GemPlus documentation.

For a Windows 95 or 98 workstation, go to Start\Settings\Control Panel\System\Devices and make sure that the GemPlus device exists and is working properly. If it does not, refer to the GemPlus documentation.

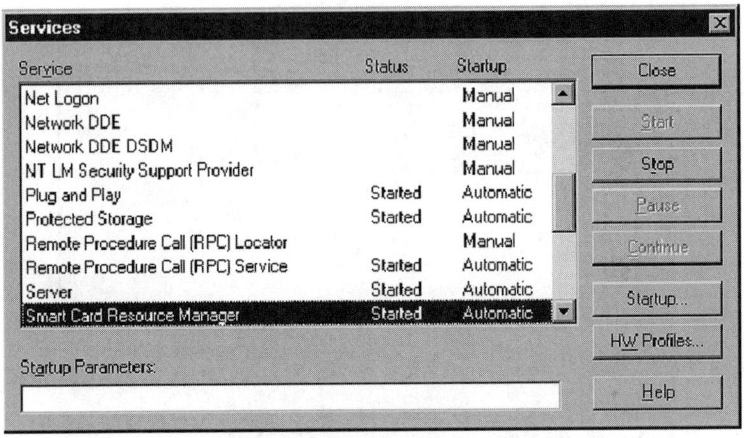

Services

Service	Status	Startup
Net Logon		Manual
Network DDE		Manual
Network DDE DSDM		Manual
NT LM Security Support Provider		Manual
Plug and Play	Started	Automatic
Protected Storage	Started	Automatic
Remote Procedure Call (RPC) Locator		Manual
Remote Procedure Call (RPC) Service	Started	Automatic
Server	Started	Automatic
Smart Card Resource Manager	Started	Automatic

Close
Start
Stop
Pause
Continue
Startup...
HW Profiles...
Help

Startup Parameters:

FIGURE 14.23

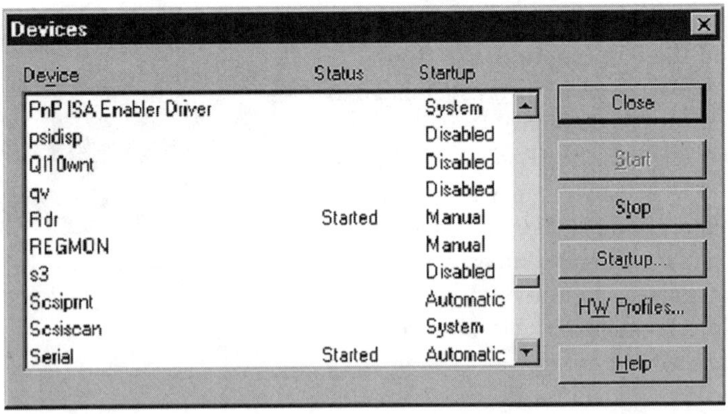

Devices

Device	Status	Startup
PnP ISA Enabler Driver		System
psidisp		Disabled
Ql10wnt		Disabled
qv		Disabled
Rdr	Started	Manual
REGMON		Manual
s3		Disabled
Scsiprnt		Automatic
Scsiscan		System
Serial	Started	Automatic

Close
Start
Stop
Startup...
HW Profiles...
Help

FIGURE 14.24

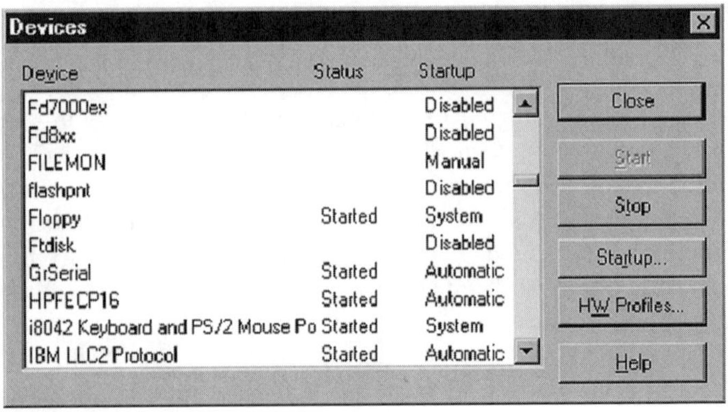

Devices

Device	Status	Startup
Fd7000ex		Disabled
Fd8xx		Disabled
FILEMON		Manual
flashpnt		Disabled
Floppy	Started	System
Ftdisk		Disabled
GrSerial	Started	Automatic
HPFECP16	Started	Automatic
i8042 Keyboard and PS/2 Mouse Po	Started	System
IBM LLC2 Protocol	Started	Automatic

Close
Start
Stop
Startup...
HW Profiles...
Help

FIGURE 14.25

PDF HINTS AND TIPS

The EPO can accept documents prepared only in the Portable Document Format (PDF) format with the correct settings. Because *epoline* requires attachments to be in PDF format, it is important to know how to prepare these documents. The following hints and tips are provided to assist you in preparing documents in PDF.

PDF documents can be created with a number of tools, including:

- Adobe Acrobat, which is an open standard for electronic document distribution. Acrobat preserves all the fonts, formatting, graphics, and color of the source document, regardless of the application and platform used to create it.
- Amyuni PDF Writer, which is delivered with the *epoline* Online Filing software. This software package is less feature-rich than Acrobat, but it is reliable and easy to use.

There are many other products on the market that generate PDF documents and you may select any tool that produces PDF documents in PDF 1.2 format. The key points to remember are

- Correct fonts must be chosen in order to display information correctly, including characters such as mathematical formulae and Greek characters.
- Paper size must be A4.
- Page orientation must be Portrait.

FONTS IN PDF DOCUMENTS

A PDF document is the electronic equivalent of a paper printout. It should be checked carefully. There are two ways of using fonts in a document, linking and embedding. There are a few areas where problems might occur, especially in the field of font embedding.

Linking Fonts

Linking references the font from where it is stored on your computer. The advantage of this is that the document file size can remain small. The disadvantage is that if you send the document to another system, as is the case with *epoline* Online Filing, the linked information cannot be referenced. Specialized fonts, e.g., ones that use mathematical symbols, Greek characters, or other non-Latin alphabets, may not be interpreted correctly.

Embedding Fonts

Embedding means that the font is included with the document, so the entire package is self-contained. This is the appropriate option when sending it outside your own system. It is strongly recommended that you use standard fonts only, i.e., fonts that are included in the set that comes with Adobe Reader. But if you must use a nonstandard font, e.g., for symbols not available otherwise, you must ensure that the font is embedded.

If you are using special copyright-protected fonts, you must also ensure that you have sufficient rights to embed the font with your document. You should note the following from the Adobe Acrobat 4.0 Guide:

> A TrueType font can contain a setting added by the font's designer that prevents the font from being embedded in PDF files. Even though you can move such a font to an embed list, Distiller does not embed it in the PDF file, but displays an error message and lists the font in the log file. You can check whether the font was embedded by opening the resulting PDF file and viewing the Font Info dialog box.

As a general rule, programs used for PDF provide an option to embed all fonts. The suggestions below describe the options for Acrobat and Amyuni. For other software products, consult the manufacturer.

Adobe

Adobe provides two ways of producing PDF documents, PDFWriter and Distiller. As a general rule of thumb, use Distiller for more complex documents that include graphics and specialized fonts. Embedding all fonts in Distiller is done in a configuration file called *epoline*.joboptions. This file must be copied into the Distiller settings directory, usually C:\Program Files\Adobe\Acrobat 4.0\Distillr\Settings.

Adobe automatically installs files for print- and screen-optimized PDF output in this directory, with default setting as shown in Figures 14.26 and 14.27. The Embed All Fonts option is selected automatically. It might be a good idea to make the *epoline*.joboptions file read-only.

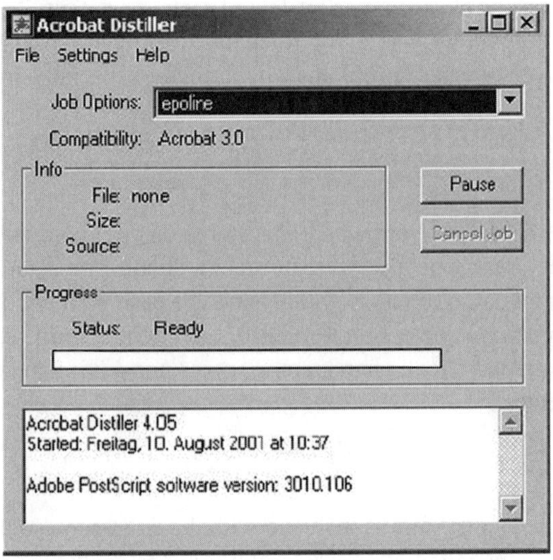

FIGURE 14.26

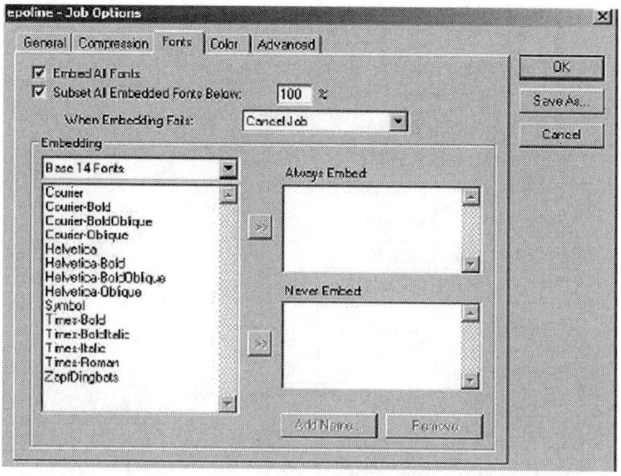

FIGURE 14.27

Amyuni

For the Amyuni PDF Converter, font embedding is done after Amyuni PDF Converter has been selected as the printer.

1. Select File, Print from the document menu.
2. Select Amyuni PDF Converter as the printer.
3. In the Print dialog window, select Properties. The Amyuni PDF Converter Printer Defaults window opens.
4. Select the Font embedding option.

We suggest that you also select the multilanguage support option, and this is mandatory if non-Latin characters are to be used. To set the Amyuni font embedding options:

1. Click the Embedding Options button (shown in Figure 14.28). The Font Embedding Options window appears (Figure 14.29).
2. Select all options.
3. Click OK.

It is recommend that you configure the Amyuni Printer settings once for all print jobs by accessing the Printers menu in the Control Panel. If Windows NT/2000 is being used, this should be done preferably via an Administrator's account.

IDENTIFICATION OF POSSIBLE PROBLEM AREAS

Identifying and testing problem areas might be useful preparatory work. There are multiple computer platforms, and virtually hundreds of applications that can generate PDFs. It is next to impossible to test all of these application/platform combinations and evaluate how they might handle certain complex document conversions. We recommend that you restrict yourself to the platform/application combination that

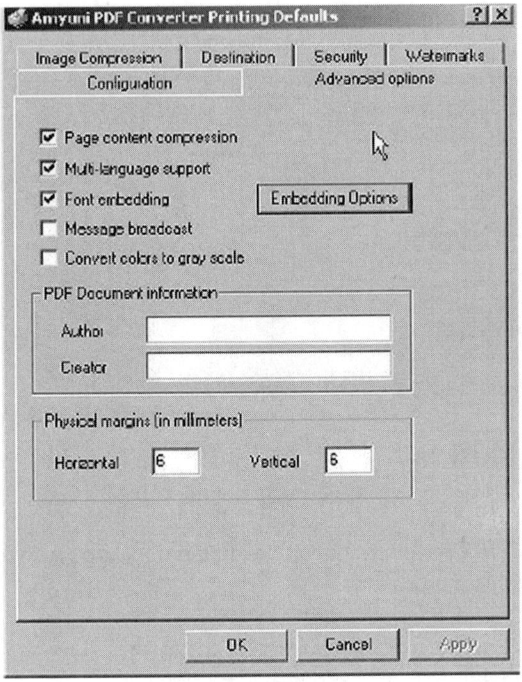

FIGURE 14.28

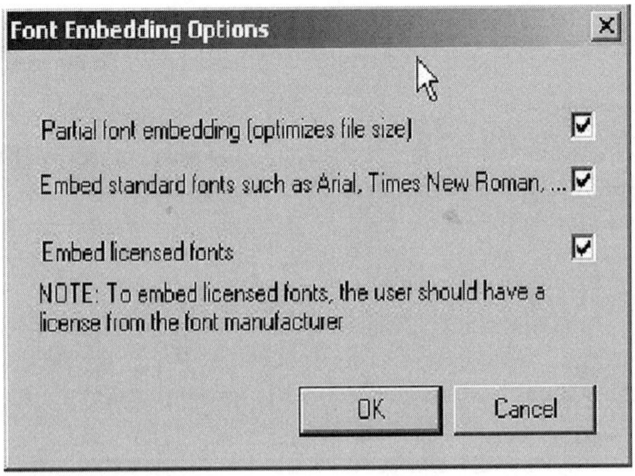

FIGURE 14.29

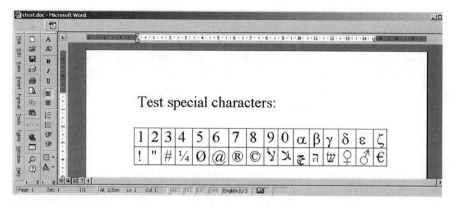

FIGURE 14.30

you plan to use for PDF conversion. Then identify any complex elements that future application documents might include. A few examples of complex elements are

- Uncommon fonts
- Non-Latin characters, e.g., the Euro symbol
- Any Greek, Russian, Hebrew, Arabic, or other characters
- Embedded mathematical formulas or other embedded objects
- Superscripts and subscripts

Once those complex elements common to the application documents are identified

1. Create a test document with the authoring tool you intend to use, for example, Microsoft Word.
2. Try converting the document to PDF. When you achieve a PDF that looks exactly like the original word-processed document, use the same settings for real online patent applications. Figure 14.30 illustrates how a test document with special characters prepared in Microsoft Word should appear identical in Adobe Acrobat Reader.

WHICH TOOL MIGHT BE THE BEST?

No statement can be made as to which of the tools might be the best. Although Abode PDF Distiller is generally considered as the reference, it should be pointed out that the test approach described earlier is recommended as a way of finding out what suits your requirements the best. In some cases, Acrobat PDF Writer with font embedding selected or any other PDF generating tool can do the job as well as the tools in the *epoline* Online Filing package.

HOW TO VERIFY THAT A PDF FILE IS SELF-CONTAINED

If a nonstandard font has been used in the creation of a technical document, then it is important to preview the file on a PC where this font is not installed in order to check whether the characters are indeed embedded. Therefore it is advisable to use different PCs at least once for the creation of the technical documents and for the electronic filing to ensure that the selected PDF generating method is working properly. Make sure that the nonstandard fonts are not installed on the PC used for electronic filing (and reviewing of the PDF files). Using a PDF viewer other than Acrobat could be an option as well. For more information, see the discussion of Ghostview later in the chapter.

PAPER SIZE

Rule 35(4) EPC requires the documents making up the European patent application to be on A4 paper (http://www.europeanpatentoffice.org/legal/epc/e/r35.html). This rule also should be followed for electronic filings, even though electronic rather than physical paper is being used. Any PDF generation software should be set to A4 paper size, i.e., 29.7×21.0 cm (or 8.267 x 11.693 in.), portrait orientation (landscape should be avoided). Set the page size to A4 in both your word processor and the PDF generator.

To set Distiller to A4 (Figure 14.31):

1. Select Printer Properties.
2. Click the Advanced option.
3. Select Portrait mode.

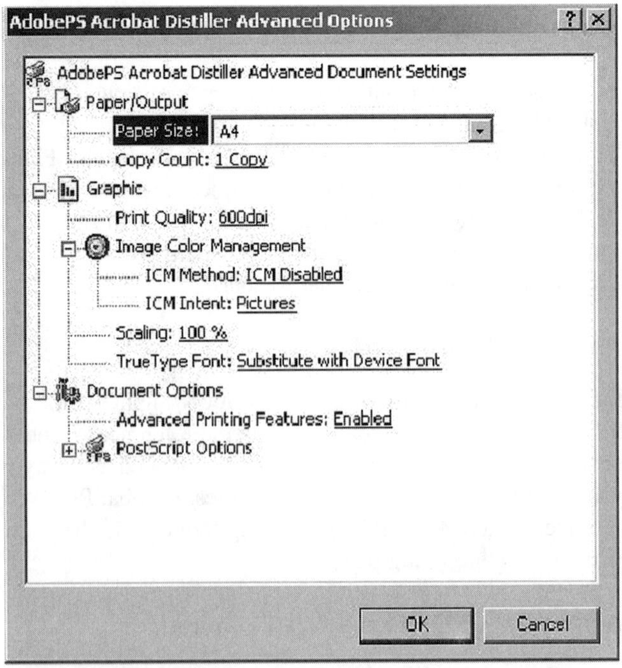

FIGURE 14.31

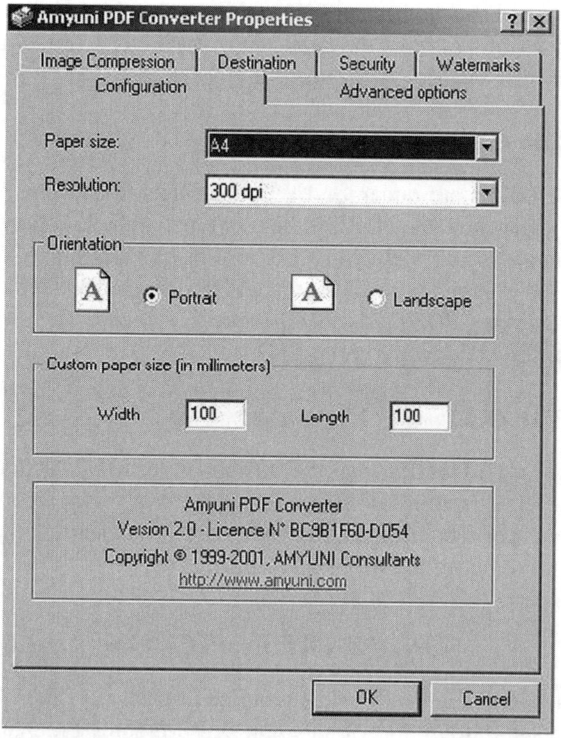

FIGURE 14.32

To set Amyuni to A4, select the A4 option directly under Printer Properties (Figure 14.32).

This seems to be especially important when drawings are not generated by graphic programs but are scanned and converted to PDF files. For any PDF filings that do not follow this rule, the EPO internal image database might then contain pages with black areas filling the remaining area between the unintentionally chosen format and A4 format.

ADDITIONAL REMARKS

ACROBAT UPGRADES

Up to and including version 1.01e of the *epoline* Online Filing software, only Acrobat 4.0x is supported as a conversion tool. The system must not be upgraded to Acrobat 5.0 or later.

POSTSCRIPT PRINTER

Installation of a Postscript (PS) printer driver is mandatory when using Acrobat Distiller, even if there is no physical printer attached to the computer system.

Version 4.0 of Acrobat which was delivered with the first *epoline* Online Filing software packages did not force the applicant to install a PS printer driver, whereas Version 4.05 (a maintenance release from Adobe) did.

GHOSTSCRIPT AND GHOSTVIEW*

Both of these products are under GNU** public license and give Windows users the ability to preview how the PDF will be converted at the European Patent Office. Ghostview is an alternative viewer that can also display PDF files. The EPO uses a Ghostscript-based program to feed incoming PDF documents into its internal image database, so previewing PDF files with Ghostview is another way to check that PDF files will be converted correctly in the EPO.

GENERATING PDF DOCUMENTS USING A SCANNER

A scanner is very useful for drawings and all sorts of technical documents. However, do not use any default settings of the scanning/capturing software that might influence the virtual paper size of the PDF documents. Before starting the scan process, the scan area has to be set to DIN A4, Portrait.

ONLINE FILE INSPECTION

The EPO has recently begun allowing an online inspection of files. You can access this at the Web site (http://pfipreview.*epoline*.org/) (Figures 14.33 and 14.34).

---

* Installation of Ghostscript 6.x first and then Ghostview 3.4. For more information on Ghostscript 6.x see the Web site at http://www.cs.wisc.edu/~ghost/doc/gnu/index.htm. For more information on Ghostview 3.4 see the Web site at http://www.cs.wisc.edu/~ghost/gsview/get36.htm.

** Acronym for GNU's Not UNIX. A collection of software based on the UNIX operating system maintained by the Free Software Foundation. GNU is distributed under the GNU General Public License, which requires that anyone who distributes GNU or a program based on GNU may charge only for distribution and support and must allow the user to modify and redistribute the code on the same terms.

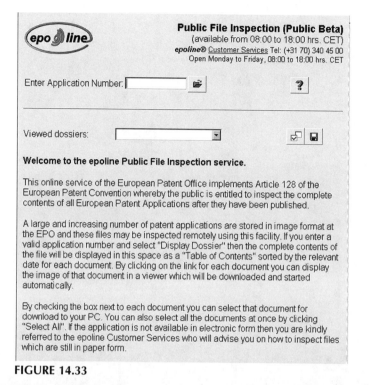

FIGURE 14.33

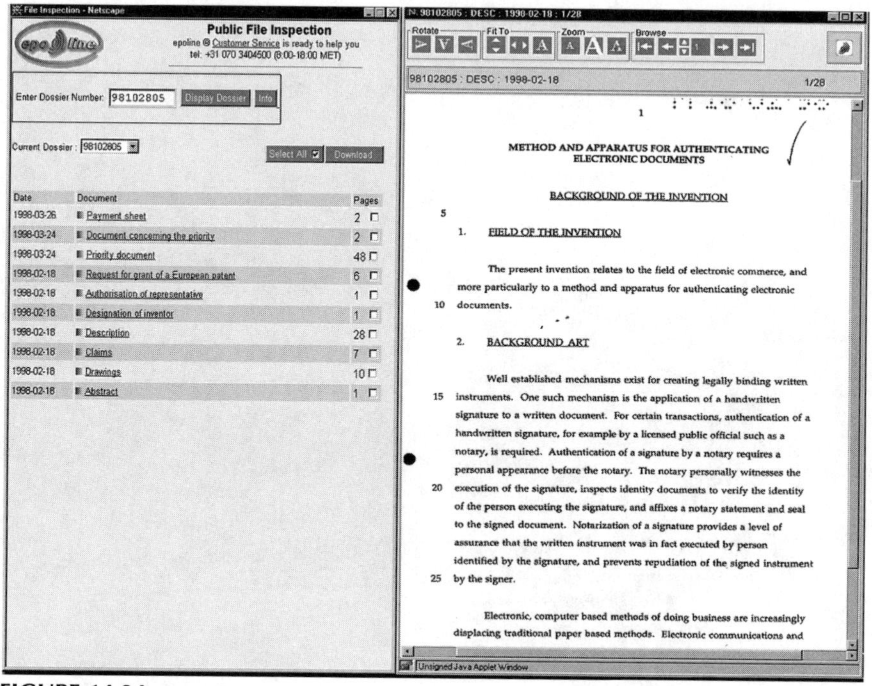

FIGURE 14.34

Appendix
Glossary of Common Terms

Abstract of the disclosure A concise statement of the technical disclosure including that which is new in the art to which the invention pertains.

Administrative Instructions Set out the provisions and requirements in relation to the filing and processing of the international (patent) application under the PCT and are established by the Director General of WIPO.

ADS Application Data Sheet

AIPA American Inventors Protection Act of 1999

Application (patent) A nonprovisional utility patent application must include a specification, including a claim or claims; drawings, when necessary; an oath or declaration; and the prescribed filing fee.

Application number (patent) The unique number assigned to a patent application when it is filed. The application number includes a two-digit series code and a six digit serial number.

BPAI Board of Patent Appeals and Interferences

CD (1) A type of form designation such as Form CD435, meaning a Commerce Department form; (2) a compact disc (electronic data storage media).

Certificate of mailing A certificate for each piece of correspondence mailed prior to the expiration of the set period of time for response, stating the date of deposit with the U.S. Postal Service and including a signature.

CFC Combined Federal Campaign

CFR Code of Federal Regulations

Chapter I The first, mandatory phase under the Patent Cooperation Treaty that includes performance of an international-type search, issuance of an International Search Report, and publication of the application and Search Report by the International Bureau of WIPO

Chapter II The second, optional phase under the Patent Cooperation Treaty that includes examination of the international application and issuance of an International Preliminary Examination Report.

CIP Continuation-in-Part. An application filed during the lifetime of an earlier nonprovisional application, repeating some substantial portion or all of the earlier nonprovisional application and adding matter not disclosed in the earlier nonprovisional application.

Claims Define the invention and are what are legally enforceable. The specification must conclude with a claim particularly pointing out and distinctly claiming the subject matter which the applicant regards as his invention or discovery. The claim or claims must conform to the invention as set forth in the remainder of the specification and the terms and phrases used in the claims must find clear support or antecedent basis in the description so that the meaning of the terms in the claims may be ascertainable by reference to the description.

Continuation A second application for the same invention claimed in a prior nonprovisional application and filed before the first application becomes abandoned or patented.

Continuing application A continuation, divisional, or continuation-in-part patent application.

Contracting State A national Office or an intergovernmental organization that is party to the Patent Cooperation Treaty.

Control No. Unique number assigned to a patent reexamination request when it is filed, having a two-digit series code (90 for *ex parte* reexamination requests; 95 for *inter partes* reexamination requests), and a six-digit control number.

copyrights Protect works of authorship, such as writings, music, and works of art that have been tangibly expressed. The Library of Congress registers copyrights which last for the life of the author plus 70 years.

CPA Continued Prosecution Application. A continuation or divisional application filed under 37 CFR 1.53(d).

CRU Central Reexamination Unit

Customer Number Number assigned to each filing candidate.

Demand Form PCT/IPEA/401, filed with an International Preliminary Examining Authority, demanding that an international application shall be the subject of an international preliminary examination.

deposit account An account established for the convenience of paying fees for any services requested from the USPTO.

design application (patent) An application for a patent to protect against the unauthorized use of new, original, and ornamental designs for articles of manufacture.

design patent May be granted to anyone who invents a new, original, and ornamental design for an article of manufacture.

designation An indication made by applicant, in the Request for an International Application filed under the Patent Cooperation Treaty, as to the Contracting States in which protection for an invention is desired.

disclosure In return for a patent, the inventor gives as consideration a complete revelation or disclosure of the invention for which protection is sought.

disclosure document A paper disclosing an invention (called a Disclosure Document) and signed by the inventor or inventors that has been forwarded to the USPTO by the inventor (or by any one of the inventors when there are joint inventors), by the owner of the invention, or by the attorney or agent of the inventor(s) or owner. The Disclosure Document will be retained for 2 years, and then be destroyed unless it is referred to in a separate letter in a related patent application filed within those 2 years.

divisional application A later application for an independent or distinct invention disclosing and claiming only subject matter disclosed in the earlier or parent application.

DO Designated Office. The national Office or intergovernmental organization of or acting for the Contracting State designated by the applicant under Chapter I of the Patent Cooperation Treaty.

EBC Electronic Business Center, also Patents EBC and Trademarks EBC. A web page containing hyperlinks to all online systems for conducting electronic commerce with the USPTO.

EFS Electronic Filing System (for patent applications). Supports secure electronic filing of patent application documents via the Internet.

election (PCT) An indication made by applicant, in the Demand for an International Application filed under the Patent Cooperation Treaty, as to the Contracting States in which applicant intends to use the results of the international preliminary examination.

EO Elected Office. The national Office or intergovernmental organization of or acting for the Contracting State elected by the applicant under Chapter II of the Patent Cooperation Treaty.

EPO European Patent Office

examination copy A copy of an international application filed under the Patent Cooperation Treaty maintained by the International Preliminary Examining Authority.

express mail mailing label Correspondence delivered to the USPTO via the "Express Mail Post Office to Addressee" service of the U.S. Postal Service (USPS) which is considered filed in the Office on the date of deposit with the USPS, shown by the "date-in" on the "Express Mail" mailing label.

FAQ Frequently Asked Questions

filing date The date of receipt in the Office of an application which includes (1) a specification containing a description and, if the application is a nonprovisional application, at least one claim, and (2) any required drawings.

FOIA Freedom of Information Act

FR Federal Register

FWC File Wrapper Continuing application. A continuation, continuation-in-part, or divisional application filed under 37 CFR 1.62, which uses the specification, drawings and oath or declaration from a prior nonprovisional application, which is complete as defined by 37 CFR 1.51(a)(1).
Note: 37 CFR 1.62 was deleted effective December 1, 1997. See 1203 OG 63, October 21, 1997.

GICP General Information Concerning Patents

home copy A copy of an international application filed under the Patent Cooperation Treaty maintained by the receiving Office where the international application was filed.

IB International Bureau. The secretariat of the WIPO which, among other functions, centralizes information of various kinds relating to the protection of intellectual property.

interference A proceeding, conducted before the Board of Patent Appeals and Interferences (Board), to determine priority of invention between a pending application and one or more pending applications and/or one or more unexpired patents.

international application An application filed under the Patent Cooperation Treaty.

IPEA International Preliminary Examining Authority. Either a national Office or an intergovernmental organization whose tasks include the establishment of examination reports on inventions which are the subject of international applications.

IPER International Preliminary Examination Report (Form PCT/IPEA/409), produced by an International Preliminary Examining Authority, is a preliminary and non-binding opinion on whether the invention claimed in an international application appears to be novel, to involve an inventive step (to be non-obvious), and to be industrially applicable.

ISA International Search Authority. Either a national Office or an intergovernmental organization whose tasks include the establishment of documentary search reports on prior art with respect to inventions, which are the subject of international applications.

ISR International Search Report (Form PCT/ISA/210), produced by an International Searching Authority, is a report listing citations of published documents that might affect the patentability of the invention claimed in an international application.

ITU Intent to Use.

joint application An application in which the invention is presented as that of two or more persons.

JPTOS *Journal of the Patent and Trademark Office Society*

kind codes WIPO Standard ST. 16 codes (kind codes) include a letter, and in many cases a number, used to distinguish the kind of patent document (e.g., publication of an application for a utility patent (patent application publication), patent, plant patent application publication, plant patent, or design patent) and the level of publication (e.g., first publication, second publication, or corrected publication). Detailed information on Standard ST. 16 and the use of kind codes by patent offices throughout the world is available on the WIPO web site at http://www.wipo.int/scit/en, under the links for WIPO standards and other documentation.

maintenance fees Fees for maintaining in force a patent based on an application filed on or after December 12, 1980.

MPEP *Manual of Patent Examining Procedure*

national stage application An application that has entered the national phase of the Patent Cooperation Treaty by the fulfillment of certain requirements in a national Office, which is an authority entrusted with the granting of national or regional patents. Such an application is filed under 35 USC 371 in the U.S. and is referred to as a "371 application."

nonprofit organization For purposes of small entity determination per MPEP 509.02 (1) a university or other institution of higher education located in any country; (2) an organization of the type described in section 501(c)(3) of the Internal Revenue Code of 1954 (26 USC 501(c)(3)) and exempt from taxation under section 501(a) of the Internal Revenue Code (26 USC 501(a)); (3) any nonprofit scientific or educational organization qualified under a non-profit organization statute of a state of this country (35 USC 201(i)); or (4) any nonprofit organization located in a foreign country which would qualify as a nonprofit organization under paragraphs (e) (2) or (3) of MPEP section 509.02 if it were located in this country.

nonprovisional application An application for patent filed under 35 USC 111(a); wherein patent application includes all patent applications (i.e., utility, design, plant, and reissue) except provisional applications. The nonprovisional application establishes the filing date and initiates the examination process.

OED Office of Enrollment and Discipline

OG Official Gazette

OGC Office of General Counsel

OIIP Office of Independent Inventors Programs

OIPE Office of Initial Patent Examination

OPLA Office of Patent Legal Administration

original application "Original" is used in the patent statute and rules to refer to an application which is not a reissue application. An original application may be a first filing or a continuing application.

PAC (1) Patent Assistance Center; (2) Public Advisory Committee

PAIR Patent Application Information Retrieval. Provides secure access for customers who want to view current patent application status electronically via the Internet.

parent application The term "parent" is applied to an earlier application of the inventor disclosing a given invention.

patent A property right granted by the Government of the United States of America to an inventor "to exclude others from making, using, offering for sale, or selling the invention throughout the United States or importing the invention into the United States" for a limited time in exchange for public disclosure of the invention when the patent is granted.

patent application publication Pre-grant publication of patent application at 18 months from priority date.

patent number The number assigned by the USPTO to an issued patent.

patent pending A phrase that often appears on manufactured items. It means that someone has applied for a patent on an invention that is contained in the manufactured item. It serves as a warning that a patent may issue that would cover the item and that copiers should be careful because they might infringe if the patent issues. Once the patent issues, the patent owner will stop using the phrase "patent pending" and start using a phrase such as "covered by U.S. Patent Number XXXXXXX." Applying the patent pending phrase to an item when no patent application has been made can result in a fine.

PBG Patent Business Goals

PBG Final Rule Patent Business Goals Final Rule was implemented to streamline patent practice; a result of the American Inventors Protection Act of 1999.

PCT Patent Cooperation Treaty. Provides a mechanism by which an applicant can file a single application that, when certain requirements have been fulfilled, is equivalent to a regular national filing in each designated Contracting State. There are currently over 112 PCT Contracting States.

PCT Regulations Provide rules concerning matters expressly referred to in the Patent Cooperation Treaty, any administrative requirements, matters, or procedures, and concerning any details useful in the implementation of the provisions of the Patent Cooperation Treaty. The Assembly of WIPO must adopt the rules.

PDF Portable Document Format. A common proprietary document format from Adobe used for documents having mixtures of text and images that preserves the look and feel of a printed page and permits the user to zoom and magnify the pages when viewing; not "archival" because of its proprietary nature.

person For purposes of small entity determination, a person is defined as any inventor or other individual (e.g., an individual to whom an inventor has transferred some rights in the invention), who has not assigned, granted conveyed, or licensed, and is under no obligation under contract or law to assign, grant, convey, or license any rights in the invention.

PG Pub Pre-grant publication of patent application at 18 months from priority date.

PKI Public Key Infrastructure. A system of administrative procedures and methods, combined with secure information technologies, that is used to manage secure electronic commerce. Provides for a means of securely identifying participants in electronic transactions as well as secure transmission and handling of data.

plant application (patent) Applications to protect invented or discovered, asexually reproduced plant varieties.

plant patent May be granted to anyone who invents or discovers and asexually reproduces any distinct and new variety of plant.

PLT Patent Law Treaty

postcard receipt A self-addressed, stamped postcard with itemized list of parts of patent application and number of pages per MPEP 503; used as a receipt for what was submitted in an application.

PPAC Patent Public Advisory Committee

PPS PowerPoint Show file. A type of encapsulated, noneditable Microsoft slideshow.

PPT PowerPoint file. A native, editable type of Microsoft slideshow file.

precautionary designation Designation of a Contracting State in an international application filed under the Patent Cooperation Treaty which must be confirmed prior to 15 months from the priority date.

primary examiner A patent examiner who is fully authorized to sign office actions (signatory authority) regarding patentability.

prior art (reference) Knowledge that is in existence or publicly available before the date of the invention or more than 1 year prior to the first patent application date.

Priority claim Claims under 35 USC 119(a)-(e) and 35 USC 120 for the benefit of the filing date of earlier filed applications.

pro se Used to designate an independent inventor who has elected to file an application by themselves without the services of a licensed representative.

Provisional patent application A provisional application for patent is a U.S. national application for patent filed in the USPTO under 35 USC 111(b). It allows filing without a formal patent claim, oath or declaration, or any information disclosure (prior art) statement. It provides the means to establish an early effective filing date in a nonprovisional patent application filed under 35 USC 111(a) and automatically becomes abandoned after 1 year. It also allows the term "Patent Pending" to be applied.

PTDL Patent and Trademark Depository Library

PTO Patent and Trademark Office. Former designation for USPTO; also a type of form designation for forms generated by the USPTO (as in PTO-892).

PTOL A type of form designation such as Form PTOL, meaning a Patent and Trademark Office Legal form.

PTOS Patent and Trademark Office Society

publication number A number assigned to the publication of patent applications filed on or after November 29, 2000. It includes the year, followed by a seven-digit number, followed by a kind code, e.g., 200011234567A1.

RCE Request for Continued Examination. A request filed in an application in which prosecution is closed (e.g., the application is under final rejection or a notice of allowance) that is filed to reopen prosecution and continue examination of the application; requires the filing of a submission and payment of a fee; see 37 CFR 1.114.

record copy Original copy of an international application filed under the Patent Cooperation Treaty maintained by the International Bureau of the World Intellectual Property Organization.

reference (prior art) Knowledge that is in existence or publicly available before the date of the invention or more than 1 year prior to the first patent application date.

reissue application An application for a patent to take the place of an unexpired patent that is defective in some one or more particulars.

Request (PCT) Form PCT/RO/101, filed with an international application in a receiving Office, which includes an indication of applicant(s) and a designation of one or more Contracting States.

RO Receiving Office. The national Office or the intergovernmental organization with which an international application has been filed.

SB A type of form designation such as Form PTO/SB/05.

search copy Copy of an international application filed under the Patent Cooperation Treaty maintained by the International Searching Authority.

serial number A number assigned to a patent application when it is filed. A serial number is usually used together with a two-digit series code to distinguish between applications filed at different times.

series code A two-digit code representing a period of time. Application Filing Date examples: 01/01/79–12/31/86 Series 06; 01/01/87–12/31/92 Series 07; 01/01/93–12/31/97 Series 08; 01/01/98–Present Series 09.

SF A type of form designation such as Form SF51, meaning a Standard Form used throughout the Federal Government.

SIR A published statutory invention registration contains the specification and drawings of a regularly filed nonprovisional application for a patent without examination if the applicant (1) meets the requirements of section 112 of this title; (2) has complied with the requirements for printing, as set forth in regulations of the Commissioner; (3) waives the right to receive a patent on the invention within such period as may be prescribed by the Commissioner; and (4) pays application, publication, and other processing fees established by the Commissioner. A request for a statutory invention registration (SIR) may be filed at the time of filing a nonprovisional application for patent, or may be filed later during pendency of the non-provisional application.

small business concern For purposes of small entity determination per MPEP 509.02, any business concern meeting the size standards set forth in 13 CFR Part 121 to be eligible for reduced patent fees. Questions related to size standards for a small business concern may be directed to: Small Business Administration, Size Standards Staff, 409 Third Street, SW, Washington, D.C. 20416.

small entity For purposes of small entity determination per MPEP 509.02, an independent inventor, a small business concern, or a nonprofit organization eligible for reduced patent fees.

specification A written description of the invention and the manner and process of making and using the same.

substitute patent application An application that is in essence a duplicate of a prior (earlier filed) application by the same applicant abandoned before the filing of the substitute (later filed) application; a substitute application does not obtain the benefit of the filing date of the prior application.

TIF A lossless, archival image file format; a type using G4 compression is used for patent images.

TMEP Trademark Manual of Examining Procedure

TPAC Trademark Public Advisory Committee

trade secret Information that companies keep secret to give them an advantage over their competitors.

Trademark Protects words, names, symbols, sounds, or colors that distinguish goods and services. Trademarks, unlike patents, can be renewed forever as long as they are being used in business.

TTAB Trademark Trial and Appeal Board

USC United States Code

USPTO United States Patent and Trademark Office, designation became effective April 3, 2000; a result of the American Inventors Protection Act of 1999.

utility patent May be granted to anyone who invents or discovers any new, useful, and nonobvious process, machine, article of manufacture, or composition of matter, or any new and useful improvement thereof.

utility patent application Protect useful processes, machines, articles of manufacture, and compositions of matter.

WIPO World Intellectual Property Organization. An intergovernmental organization of the United Nations system. WIPO is responsible for the promotion of the protection of intellectual property throughout the world and for the administration of various multilateral treaties dealing with the legal and administrative aspects of intellectual property.

Index

D

E

transmission of, 378–382
International classification searches, 37
International PCT application, 31
International Preliminary Examination
  Report. *See* IPER
International Preliminary Examining
  Authority. *See* IPEA
International Search Report, 384
International Searching Authority, 6, 384
Internet, history of, 1–3
Internet Explorer, changing browser display
  font, 175–177
Internet search engines, 70
Invention, 13
  date of, 22
  manner of, 28
  patentability search for, 35
  status of, 22
Invention disclosure statement, 92–93
Inventor's certificate, 326
Inventor's certificate of addition, 327
Investor's Digest, 71
IPEA, 384
  written opinion from, 6
IPER, 6

J

Jepson-type claims, 22, 30
JFIF images, 375
Joint patent protection agreements, 4
Journal publication data, 228

K

Keyword, selection and searching, 41–46
Knowledge, 22

L

Lexis-Nexis, 71
Low-level digital certificates, 381

M

Machine, 35
  as defined by patent law, 11
Manner of invention, 28

Manual of Classification, 49–50
Manual of Patent Examining Procedure.
  See MPEP
Manufacture, 35
  as defined by patent law, 12
Markush alternates, 21
Markush group, 21
Mathematical equations, in patent
  applications, 106–109
Mayall, 71
Means-plus-function clauses, 20
Microorganisms, deposited, 339–341
Micropatent, 71
Microsoft Word. *See also* PASAT
  changes when copying into PASAT,
    105–106
  correcting, 169–171
  features disabled in PASAT, 160
MIT, invention development URL, 71
Mixed-class claims, 22
MPEP, 8–9, 15, 91
Multiple assignment transfer, 100
Multiple concurrent national filings, 31
Multiple dependent claims, 19
Multisequence data files, importing into
  PatentIn, 218

N

NAFTA, 15
Narrowing of a claim, 19
National application, 31
National filings, multiple concurrent, 31
National Institutes of Health, technical
  database, 71
National patents, 325
National security, submitting patents related
  to, 100–101
National stage application, 31
Negative limitations, 21
Nerac, technical database, 71
Nested search operators, 42–43
Nondisclosure Agreements, 14
Nonobviousness, 28–30
Nonprovisional applications, 15
North American Free Trade Agreement. *See*
  NAFTA
Novelty and loss of right to patent, 22–28
Nucleic acids

V

W